AF251893

1994
YEAR BOOK OF
ORTHOPEDICS®

Statement of Purpose

The YEAR BOOK Service

The YEAR BOOK series was devised in 1901 by practicing health professionals who observed that the literature of medicine and related disciplines had become so voluminous that no one individual could read and place in perspective every potential advance in a major specialty. In the final decade of the 20th century, this recognition is more acutely true than it was in 1901.

More than merely a series of books, YEAR BOOK volumes are the tangible results of a unique service designed to accomplish the following:

- to *survey* a wide range of journals of proven value
- to *select* from those journals papers representing significant advances and statements of important clinical principles
- to provide *abstracts* of those articles that are readable, convenient summaries of their key points
- to provide *commentary* about those articles to place them in perspective

These publications grow out of a unique process that calls on the talents of outstanding authorities in clinical and fundamental disciplines, trained literature specialists, and professional writers, all supported by the resources of Mosby, the world's preeminent publisher for the health professions.

The Literature Base

Mosby subscribes to nearly 1,000 journals published worldwide, covering the full range of the health professions. On an annual basis, the publisher examines usage patterns and polls its expert authorities to add new journals to the literature base and to delete journals that are no longer useful as potential YEAR BOOK sources.

The Literature Survey

The publisher's team of literature specialists, all of whom are trained and experienced health professionals, examines every original, peer-reviewed article in each journal issue. More than 250,000 articles per year are scanned systematically, including title, text, illustrations, tables, and references. Each scan is compared, article by article, to the search strategies that the publisher has developed in consultation with the 270 outside experts who form the pool of YEAR BOOK editors. A given article may be reviewed by any number of editors, from one to a dozen or more, regardless of the discipline for which the paper was originally published. In turn, each editor who receives the article reviews it to determine whether or not the article should be included in the YEAR BOOK. This decision is based on the article's inherent quality, its probable usefulness to readers of that YEAR BOOK, and the editor's goal to represent a balanced picture of a given field in each volume of the YEAR BOOK. In addition, the editor indicates when to include figures and tables from the article to help the YEAR BOOK reader better understand the information.

Of the quarter million articles scanned each year, only 5% are selected for detailed analysis within the YEAR BOOK series, thereby assuring readers of the high value of every selection.

The Abstract

The publisher's abstracting staff is headed by a physician-writer and includes individuals with training in the life sciences, medicine, and other areas, plus extensive experience in writing for the health professions and related industries. Each selected article is assigned to a specific writer on this abstracting staff. The abstracter, guided in many cases by notations supplied by the expert editor, writes a structured, condensed summary designed so that the reader can rapidly acquire the essential information contained in the article.

The Commentary

The YEAR BOOK editorial boards, sometimes assisted by guest commentators, write comments that place each article in perspective for the reader. This provides the reader with the equivalent of a personal consultation with a leading international authority—an opportunity to better understand the value of the article and to benefit from the authority's thought processes in assessing the article.

Additional Editorial Features

The editorial boards of each YEAR BOOK organize the abstracts and comments to provide a logical and satisfying sequence of information. To enhance the organization, editors also provide introductions to sections or individual chapters, comments linking a number of abstracts, citations to additional literature, and other features.

The published YEAR BOOK contains enhanced bibliographic citations for each selected article, including extended listings of multiple authors and identification of author affiliations. Each YEAR BOOK contains a Table of Contents specific to that year's volume. From year to year, the Table of Contents for a given YEAR BOOK will vary depending on developments within the field.

Every YEAR BOOK contains a list of the journals from which papers have been selected. This list represents a subset of the nearly 1,000 journals surveyed by the publisher and occasionally reflects a particularly pertinent article from a journal that is not surveyed on a routine basis.

Finally, each volume contains a comprehensive subject index and an index to authors of each selected paper.

The 1994 Year Book Series

Year Book of Allergy and Clinical Immunology: Drs. Rosenwasser, Borish, Gelfand, Leung, Nelson, and Szefler

Year Book of Anesthesiology and Pain Management: Drs. Tinker, Abram, Kirby, Ostheimer, Roizen, and Stoelting

Year Book of Cardiology®: Drs. Schlant, Collins, Engle, Gersh, Kaplan, and Waldo

Year Book of Chiropractic: Dr. Lawrence

Year Book of Critical Care Medicine®: Drs. Rogers and Parrillo

Year Book of Dentistry®: Drs. Meskin, Currier, Kennedy, Leinfelder, Berry, and Roser

Year Book of Dermatologic Surgery: Drs. Swanson, Glogau, and Salasche

Year Book of Dermatology®: Drs. Sober and Fitzpatrick

Year Book of Diagnostic Radiology®: Drs. Federle, Clark, Gross, Madewell, Maynard, Sackett, and Young

Year Book of Digestive Diseases®: Drs. Greenberger and Moody

Year Book of Drug Therapy®: Drs. Lasagna and Weintraub

Year Book of Emergency Medicine®: Drs. Wagner, Burdick, Davidson, McNamara, and Roberts

Year Book of Endocrinology®: Drs. Bagdade, Braverman, Poehlman, Kannan, Landsberg, Molitch, Morley, Odell, Rogol, Ryan, and Nathan

Year Book of Family Practice®: Drs. Berg, Bowman, Davidson, Dietrich, and Scherger

Year Book of Geriatrics and Gerontology®: Drs. Beck, Reuben, Burton, Small, Whitehouse, and Goldstein

Year Book of Hand Surgery®: Drs. Amadio and Hentz

Year Book of Hematology®: Drs. Spivak, Bell, Ness, Quesenberry, and Wiernik

Year Book of Infectious Diseases®: Drs. Keusch, Wolff, Barza, Bennish, Gelfand, Klempner, and Snydman

Year Book of Infertility and Reproductive Endocrinology: Drs. Mishell, Lobo, and Sokol

Year Book of Medicine®: Drs. Bone, Cline, Epstein, Greenberger, Malawista, Mandell, O'Rourke, and Utiger

Year Book of Neonatal and Perinatal Medicine®: Drs. Klaus and Fanaroff

Year Book of Nephrology®: Drs. Coe, Favus, Henderson, Kashgarian, Luke, Myers, and Curtis

Year Book of Neurology and Neurosurgery®: Drs. Bradley and Crowell

Year Book of Neuroradiology: Drs. Osborn, Eskridge, Grossman, and Harnsberger

Year Book of Nuclear Medicine®: Drs. Hoffer, Gore, Gottschalk, Rattner, Zaret, and Zubal

Year Book of Obstetrics and Gynecology®: Drs. Mishell, Kirschbaum, and Morrow

Year Book of Occupational and Environmental Medicine: Drs. Emmett, Frank, Gochfeld, and Hessl

Year Book of Oncology®: Drs. Simone, Longo, Ozols, Steele, Glatstein, and Bosl

Year Book of Ophthalmology®: Drs. Laibson, Adams, Augsburger, Benson, Cohen, Eagle, Flanagan, Nelson, Rapuano, Reinecke, Sergott, and Wilson

Year Book of Orthopedics®: Drs. Sledge, Poss, Cofield, Frymoyer, Griffin, Springfield, Swiontkowski, and Wilson

Year Book of Otolaryngology–Head and Neck Surgery®: Drs. Paparella and Holt

Year Book of Pain: Drs. Gebhart, Haddox, Jacox, Payne, Rudy, and Shapiro

Year Book of Pathology and Clinical Pathology®: Drs. Gardner, Bennett, Cousar, Garvin, and Worsham

Year Book of Pediatrics®: Dr. Stockman

Year Book of Plastic, Reconstructive, and Aesthetic Surgery: Drs. Miller, Cohen, McKinney, Robson, Ruberg, and Whitaker

Year Book of Podiatric Medicine and Surgery®: Dr. Kominsky

Year Book of Psychiatry and Applied Mental Health®: Drs. Talbott, Frances, Breier, Meltzer, Perry, Schowalter, and Yudofsky

Year Book of Pulmonary Disease®: Drs. Bone and Petty

Year Book of Rheumatology: Drs. Sergent, LeRoy, Meenan, Panush, and Reichlin

Year Book of Sports Medicine®: Drs. Shephard, Drinkwater, Eichner, Torg, Col. Anderson, and Mr. George

Year Book of Surgery®: Drs. Copeland, Deitch, Eberlein, Howard, Luce, Ritchie, Seeger, Souba, and Sugarbaker

Year Book of Thoracic and Cardiovascular Surgery: Drs. Ginsberg, Lofland, and Wechsler

Year Book of Transplantation®: Drs. Sollinger, Eckhoff, Hullett, Knechtle, Longo, Mentzer, and Pirsch

Year Book of Ultrasound: Drs. Merritt, Babcock, Carroll, Goldstein, and Mittelstaedt

Year Book of Urology®: Drs. Gillenwater and Howards

Year Book of Vascular Surgery®: Dr. Porter

Editor
Clement B. Sledge, M.D.
Chairman, Department of Orthopedic Surgery, Brigham and Women's Hospital; Professor of Orthopedic Surgery, Harvard Medical School, Boston, Massachusetts

Co-Editor
Robert Poss, M.D.
Vice Chairman, Department of Orthopaedic Surgery, Brigham and Women's Hospital; Professor of Orthopaedic Surgery, Harvard Medical School, Boston, Massachusetts

Associate Editors
Robert H. Cofield, M.D.
Professor of Orthopedic Surgery, Mayo Medical School; Vice-Chairman, Department of Orthopaedics, Mayo Clinic, Rochester, Minnesota

James H. Dobyns, M.D.
Emeritus Professor of Orthopedic Surgery, Mayo Foundation, Rochester, Minnesota; Clinical Professor, University of Texas Health Sciences Center, San Antonio, Texas

John W. Frymoyer, M.D.
Dean of the College of Medicine, Professor of Orthopedic Surgery, University of Vermont; Director, McClure Musculoskeletal Research Center, Burlington, Vermont

Paul P. Griffin, M.D.
Professor of Orthopaedic Surgery, Medical University of South Carolina, Charleston, South Carolina

Dempsey S. Springfield, M.D.
Associate Professor of Orthopaedic Surgery, Harvard Medical School; Visiting Orthopaedic Surgeon, Massachusetts General Hospital, Boston, Massachusetts

Marc F. Swiontkowski, M.D.
Chief, Department of Orthopaedics, Harborview Medical Center; Professor of Orthopaedics, University of Washington School of Medicine, Seattle, Washington

Michael G. Wilson, M.D.
Director, Foot and Ankle Surgery Service, Brigham and Women's Hospital; Problem Foot Service, Massachusetts General Hospital; Clinical Instructor of Orthopedic Surgery, Harvard Medical School, Boston, Massachusetts

1994

The Year Book of ORTHOPEDICS®

Editor
Clement B. Sledge, M.D.

Co-Editor
Robert Poss, M.D.

Associate Editors
Robert H. Cofield, M.D.
James H. Dobyns, M.D.
John W. Frymoyer, M.D.
Paul P. Griffin, M.D.
Dempsey S. Springfield, M.D.
Marc F. Swiontkowski, M.D.
Michael G. Wilson, M.D.

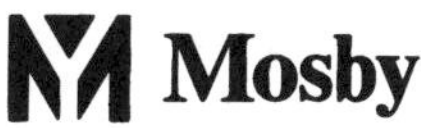 **Mosby**

St. Louis Baltimore Boston Chicago London Madrid Philadelphia Sydney Toronto

Vice President and Publisher, Continuity Publishing: Kenneth H. Killion
Director, Editorial Development: Gretchen C. Murphy
Developmental Editor: Cathy Flanagan
Acquisitions Editor: Linda Steiner
Illustrations and Permissions Coordinator: Lois M. Ruebensam
Director of Editorial Services: Edith M. Podrazik, R.N.
Senior Information Specialist: Terri Santo, R.N.
Information Specialist: Nancy Dunne, R.N.
Senior Medical Writer: David A. Cramer, M.D.
Senior Project Manager: Max F. Perez
Project Manager: Tamara L. Smith
Project Supervisor: Rebecca Nordbrock
Senior Production Editor: Wendi Schnaufer
Production Coordinator: Sandra Rogers
Proofroom Supervisor: Barbara M. Kelly
Vice President, Professional Sales and Marketing: George M. Parker
Marketing and Circulation Manager: Barry J. Bowlus
Marketing Coordinator: Lynn Stevenson

1994 EDITION

Printed in the United States of America
Composition by International Computaprint Corporation
Printing/binding by Maple-Vail

Mosby–Year Book, Inc.
11830 Westline Industrial Drive
St. Louis, MO 63146

Editorial Office:
Mosby–Year Book, Inc.
200 North LaSalle St.
Chicago, IL 60601

International Standard Serial Number: 0276-1092
International Standard Book Number: 0-8151-7811-5

Table of Contents

Mosby Document Express

Copies of the full text of the original source documents of articles abstracted or referenced in this publication are available by calling Mosby Document Express, toll-free, at **1 (800) 55-MOSBY.**

With Mosby Document Express, you have convenient, 24-hour-a-day access to literally every article on which this publication is based. In fact, through Mosby Document Express, virtually any medical or scientific article can be located and delivered by FAX, overnight delivery service, international airmail, electronic transmission of bitmapped images (via Internet), or regular mail. The average cost of a complete, delivered copy of an article, including up to $4 in copyright clearance charges and first-class mail delivery, is $12.

For inquiries and pricing information, please call the toll-free number shown above. To expedite your order for material appearing in this publication, please be prepared with the code shown next to the bibliographic citation for each abstract.

Journals Represented

Mosby subscribes to and surveys nearly 1,000 U.S. and foreign medical and allied health journals. From these journals, the Editors select the articles to be abstracted. Journals represented in this YEAR BOOK are listed below.

Acta Neurologica Scandinavica
Acta Orthopaedica Scandinavica
American Journal of Epidemiology
American Journal of Public Health
American Journal of Roentgenology
American Journal of Sports Medicine
Anaesthesia
Annals of Rheumatic Diseases
Archives of Orthopaedic and Trauma Surgery
Arthritis and Rheumatism
Arthroscopy
British Journal of Plastic Surgery
British Journal of Radiology
British Medical Journal
Calcified Tissue International
Canadian Journal of Surgery
Cancer
Clinical Orthopaedics and Related Research
Foot and Ankle
Human Pathology
Injury
International Journal of Radiation, Oncology, Biology, and Physics
International Orthopaedics
Investigative Radiology
Italian Journal of Orthopaedics and Traumatology
Journal of Applied Physiology: Respiratory, Environmental and Exercise
    Physiology
Journal of Arthroplasty
Journal of Biomechanics
Journal of Bone and Joint Surgery (American Volume)
Journal of Bone and Joint Surgery (British Volume)
Journal of Bone and Mineral Research
Journal of Hand Surgery (American)
Journal of Hand Surgery (British)
Journal of Neurosurgery
Journal of Orthopaedic Research
Journal of Orthopaedic Trauma
Journal of Orthopaedic and Sports Physical Therapy
Journal of Pediatric Orthopedics
Journal of Rheumatology
Journal of Shoulder and Elbow Surgery
Journal of Spinal Disorders
Journal of Trauma
Journal of Vascular Surgery
Journal of the American Geriatrics Society
Journal of the Royal College of Surgeons of Edinburgh
Journal of the Royal Society of Medicine
Lancet
Medical Journal of Australia
Microsurgery

Neuro-Chirurgie
Orthopaedic Review
Pediatric Radiology
Plastic and Reconstructive Surgery
Postgraduate Medical Journal
Prosthetics and Orthotics International
Radiology
Science
Skeletal Radiology
Spine
Transfusion

STANDARD ABBREVIATIONS

The following terms are abbreviated in this edition: acquired immunodeficiency syndrome (AIDS), the central nervous system (CNS), cerebrospinal fluid (CSF), computed tomography (CT), electrocardiography (ECG), human immunodeficiency virus (HIV), and magnetic resonance (MR) imaging (MRI).

Dedication

When trying to put down on paper the significant events that occurred in 1993 relative to orthopedic surgery and the YEAR BOOK OF ORTHOPEDICS, it is difficult to think of anything other than the death of Kenneth Johnson. Kenneth had been a part of the editorial team since I took over the YEAR BOOK OF ORTHOPEDICS in 1989, and his selections and comments made the Foot and Ankle section outstanding. In a broader sense, Ken was clearly one of the fathers of modern foot and ankle surgery in orthopedics and was widely recognized as such throughout the United States and the English-speaking world. We will all miss him very much.

Clement B. Sledge, M.D.

Introduction

This year's edition includes 3 new contributors. Marc Swiontkowski takes over the Trauma section from Sig Hansen, James Dobyns takes over the Hand section from Barry Simmons, and Michael Wilson has stepped in to take over the section on the Foot and Ankle. I thank Drs. Simmons and Hansen for their excellent contributions to the YEAR BOOK OF ORTHOPEDICS during the past 4 years, and I welcome Drs. Dobyns, Swiontkowski, and Wilson to the group.

This year, as in the past several years, readers will find a broad spectrum of offerings from the literature, with critical analyses by the editors. Although there are no major new trends, there continues to be an increased interest in long-term studies coupled with the use of patient-derived measures of satisfaction as we enter the era of accountability and the growth of contractual medicine. Under this new approach to the delivery of health care in this country, there will be increased emphasis on proving the efficacy of treatment. Part of that proof will be the demonstration that patients' expectations are met by their treatment. There is also increasing awareness of the necessity to evaluate the cost-effectiveness of health care, and this is beginning to be reflected in the orthopedic literature.

These new dimensions of medicine make it all the more important to have a service like that provided by the YEAR BOOK OF ORTHOPEDICS; no single individual can read, let alone analyze, the tremendous volume of literature that is presented in the YEAR BOOK. It would be difficult, if not impossible, merely to keep up with the traditional orthopedic literature. Now journals outside the usual realm of orthopedics are beginning to publish articles dealing with the issues of delivery of health care, outcome assessment, and cost-effectiveness. I look forward to a time when we will have to add a new editor just to cover literature in these fields, the impact of which is just beginning to be seen in orthopedic surgery.

Clement B. Sledge, M.D.

1 Pediatrics

Introduction

The articles selected for the pediatric section are about conditions of the hip and spine and trauma. Several interesting studies that could not be easily grouped by diagnosis or treatment are included under a general group.

Developmental dysplasia of the hip continues to be of great interest. I have included studies on the value of ultrasound in management and prognosis (Abstracts 129-94-1-8 through 129-94-1-10). There is little that is new about the standard treatment of developmental dysplasia of the hip, but I have selected several good studies of closed and open reductions. There is no absolute evidence that we can use to comfortably prognosticate outcome in the late-treated patient, but 1 or 2 studies included give us some guidelines.

In the subsection on trauma there are several articles on interesting fractures and their diagnosis and treatment. Techniques useful in treating fractures of the proximal metaphysis of the radius and radial head appear in 2 of the papers selected (Abstracts 129-94-1-15 and 129-94-1-16). One paper addresses the issue of age in the use of intramedullary rod fixation in fractures of the femur (Abstract 129-94-1-18). A study on hemarthrosis of the knee revealed some statistics that will cause concern for those who treat knee injuries in children (Abstract 129-94-1-19).

A number of papers on treatment of scoliosis have been included. The use of rib resection to reduce the rib hump is well presented in Abstract 129-94-1-22. The value of bracing in adolescent scoliosis is still questioned by some orthopedists. We present papers on this subject (Abstracts 129-94-1-23 and 129-94-1-24).

In the general group, articles were selected to address subjects such as latex allergy (Abstract 129-94-1-29) and the use of electrical stimulation in patients with cerebral palsy (Abstract 129-94-1-30) among several other subjects. One particularly interesting study showed the value of a bone scan for early decision-making in patients with gangrene from meningococcemia (Abstract 129-94-1-34).

In general, articles have been chosen that add new thoughts on the diagnosis and treatment of pediatric problems, as well as studies that further support older concepts and ideas.

Paul P. Griffin, M.D.

1

Hip

Comparison of Inpatient and Outpatient Traction in Developmental Dislocation of the Hip

Camp J, Herring JA, Dworezynski C (Desert Orthopaedic Ctr Research Found, Las Vegas, Nev; Texas Scottish Rite Hosp, Dallas)
J Pediatr Orthop 14:9–12, 1994   129-94-1–1

Introduction.—In 1986, Mubarak et al. proposed further simplification of prereduction traction for the treatment of developmental dysplasia of the hip (DDH), using outpatient skin traction without radiographic assessment of hip station. The effectiveness and safety of this outpatient traction program were compared with those of an identically instituted inpatient program.

Treatment.—Eighty-three hips in 72 children with DDH were treated in simple vertical skin traction as described by Mubarak et al. Forty hips were treated on an inpatient basis and 43 on an outpatient basis for an average of 17 days (range, 8–27 days). No routine in-traction radiographs were taken in either group. The average follow-up was 51 months (range, 24–169 months).

Outcome.—After traction, 55 hips achieved a stable closed reduction whereas 28 hips required open reduction. Severe avascular necrosis (AVN), defined as Bucholz and Ogden types II–IV, occurred in 4 hips (5%), including 1 (2.5%) in the outpatient group and 3 (7.5%) in the inpatient group; the difference was not statistically significant. The incidence of total AVN was essentially equal in both groups. Open reduction was performed in 28 hips (34%) after failed closed reduction.

Conclusion.—An outpatient traction program instituted before reduction without attention to radiographic hip station is as safe as an identically instituted inpatient program. Despite the high incidence of open reduction, this outpatient traction protocol appears to be the least expensive and most convenient alternative for the patient, while maintaining a low risk of AVN.

Open Reduction Through a Medial Approach for Congenital Dislocation of the Hip: A Critical Review of the Ludloff Approach in Sixty-Six Hips

Mankey MG, Arntz CT, Staheli LT (Orthopedic Physicians, Seattle; Valley Orthopedic Assoc, Renton, Wash; Children's Hosp and Med Ctr, Seattle)
J Bone Joint Surg (Am) 75-A:1334–1344, 1993   129-94-1–2

Background.—There is no agreement on the best surgical approach for reducing congenital hip dislocation. The outcomes of open reduction through the medial approach of Ludloff in 1 series were analyzed.

Data On Patients Who Had the Development of or Had Preexisting Avascular Necrosis

Case	Sex	Side	Age at Diagnosis (Mos.)	Preop. Treatment	Age at Op. (Mos.)	Est. Blood Loss (ml)	Op. Time (Mins.)	Duration in Cast (Wks.)	Duration of Follow-up (Yrs.)	Grade of Avasc. Necros.[23]	Subsequent Treatment	Preop. Acetab. Index/ Center-Edge Angle (Degrees)	Follow-up Acetab. Index/ Center-Edge Angle (Degrees)	Range of Motion	Fem. Head Diameter (mm)	Limb Lengths
1	M	L	16	Skin tract., 18 days	25	50	120	16	10	5	Salter osteot., varus derot. osteot.	33/0	20/18	Full	52	Equal
		R	16	Skin tract., 18 days	25	50	120	16	10	5	Salter osteot., varus derot. osteot.	30/0	10/27	Full	51	Equal
2*	F	L	62	Skin tract., closed reduct., cast	63	40	105	9	8	4	Pemberton osteot.	40/0	15/26	Full	44, R; 44, L	Equal
3*	F	L	16	Skin tract., closed reduct., cast	26	250	175	16	5	5	None	20/0	9/40	Full	31, R; 33, L	Equal
4	F	R	1	Abduct. splint., closed reduct., cast, skin tract.	10	5	30	16	8	4	None	25/0	18/19	Full	29, R; 30, L	R > L, 1 cm

(continued)

Table *(continued)*

5	F	R	11	Skin tract., 16 days	14	10	30	16	5	4	Salter osteot.	40/0	10/34	Full	31, R; 29, L	Equal
6	F	R	15	Bone tract., closed reduct., skin tract., cast, adduct. tenot.	18	60	60	16	10	5	Salter osteot.	34/0	8/40	Full	48, R; 45, L	L > R, approx. 2 cm
7	M	R	1	Pavlik harness, closed reduct., cast, skin tract.	12	50	80	32	3.3	2	None	30/0	21/24	Full	26	Equal
		L	1	Pavlik harness, closed reduct., cast, skin tract.	14	50	60	16	3.1	3	None	30/0	27/14	Full	30	Equal

* Avascular changes preceded the procedure through the Ludloff approach
(Courtesy of Mankey MG, Arntz CT, Staheli LT: *J Bone Joint Surg (Am)* 75-A:1334–1344, 1993.)

Patients and Outcomes.—Sixty-six hips in 63 children were treated for congenital dislocation. The mean age at surgery was 12 months. The mean duration of follow-up was 6 years. Avascular necrosis was evident before surgery in 3% of the hips and postoperatively in 11%. Patient age at the time of surgery was correlated with postoperative avascular necrosis. The prevalence of this complication was increased in patients managed with open reduction after 24 months of age. One redislocation and 2 subluxations were found at the time of the first cast change 4 weeks after surgery. The acetabular index improved from a mean of 38 degrees preoperatively to 16 degrees at follow-up assessment. Acetabular dysplasia did not resolve in 33% of the hips, and pelvic osteotomy was needed (table).

Conclusion.—The Ludloff approach is a safe, effective technique for treating congenital hip dislocation in infants younger than 24 months of age and in whom a concentric reduction with less than 60 degrees of abduction was not achieved after closed reduction. This approach has the advantages of direct access to the iliopsoas, the transverse acetabular ligament, and the constricted capsule; minimal blood loss; and an aesthetically acceptable scar.

▶ I believe that after 12 months, the acetabular dysplasia is too severe to expect the hip to develop satisfactorily after the Ludloff approach. The high percentage of patients (33%) who required further surgery would seem to support this concept; however, in this study, age was not evaluated. The position of the hip in flexion and abduction is important for maintaining the reduction. This position should be one in which the hip is maximally stable but without excessive abduction and flexion.—P.P. Griffin, M.D.

Effect of Effusion on Hip Joint Stability in the Newborn: A Postmortal Study
Hinderaker T, Udén A, Reikerås O (Univ Hosp, Tromsø, Norway)
Acta Orthop Scand 64:64–66, 1993   129-94-1–3

Objective.—Previous reports have suggested that repeated clinical assessments for hip joint instability in the newborn may be harmful. One study demonstrated that instability can actually result from stretching of the joint capsule during Barlow's test. A postmortem study was performed to determine whether effusion could be a cause of hip instability.

Methods.—Experiments were performed in 1 stillborn neonate and 1 infant who died at 3 days of age. Fluid was injected into the hip joints via the triradiate cartilage, then the hips were evaluated by Ortolani's and Barlow's tests. In the latter child, clinical and dynamic sonographic examinations were performed as increasing amounts of fluid were injected.

Findings.—Both hips were clinically stable before the experiment. Both clinical tests were positive after injection of 1 mL of fluid. The instability was readily apparent sonographically, although there was no change in bony rim percentage. The instability persisted even after aspiration of the fluid without air leakage. The joints held a maximum of about 3 mL of fluid.

Conclusion.—These experimental results suggest that effusion is a possible mechanism of hip joint instability in the newborn. Repeated assessments may cause distention of the joint capsule, which, along with a vacuum effect, may explain the increased stability observed a few days after birth.

▶ This study raises questions about possible harm in performing Barlow's test. Most orthopedists do Barlow's test, but I have always objected on the grounds that a joint should not be forcefully dislocated. To do so stretches the capsule.—P.P. Griffin, M.D.

Improvement in Acetabular Index After Reduction of Hips With Developmental Dysplasia

Tasnavites A, Murray DW, Benson MKD'A (Bhumibol Adulyadej Hosp, Bangkok, Thailand; Nuffield Orthopaedic Centre, Oxford, England)
J Bone Joint Surg (Br) 75-B:755–759, 1993   129-94-1-4

Introduction.—When treatment is delayed in children with developmental dysplasia of the hip (DDH), it is difficult to know if and when acetabular reconstruction is required. Acetabular development was studied in a group of patients who had late reduction of the femoral head and no pelvic surgery.

Patients and Methods.—Twenty patients fulfilled criteria for study entry. Each had only 1 unstable hip and all were between 12 and 24 months of age at the time of reduction. Nineteen patients (17 girls and 2 boys) were available for follow-up. Twelve hips were treated with closed and 7 with open reduction. Ten patients underwent percutaneous adductor tenotomy. After reduction, the hip was immobilized in a spica cast for 6–12 weeks. The children were assessed clinically and radiographically during follow-up.

Results.—All patients experienced steady improvement during the first 3 years after reduction; none were dysplastic at this time as measured by the acetabular index (AI). There were 2 cases of dysplasia, as assessed by the more sensitive center-edge angle (CEA), after the age of 10 years. When these 2 dysplastic hips were excluded, the mean CEA of the affected hips was not significantly different from that of unaffected or normal hips. After 5 years the mean AI of the unaffected and normal hips became the same. No factors were found to identify which hips would become dysplastic, and no correlation was found between the cartilaginous AI and postoperative hip development.

Conclusion.—Dysplasia may be difficult to confirm or exclude during the first 3 years after reduction of hips with DDH. During this period, there is potential for improvement in the acetabulum, and reconstruction should not be immediately undertaken. Some hips that appear to be developing normally will become dysplastic despite good reduction and careful follow-up. The CEA should be used to evaluate the hip in children 10 years of age and older.

▶ Acetabular development after reduction is greatest during the first year after reduction. Criteria to predict which hips will continue to improve and become normal are not clear. Dysplasia without subluxation can improve for a number of years. Those with subluxations are not likely to improve. The hip that shows no improvement in AI or CEA for 12–18 months is not only unlikely to improve, the dysplasia may actually increase.—P.P. Griffin, M.D.

Acetabular Development After Closed Reduction of Congenital Dislocation of the Hip

Noritake K, Yoshihashi Y, Hattori T, Miura T (Nagoya Univ, Japan; Aichi Prefectural Hosp and Rehabilitation Centre for Disabled Children, Okazaki City, Japan)
J Bone Joint Surg (Br) 75-B:737–743, 1993

129-94-1–5

Introduction.—Many orthopedic surgeons in Japan have adopted overhead traction (OHT) before closed reduction of congenital dislocation of the hip (CDH). In a previous article, long-term results, using Severin's classification, were reported in 109 hips treated by OHT. Only 34% of the hips attained Severin group I (normal). The causes of acetabular dysplasia in hips treated by closed reduction after OHT were determined.

Patients and Methods.—Excluded from analysis were hips with femoral head deformity or residual subluxation. Also excluded were male patients because gender can influence development. Forty-seven female patients (54 hips) met the study criteria. These patients were reviewed for long-term outcome and the results were compared with those from a control series of unaffected hips of patients with unilateral CDH. The average age at treatment by OHT in the 47 patients was 11 months; at most recent follow-up, their average age was 17 years. Measurements were made on pelvic radiographs taken at 2 or 3 years of age, 5 or 6 years of age, 8 or 9 years of age, 11 or 12 years of age, and at the most recent follow-up. The 54 previously dislocated hips and the 79 unaffected control hips were classified according to the Severin group at most recent follow-up.

Results.—Twenty-four of the 54 dislocated hips (44.4%) and 13.9% of the control hips were rated as Severin group III (dysplastic but without subluxation). After the age of 11 or 12 years, acetabular development was significantly worse in Severin group III than in Severin group I hips on the affected side or Severin group III in unaffected control hips. The affected side showed a significant degree of change in the center-edge angle (CEA) during the final interval before the most recent follow-up. The unaffected control group had no such changes at any of the follow-up periods.

Conclusion.—Comparison of the 2 groups of patients showed that on the affected side, in the interval from 11 to 12 years to the most recent follow-up, improvement in the CEA of group III hips was significantly worse than that of group I hips. Thus, acetabular dysplasia after treatment by closed reduction is related to poor improvement in the CEA after 11 or 12 years, perhaps attributable to impaired secondary ossification in the acetabular rim. The findings emphasize the need to continue follow-up for CHD until full skeletal maturity.

▶ After closed reduction, hips that do not have good acetabular development (CEA > 15–20 degrees) by 12 years of age are not likely to improve. In a unilateral dislocation, it is not uncommon for the acetabulum on the contralateral side to have dysplasia. I believe it is prudent to continue to observe all children with a dislocated hip until maturity, because a hip that appears "almost" normal at 4 or 5 years of age may be a Severin III or IV by 13–14 years of age.—P.P. Griffin, M.D.

Failures of Screening and Management of Congenital Dislocation of the Hip

Lennox IAC, McLauchlan J, Murali R (Royal Aberdeen Children's Hosp, Scotland)

J Bone Joint Surg (Br) 75-B:72–75, 1993   129-94-1-6

Background.—With neonatal diagnosis and simple splinting, congenital dislocation of the hip (CDH) can be treated successfully. In 1960, a screening program was begun for all children born in the Grampian region of Scotland. However, some cases of CDH are still missed, and the prognosis for these children may be worse than before the program was started, because the diagnosis is not suspected by health care providers who believe that neonatal screening is fully effective. The Grampian experience was further assessed.

Methods and Findings.—Between 1980 and 1989, 67,093 infants were screened for CDH. The results in these patients were compared with those of children screened in the 2 preceding decades. More dislocations were missed at neonatal examination between 1980 and 1989 (.13% of live births) than in preceding decades. A total of 163 children received diagnoses after the neonatal period and needed surgery. One hundred nine were screening failures, 10 of whom were born outside the Grampian region. The mean age at presentation was 11 months.

Conclusion.—After 30 years of screening in the Grampian region, the late presentation of CDH has actually increased in incidence. Forty percent more children underwent surgery in 1980–1989 than in the decade before screening was begun. In addition, a subgroup of patients in whom the condition was diagnosed at birth are probably resistant to treatment with splinting.

▶ Hip screening in newborns is effective in diagnosing dislocatable hips. However, the physician who follows a patient with a reported normal screen must continue to evaluate the hip at each newborn examination. Hips that are eventually diagnosed as dislocated or dysplastic are not all detected in the newborn exam. This study also identified a group of patients who failed to respond to splinting and another group who, after treatment with splinting, appeared normal but were subsequently found to be dysplastic.—P.P. Griffin, M.D.

Open Reduction of CDH Before One Year of Age: 69 Hips Followed for 13 (10–19) Years

Doudoulakis JK, Cavadias A (Agia Sofia Children's Hosp, Athens, Greece)
Acta Orthop Scand 64:188–192, 1993   129-94-1–7

Background.—Congenital dislocation of the hip (CDH) is common in Greece. Surgery may be needed in cases of irreducible or unstable hips. The results of open reduction in a large series of patients with CDH treated at a children's hospital in Athens were reported.

Patients and Outcomes.—Fifty infants, aged 2–12 months, with 69 affected hips underwent open reduction. In 4 hips, the result was poor because of severe necrosis of the femoral head. In another 5 hips with less severe necrosis, the outcome was fair. Seven of the 9 hips with avascular necrosis were in children younger than 6 months of age at surgery. Thirteen hips in 9 children needed complementary surgery to establish congruous hip reduction. At a mean follow-up of 13 years, successful outcomes were noted in 53 hips. There were no differences between unilaterally and bilaterally operated hips. In most hips, anteversion eventually corrected itself. Coxa magna disappeared when hips reached maturity. The condition of hips with good results continued to be good, whereas that of hips with poor outcomes worsened.

Conclusion.—In this series, the results in 42 of 69 hips were very good; they were good in 11, fair in 12, and poor in 4. Results were, therefore, unacceptable at follow-up in one fourth of the hips. Younger infants appear to be more susceptible to necrosis.

▶ This study, like that of Kalamchi and MacEwen (1), found that infants under 6 months of age are more likely to have necrosis of the hip after open reduction than are older infants. The surgeon excised the limbus, which I think should not be done, but it should have no bearing on the incidence of necrosis.—P.P. Griffin, M.D.

Reference

1. Kalamchi A, MacEwen AD: *J Bone Joint Surg (Am)* 62-A:876, 1980.

Development of Late Congenital Hip Dysplasia: Significance of Ultrasound Screening

Stöver B, Brägelmann R, Walther A, Ball F (Albert Ludwig Univ, Freiburg, Germany; Johann Wolfgang Goethe Univ, Frankfurt, Germany)
Pediatr Radiol 23:19–22, 1993   129-94-1-8

Background.—Ultrasound has been valuable in diagnosing congenital hip dysplasia. Originally, it was thought that hip dysplasia could not develop in the first weeks of life. However, research has indicated deterioration in the hips of infants of this age. Whether hip dysplasia can develop in the first weeks of life and whether ultrasound screening of newborns can detect congenital hip dysplasia that would have been missed by clinical assessment alone were determined.

Methods.—A total of 5,970 infants undergoing ultrasound for the detection of congenital hip dysplasia were included in the study. Repeat assessment was performed in 2,121. Of those reassessed, 726 were not at risk as newborns, 70 were at risk when first investigated as newborns, and 363 were at risk when first assessed after the newborn period. The rest were not at risk when first examined after the newborn period.

Findings.—Abnormalities were found in 7.7% of the overall group. Four percent of children not at risk and 5% of those at risk had pathologic results. Three percent had deterioration of Graf's classification of types. None of the 13 children experiencing hip dysplasia would have been missed, as they were borderline type IIA on at least 1 side, which indicates mandatory follow-up.

Conclusion.—Screening is desirable in newborns with no risk factors for congenital hip dysplasia and is mandatory in newborns with risk factors. Screening should be done at 6–10 weeks of age in case there are anatomical changes in the hip joints. Late hip dysplasia can develop in some infants, independent of risk.

▶ Screening of hips by ultrasound is an effective method for detecting early hip dysplasia. The natural history of dysplasia in the neonate and infant, as defined by ultrasound, is not yet clear. Some infants improve but others deteriorate. Cost and effectiveness must be considered in ordering ultrasound of the hip. The physical signs of dysplasia are not present at birth, but by 6 weeks a patient with a unilateral dislocation or dysplasia would have a pelvic obliquity with asymmetry of the gluteal folds.—P.P. Griffin, M.D.

Ultrasound and the Pavlik Harness in CDH

Suzuki S (Shiga Med Ctr for Children, Japan)
J Bone Joint Surg (Br) 75-B:483–487, 1993   129-94-1–9

Background.—By studying the spatial relationship between the acetabulum and the dislocated femoral head in infants treated by the Pavlik harness, it was possible to establish ultrasonographic criteria for the use of the harness. Sixty-two patients with 69 congenitally dislocated hips were treated by the Pavlik harness from December 1988 to April 1992.

Patients and Methods.—Fifty-seven of the infants were girls and 5 were boys; at the start of treatment, they ranged in age from 8 days to 10 months. Congenital dislocation of the hip (CDH) had been diagnosed by both ultrasonography and radiography. Before application of the Pavlik harness, the infants were placed in skin traction for a mean of 22 days until adduction contracture of the hip had disappeared. The harness was then applied with the hip in 100 degrees of flexion. Ultrasonography was used to grade the residual displacement in the flexed and abducted position.

Results.—Based on the relationship between the femoral head and the acetabulum, 3 degrees of displacement were observed (Fig 1–1). Fifty-one of the 69 hips showed type A displacement, in which the femoral head was within the socket and in contact with the posterior inner wall of the acetabulum. The harness achieved reduction in all these cases. In type B the femoral head contacted the posterior margin of the socket; 5 of 9 type B hips were reduced. None of the 9 hips with type C displacement, with the femoral head outside the socket, were reduced. Other methods of treatment will be needed for such cases.

Conclusion.—The position of the femoral head when the hip was in flexion and abduction was a major factor in the ultimate success of re-

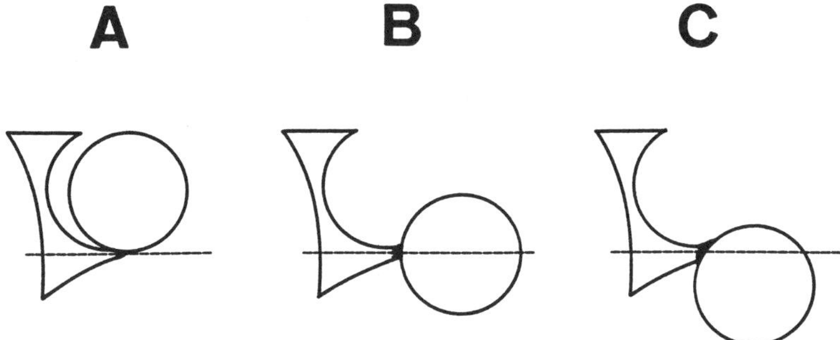

Fig 1–1.—Types of displacement. **A,** the femoral head is displaced posteriorly, but it is in contact with the inner wall of the acetabulum. **B,** the femoral head is in contact with the posterior margin of the socket, with its center at or anterior to the edge of the acetabulum. **C,** the femoral head is displaced outside the socket, with its center posterior to the acetabular edge. (Courtesy of Suzuki S: *J Bone Joint Surg (Br)* 75-B:483–487, 1993).

duction. Ultrasonography with the anterior approach is recommended for determining the indication for use of the Pavlik harness and to monitor progress in infants with CDH. Ultrasound is superior to radiography, CT, and MRI because it can be performed quickly, is harmless, and requires no sedation.

The Reliability of Ultrasonographic Assessment of Neonatal Hips

Dias JJ, Thomas IH, Lamont AC, Mody BS, Thompson JR (Leicester Royal Infirmary, England)
J Bone Joint Surg (Br) 75-B:479–482, 1993 129-94-1–10

Background.—The basic methods of Graf and Schuler are widely used for ultrasound examination of the infant hip and for classification and management of dysplasia. The reproducibility of ultrasound images and the reliability of measurements from the images were assumed. The interobserver and intraobserver reliability of ultrasound assessments of the neonatal hip was examined.

Methods.—Four hundred eighteen ultrasound images were made of the hips of 209 consecutively born neonates during a 2-week period at a single hospital. A sample of 62 scans were selected randomly, and 25 were duplicated to provide a study set of 87 scans. Five experienced observers reviewed the entire set of static images, on which they made 9 different assessments and measurements.

Results.—Agreement was insufficient for all 7 categorical assessments studied: appearance of the bony promontory and bony molding, baseline shape of the ilium, shape and appearance of the cartilaginous acetabular rim, appearance of the labrum, and appearance of the femoral head cover. Intraobserver agreement was better, but not good enough for assessment of changes in hip morphology. Measurement of the alpha angle had fairly good interobserver and intraobserver reproducibility, but interobserver reproducibility of the beta angle was poor.

Conclusion.—Poor interobserver and intraobserver reliability for static ultrasound assessment of the neonatal hip was found. Although dynamic screening can demonstrate movement and laxity of the hip, conclusions should not be reached solely on the basis of static images.

▶ The descriptive classification of the shape of the acetabular rim and labrum from a sonogram is inconsistent and of little value in selecting patients for the treatment of dysplasia. The reproducibility of the measurement of the alpha and beta angles is better, both for intraobservations and interobservations. Dynamic ultrasonography is more reliable than static measurements for showing laxity of the hip. This variability of interpretations of a static sonogram may explain why some "dysplastic" hips improve with treatment, some do not improve with treatment, and others improve only to deteriorate later.—P.P. Griffin, M.D.

Classification in Slipped Capital Femoral Epiphysis: Sonographic Assessment of Stability and Remodeling

Kallio PE, Paterson DC, Foster BK, Lequesne GW (Adelaide Children's Hosp, Australia)

Clin Orthop 294:196–203, 1993   129-94-1-11

Background.—The traditional classification of slipped capital femoral epiphysis (SCFE) is based on the duration of symptoms before treatment. This system is prone to inaccuracy, however, because it is based

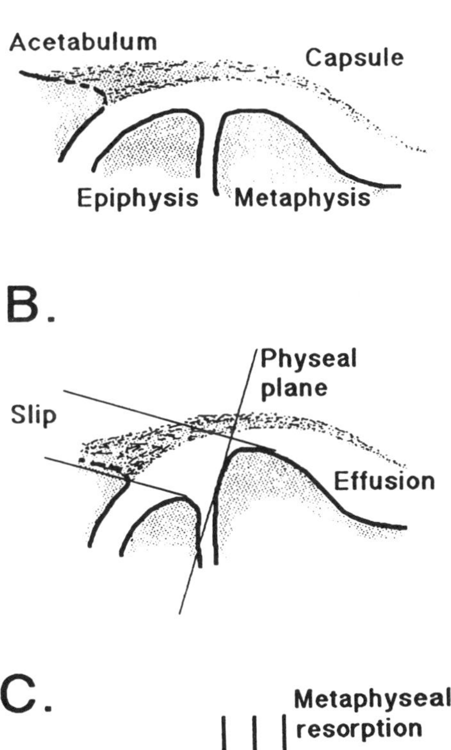

Fig 1–2.—**A,** anatomical structures of the adolescent hip joint as seen in sonographic examination; **B,** posterior displacement of the proximal femoral epiphysis and effusion in acute slipped capital femoral epiphysis; **C,** irregular and rounded metaphyseal outline indicating metaphyseal resorption in early remodeling. (Courtesy of Kallio PE, Paterson DC, Foster BK, et al: *Clin Orthop* 294:196–203, 1993.)

on the patient's recollections rather than objective data. An ideal classification of SCFE would reflect the duration of the slip, the amount of most recent displacement, the amount of total epiphyseal displacement since the first slip episode, and the stability of the slip. Sonography of the hip was used to develop a new, objective classification of SCFE.

Patients and Methods.—Twenty-one consecutive patients (26 hips) with SCFE who were admitted to a children's hospital from October 1988 to May 1991 were reviewed. The slip was considered acute if symptoms were of no more than 3 weeks' duration and chronic if of more than 3 weeks' duration. Acute-on-chronic slips were characterized by a recent deterioration of symptoms after a history of longer than 3 weeks or by acute progression in a hip with radiographic evidence of chronicity. Serial sonographic assessment of hips was carried out before and immediately after surgery, then at 3, 6, 12, and 24 weeks. Each of those examinations included assessment of effusion, measurement of physeal displacement at the anterior outline of the femoral neck, and evaluation of metaphyseal remodeling (Fig 1–2).

Results.—Eleven of the 26 hips, all with relatively recent slips, had joint effusion on admission. With one exception, effusions occurred only in the acute or acute-on-chronic slips of the traditional classification. The average duration of symptoms was 4.8 weeks for hips with effusion and 57.6 weeks for hips without effusion. Only 1 hip had an effusion after operative stabilization of the physis; the effusion did not recur after 3-week follow-up. Sonography accurately visualized the early stage of remodeling in SCFE, characterized by bony resorption at the anterior metaphysis, and was extremely sensitive to slight changes in the epiphyseal position.

Conclusion.—Objective sonographic data can be used to classify SCFEs. An acute SCFE is characterized by effusion and a chronic SCFE by remodeling but no effusion. Both effusion and remodeling are present in an acute-on-chronic SCFE. The presence of joint effusion suggests that SCFEs are unstable and should be fixed operatively.

▶ The number of skeletal conditions for which ultrasound has been used in diagnosis and/or classification seems endless. Ultrasound classification or the presence of fluid will not change the necessity for surgical treatment in SCFE, but it will add extra expense. A SCFE with an immature physis should be stabilized with pin fixation (1). The improvement in range of motion of the hip after pin fixation is not related to remodeling. The range of motion in the hip that has a slip will improve to the point at which it is very similar to that of the contralateral hip.—P.P. Griffin, M.D.

Reference

1. Gelberman R, et al: *J Bone Joint Surg* (Am) 68-A:1000, 1986.

Comparison of Lateral Pillar Classification and Catterall Classification of Legg-Calvé-Perthes' Disease

Ritterbusch JF, Shantharam SS, Gelinas C (Univ of New Mexico, Albuquerque)
J Pediatr Orthop 13:200–202, 1993   129-94-1–12

Background.—The extent of femoral head involvement affects the radiographic outcome of the hips in patients with Legg-Calvé-Perthes disease. A classification system described by Catterall has been used to evaluate the effects of treatment for Legg-Calvé-Perthes disease but has shown poor interobserver agreement. A system recently described by Herring, based on involvement of the lateral pillar of the femoral head, has been useful in predicting outcome and has shown better interobserver agreement.

Methods.—The interobserver agreement and predictive value of the Catterall and Herring classifications of Legg-Calvé-Perthes disease were compared. Seventy-one affected hips with radiographic follow-up from fragmentation stage to skeletal maturity were studied. The films were reviewed by 3 observers of varying orthopedic experience: a medical student, an orthopedic resident, and a pediatric orthopedic surgeon. Outcome films were assessed by the classification of Stulberg et al.

Results.—The Stulberg outcome was significantly better predicted by the Herring classification than by the Catterall classification. The Spearman correlation between Herring and Stulberg was .64; between Catterall and Stulberg it was only .38. All 3 observers agreed as to the Herring classification for 72% of hips, compared with 41% for the Catterall classification.

Conclusion.—This study demonstrates the better predictive outcome and interobserver agreement of the Herring classification for Legg-Calvé-Perthes disease vs. the Catterall classification. The authors have adopted the Herring classification at their institution and believe that it has the potential to improve communication regarding Legg-Calvé-Perthes disease.

▶ Dr. Arthur Legg (*Boston Medical Journal*, 1910) described the "mushroom" head (a good lateral column), which did well without treatment, and a "cap" type (lateral column collapse), which had a poor prognosis. When the lateral part of the head is not necrotic, collapse is slight, and motion is sufficient for the lateral part of the head to work beneath the acetabulum, remodeling will usually be sufficient to give a good result. Catterall's classification is difficult and it requires extensive experience for one to become comfortable with its use.—P.P. Griffin, M.D.

Trauma

Late-Onset Pseudarthrosis of the Dysplastic Tibia
Roach JW, Shindell R, Green NE (Cook-Fort Worth Children's Clinic, Fort Worth, Tex; Phoenix, Ariz; Vanderbilt Univ, Nashville, Tenn)
J Bone Joint Surg (Am) 75-A:1593–1601, 1993   129-94-1–13

Introduction.—Compared with congenital pseudarthrosis of the tibia in infants, little is known about older children who initially are thought to be normal but later have a fracture of a dysplastic tibia. Eleven such patients were treated for late-onset pseudarthrosis of the tibia. All of them had preexisting dysplastic changes and were seen with a fracture after minor trauma.

Clinical Features.—Nine patients were first seen at an average age of 7 years with a complete tibial fracture. Two others had gradually increasing tibial pain and radiographic signs of a propagating stress fracture. All the children had preexisting dysplastic changes that included cortical tapering, sclerosis, and cyst formation in the medullary canal. Three of the patients with a complete tibial fracture also had a complete fibular fracture.

Treatment and Outcome.—The patients were variably managed by immobilization in a cast, with or without preliminary bone grafting; electrical stimulation after grafting and cast immobilization; and intramedullary fixation with bone grafting, followed by cast immobilization. Fractures were fixed with a Williams rod or a Steinmann pin. Ten of the 11 patients had had no further fractures on follow-up an average of 15 years after the most recent injury. Several tibias that were immobilized for a prolonged time in a cast became abnormally bowed anteriorly and were considered to be at risk of stress fracture. Corrective osteotomy, intramedullary fixation, bone grafting, and prolonged cast immobilization yielded a clinically straight tibia with radiographically thick cortices. One patient had a persistent pseudarthrosis despite several attempts at operative repair.

Conclusion.—This experience suggests that late-onset tibial pseudarthrosis is a more benign condition and has a better prognosis than congenital pseudarthrosis of infancy. Tibial straightening, intramedullary fixation, and bone grafting are indicated if healing fails to take place during prolonged cast immobilization.

▶ A late fracture in a dysplastic tibia will usually heal with optimal treatment. An intramedullary rod plus an autograft is my preferred treatment. Delay by prolonged immobilization in a cast does not seem warranted.—P.P. Griffin, M.D.

Galeazzi-Equivalent Injuries of the Wrist in Children

Letts M, Rowhani N (Univ of Ottawa, Ont, Canada)
J Pediatr Orthop 13:561–566, 1993   129-94-1–14

Objective.—The Galeazzi fracture—a fracture of the distal radius combined with a dislocation of the distal ulna—is rare in children. However, a variant may occur in which the radial fracture is accompanied by a fracture through the distal growth plate of the ulna. A retrospective study clarified the diagnosis, treatment, and classification of the "Galeazzi-equivalent fracture" in children.

Patients.—A 15-year review of the records of a children's hospital revealed 4 children with the classic Galeazzi fracture and 6 with a Galeazzi-equivalent fracture. The children ranged in age from 7 to 14 years; most injuries occurred when the child fell during play. Two cases of Galeazzi-equivalent fracture were unrecognized. Treatment was closed reduction with general anesthesia in 7 patients, 1 of whom eventually required open reduction and internal fixation; closed reduction with local anesthesia in the emergency department in 2 patients, both of whom sustained a repeat fracture at the same site; and open reduction in 1 patient with an open fracture.

Outcome.—Results were excellent in 4 patients, fair in 5, and poor in 1. The child with poor results had ulnar shortening and deformity of the distal end because of growth-plate arrest of the distal ulnar physis. Results were less favorable in the Galeazzi-equivalent fractures than in the classic Galeazzi fractures.

Classification.—A classification system for pediatric Galeazzi fractures was devised to emphasize the importance of anatomical variations and to facilitate proper recognition and follow-up. Fractures of the radius at the junction of the middle and distal thirds are classified as type A injuries; those of the distal third of the radius, type B; greenstick fracture of the radius with distal bowing, type C; and fractures of the distal radius with volar bowing, type D.

Conclusion.—Although both classic Galeazzi and Galeazzi-equivalent injuries are uncommon in children, many of the latter are probably misinterpreted as simple fractures of the distal radius and ulna. Galeazzi-equivalent fractures carry the risk of growth-plate arrest or persistent subluxation of the distal ulna causing long-term wrist disability. All types of Galeazzi injuries are best managed with the forearm in full supination in an above-elbow cast.

▶ The importance of this study is that it brings attention to an injury that includes a fracture of the distal ulnar epiphysis as well as a fracture of the distal radius. Always identify the ulnar epiphysis when there is a fracture of the distal radius.—P.P. Griffin, M.D.

Reduction and Fixation of Displaced Radial Neck Fractures by Closed Intramedullary Pinning

Metaizeau J-P, Lascombes P, Lemelle J-L, Finlayson D, Prevot J (Hôpital Belle-Isle, Metz, France; Hôpital d'Enfant Allée du Morvan, Vandoeuvre, France; Raigmore Hosp, Inverness, Scotland)
J Pediatr Orthop 13:355–360, 1993   129-94-1-15

Background.—Radial neck fractures in children are serious. When the tilt exceeds 60 degrees, sequelae are frequent. In these patients, conservative treatment often fails, and open reduction can result in iatrogenic injury. An experience with an original technique—closed intramedullary pinning—was described.

Technique.—With the patient under general anesthesia, the upper limb is prepared and draped from the axillary fold to the hand and put on a hand table. An image intensifier is then placed perpendicular to the limb. Through a short lateral incision 1 or 2 cm above the epiphyseal plate, the inferior radial metaphysis is exposed, and the soft tissues are carefully separated. The surgeon then perforates the cortex with a drill and introduces the prepared wire into the medullary canal. A Kirschner wire is inserted into the medullary canal of the radius, and the

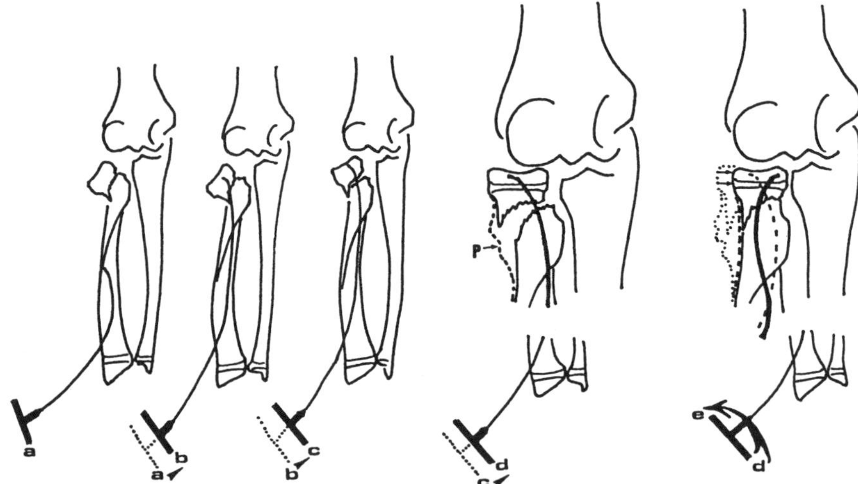

Fig 1–3.—The Kirschner wire is introduced into the lower metaphysis of the radius (*a*). It is then hammered upward, directed so that its point approaches the inferior aspect of the fracture where the tilt is the greatest, most often laterally or laterally and posteriorly (*a and b*). At this stage, the wire is advanced by gentle taps of the mallet so that the point fixes in the epiphysis and then elevates it until it is replaced under the lateral condyle, which acts as a buffer to prevent overcorrection (*c and d*). Once the tilt is corrected and the opposing epiphyseal surfaces are horizontal, a lateral shift of a few millimeters often remains (*d*). Therefore, the pin is turned around its long axis through 180 degrees (*d and e*) so that it points face inward. This produces a medial shift of the radial head and reduces it. The tension produced in the lateral intact periosteum prevents overcorrection medially (*e*). The lower metaphyseal end of the pin is then cut and the skin is closed. (Courtesy of Metaizeau J-P, Lascombes P, Lemelle J-L, et al: *J Pediatr Orthop* 13:355–360, 1993.)

pin is hammered upward until its point is at the inferior aspect of the displaced epiphysis. This allows it to be manipulated and reduced (Fig 1–3).

When the tilt exceeds 80 degrees and the epiphysis cannot be reached with the point of the intramedullary wire, the surgeon can obtain at least a partial reduction by external manipulations or percutaneous pinning. The surgeon can then perform a further reduction using the intramedullary wire. If the reduction is not perfect in the end, a second wire is introduced and fixed in the epiphysis. The surgeon then withdraws the first wire and uses the second wire as if the initial tilt had been slight. After 2–3 weeks of plaster immobilization, the elbow is gently mobilized. The wire is removed at about the eighth week when the fracture has consolidated.

Patients and Outcomes.—Thirty-one fractures with tilts of 30–80 degrees and 16 exceeding 80 degrees were treated with this technique. In the first group, the results were excellent or good in 30 fractures. In the second group, 11 fractures had excellent or good outcomes.

Conclusion.—Closed intramedullary pinning is an original technique in which the wire, introduced from below and projected upward, permits reduction of the displacement and maintenance of the correction without infringing the joint. In most fractures with tilts of 30 degrees or more, the results of this procedure are good or excellent.

▶ Insertion of a wire from the distal metaphysis to the radial head seems difficult. If the fracture is through the metaphysis in juxtaposition to the physis, manipulation as described by Bernstein, McKeever, and Bernstein (Abstract 129-94-1–16) is easier. However, if the fracture is a centimeter or more from the physis, this technique may prevent the need for an open reduction.—P.P. Griffin, M.D.

Percutaneous Reduction of Displaced Radial Neck Fractures in Children

Bernstein SM, McKeever P, Bernstein L (Univ of Southern California, Los Angeles)

J Pediatr Orthop 13:85–88, 1993   129-94-1–16

Background.—A variety of methods have been used to reduce displaced radial neck fractures in children. Open reduction of radial neck fractures is indicated in patients with severe angulation and displacement and failure of closed reduction. Percutaneous reduction with a single smooth Steinmann pin was performed in a group of patients with moderate to severe angulation to improve on the unsatisfactory results of standard radial neck fracture treatment.

Methods.—Eighteen children with displaced radial neck fractures were treated and assessed. All patients had an open physis, had sustained a fracture of the radial neck with at least 35 degrees of angulation, and had a failed attempt at closed reduction. All children were treated in the operating room, with radiographic control. Image intensification and general anesthesia were used. The technique involved a 2–3 mm stab wound dorsally on the ulnar side of the radius about 2 cm distal to the fracture. The ulnar side of the radius was chosen for the approach to avoid the arcade of Frohse, through which the deep branch of the radial nerve traverses. A Steinmann pin was then inserted and passed through the subcutaneous tissue and muscle to the radial head and neck. The radial head and neck were pushed gradually back into place, and the forearm was rotated for acceptable reduction in all planes.

Outcomes.—In 15 children, reduction was successful. The 3 treatment failures included 2 with comminuted radial head and neck fractures and 1 with a completely rotated, displaced radial head. Complications associated with the procedure were minimal.

Conclusion.—Percutaneous pin reduction in children with angulated and displaced radial neck fractures is a simple alternative to open reduction. The procedure is safe and is associated with a low complication rate.

▶ Percutaneous reduction of radial neck fractures is not new. The technique used in these patients is different from what I have used in the past, but it is shown to be very effective.—P.P. Griffin, M.D.

Treatment of Chronic Post-Traumatic Dislocation of the Radial Head in Children
Oner FC, Diepstraten AFM (Univ Hosp, Rotterdam, The Netherlands; Sophia Children's Hosp, Rotterdam, The Netherlands)
J Bone Joint Surg (Br) 75-B:577–581, 1993   129-94-1–17

Introduction.—Chronic dislocation of the radial head in children rarely results from unrecognized Monteggia lesions. A number of operative techniques have been recommended, including osteotomy of the ulna, which appears to carry a high complication rate. The small number of reported cases has made it impossible to tell whether osteotomy is necessary.

Methods.—The results with open reduction and ligament reconstruction by a triceps tendon slip were reported for 6 girls and 1 boy with chronic post-traumatic dislocation of the radial head. The patients were 4–9 years of age, and symptoms included decreased range of motion, valgus deformity, and pain. Three patients had anterior dislocation with ulnar fracture (the Bado type I dislocation); 2 had anterolateral dislocation without ulnar fracture (type I equivalent); and 2 had anterolateral dislocation with ulnar fracture. All of the operations were performed by the same surgeon using the technique of Lloyd-Roberts and Bucknill.

Results.—In each case, the radial head was easily reduced after excision of the interposed capsule. Four of the 5 patients with anterior dislocations had good results, achieving maximal range of motion within 1 year after surgery and with no complaints related to their elbows. The other patient with a type I dislocation had sickle-cell disease, preventing the use of a tourniquet. A proximal radioulnar synostosis developed, which was untreated because her arm function was satisfactory. The 2 patients with anterolateral dislocations were left with persistent bowing of the ulna; in both, subluxation of the radial head developed within 6 months. The lateral bowing was unchanged during follow-up, but the sagittal angulation of the ulna remodeled progressively.

Conclusion.—Open reduction and ligament reconstruction is an effective procedure for children with chronic post-traumatic anterior dislocations of the radial head. Children with anterolateral dislocations should have a combination of open reduction and ligament reconstruction with osteotomy of the ulna. Osteotomy should be done only for patients in whom stable reduction is otherwise impossible or for those in whom the deformity may cause later subluxation, as in patients with anterolateral dislocation.

► When the ulna is malunited and has plastic deformation with the apex of the angulation (anterior or lateral), the radial head cannot be anatomically reduced. If the radial head is reduced and held with a pin, it will very likely gradually become subluxated. When in doubt, osteotomize the ulna, reduce the head, and internally stabilize the osteotomy.—P.P. Griffin, M.D.

Premature Greater Trochanteric Epiphysiodesis Secondary to Intramedullary Femoral Rodding

Raney EM, Ogden JA, Grogan DP (Shriners Hosp for Crippled Children, Tampa, Fla)
J Pediatr Orthop 13:516–520, 1993   129-94-1-18

Introduction.—Intramedullary rod treatment is often recommended for children in their second decade of life for femoral subtrochanteric and diaphyseal fractures. Five young patients in whom premature closure of the greater trochanteric physis developed after treatment with the rods for femoral diaphyseal fractures were reported.

Patients and Findings.—The patient group included 3 boys aged 11–13 years and 2 girls aged 9 and 11 years. Three of the children had closed reduction and fluoroscopic femoral rodding (Fig 1–4, A and B), and 2 had open reduction and open placement of the femoral rod. Evidence of closure appeared 5–8 months after the operation in 4 patients and 3 years later in the fifth patient. In 4 children, an increased valgus position of the femoral neck developed progressively as compared with the contralateral hip (Fig 1–4, C). Despite an obvious morphological difference between the operated and contralateral hips, none of the patients had any functional deficit at a follow-up of 2–7 years.

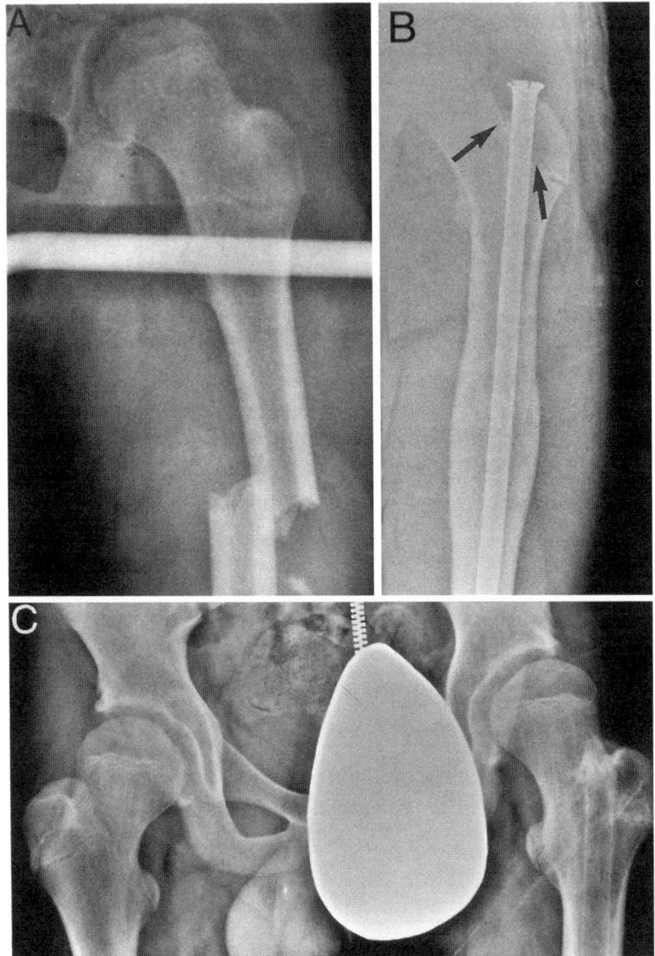

Fig 1–4.—Boy, 14 years 10 months of age, who underwent femoral rodding at age 12 years 1 month. **A,** appearance of the hip and femoral fracture at time of injury. The femoral head is located and covered. **B,** healed fracture 9 months after intramedullary rodding with osseous bridging on either side of the medullary rod (*arrows*), although the lateral portion of the trochanteric physis is open. The femoral head is well covered. **C,** radiograph taken 7 months after removal of the rod shows increased articulotrochanteric distance of the left femur vs. the uninjured right femur, which still had an open greater trochanteric physis. In contrast, the left femur had premature closure of the trochanteric physis, whereas the capital femoral physis was still open. There was lateral uncovering of the femoral head 27 months after the injury. (Courtesy of Raney EM, Ogden JA, Grogan DP: *J Pediatr Orthop* 13:516–520, 1993.)

Discussion.—Examination of 16 proximal femurs from cadavers or hip amputations of patients aged 8–14 years confirmed that a rod placed across the cartilage connecting the greater trochanter and the capital femur could affect the growth potential of both the femoral neck and greater trochanter. Premature fusion and deformity may also occur if smooth pins with a diameter significantly smaller than the intramedullary rod are placed across the physis.

Conclusion.—Skeletally immature patients with the type of fractures described should be considered for alternative methods of treatment, either operative or nonoperative. The rods can be safely used in children who are in the middle or at the end of the growth spurt and who have subchondral "sclerosis" along the greater trochanteric physis. Because neither the patients reported here nor those described in the literature have had long-term follow-up, it is not known whether the increased valgus will result in lasting consequences.

▶ In the immature patient, coxa valga and overgrowth of the femur may interfere with normal growth of the lateral acetabulum that could result in acetabular dysplasia. In patients with developmental dysplasia of the hip in whom a long leg develops after an open reduction and femoral osteotomy, the acetabular dysplasia will frequently be maintained or increased if, in addition to the long leg, femoral neck valgus redevelops.—P.P. Griffin, M.D.

Observations on Acute Knee Hemarthrosis in Children and Adolescents

Stanitski CL, Harvell JC, Fu F (Wayne State Univ, Detroit; East Carolina Univ, Greenville, NC; Univ of Pittsburgh, Pa)
J Pediatr Orthop 13:506–510, 1993   129-94-1-19

Purpose.—Most studies of hemarthrosis in acute knee injuries have focused on adult patients. Traditionally, intra-articular injury in the knees of children and adolescents has been considered rare. The findings of 70 pediatric patients with acute knee injury and hemarthrosis were reviewed.

Patients.—Fifteen of the children were preadolescent (10 girls and 5 boys) and 55 were adolescent (37 boys and 18 girls). More than 70% were injured during sports participation. All underwent systematic diagnostic arthroscopy for evidence of injuries to various structures.

Findings.—Meniscal tears were noted in 47% of the preadolescents and 45% of the adolescents. The incidences of anterior cruciate ligament tears were 47% and 65%, respectively. Combination meniscal and anterior cruciate ligament tears were present in 1 member of the preadolescent group and in 18% of the adolescent group. Osteochondral injuries were noted in 7% of patients overall.

Conclusion.—Children and adolescents with acute knee hemarthrosis commonly have meniscal and anterior cruciate ligament injury, particularly adolescents. Contrary to traditional teaching, this age group can and does sustain intra-articular injuries. Arthroscopy is an effective means of diagnosis and specific treatment.

▶ This study identified the frequency of meniscal and anterior cruciate ligament tears in children with hemarthrosis. Traditionally, most young children with hemarthrosis of the knee appear to do well with protection followed by rehabilitation. However, the question remains whether these children need acute surgical treatment. I tremble at the thought of the number of patients with hemarthrosis that I have treated without arthroscopic diagnosis. The author needs to report on the treatment and outcome of these patients.—P.P. Griffin, M.D.

Long-Term Follow-Up of Anterior Tibial Eminence Fractures
Willis RB, Blokker C, Stoll TM, Paterson DC, Galpin RD (Univ of Western Ontario, London, Ont, Canada; Adelaide Children's Hosp, North Adelaide, Australia)
J Pediatr Orthop 13:361–364, 1993   129-94-1–20

Background.—In a recent long-term assessment of children with anterior tibial eminence fractures, chronic anterior instability of the knee was found to be a common sequela unrelated to the type of treatment used for reduction. Another assessment was done to determine the clinical signs of anterior laxity and to quantify the degree of anterior instability with a KT-1000 arthrometer, which is commonly used to evaluate knee ligament function.

Patients and Findings.—Of 97 patients treated at 2 centers for fractures of the anterior intercondylar eminence of the tibia, 50 agreed to return at least 2 years after injury for a detailed follow-up assessment. At the time of injury, the average patient age was 13 years. Twenty-nine patients had type III injuries; 18 had type II; and 3 had type I. At a mean follow-up of 4 years, 64% had clinical signs of anterior instability. Seventy-four percent had objective evidence of laxity as determined by the KT-1000 arthrometer. Ten percent of the patients reported pain. None complained of instability. The method of treatment—open or closed—had no effect on eventual outcome.

Conclusion.—In the long term, most children sustaining a tibial eminence fracture have objective evidence of anterior cruciate ligament laxity; however, few have subjective complaints. Closed reduction and immobilization in extension should be performed in children with anterior tibial eminence fractures. Clinicians may use arthroscopy to ensure adequate fragment reduction. Open reduction and internal fixation should be used only for patients with irreducible tibial eminence fractures. In light of the persistent anterior cruciate ligament laxity found in this series, the long-term prognosis for patients with this injury must remain guarded.

▶ This is another report that supports the nonoperative treatment of fractures of the tibial eminence. The knee laxity that occurs in most children as a sequela to this fracture will not alter function. Loss of extension can be prevented if the fracture is treated with the knee extended. If the knee cannot be fully extended, open reduction or arthroscopic reduction is indicated.—P.P. Griffin, M.D.

Spine

Correlation Between Bone Age and Risser's Sign in Adolescent Idiopathic Scoliosis

Dhar S, Dangerfield PH, Dorgan JC, Klenerman L (Royal Liverpool Childrens Hosp, England; Univ of Liverpool, England)
Spine 18:14–19, 1993   129-94-1-21

Objective.—Two ways of estimating skeletal maturity in adolescent idiopathic scoliosis—determining bone age at the hand and wrist and evaluating the degree of development of the iliac apophysis (Risser's sign)—were compared in 86 affected girls.

Subjects and Methods.—The chronological age range was 10–18 years. When radiographs of the hand and wrist were rated by 2 observers, agreement within and between the observers ranged from 84% to 86%. For pelvic radiographs, levels of agreement ranged from 89% to 93%.

Findings and Implications.—The 2 methods of estimating skeletal maturity correlated to a significant degree. The development of the iliac apophysis is a sensitive and convenient measure of skeletal maturity in adolescent girls with idiopathic scoliosis.

▶ It is easier to read the Risser sign on appropriate radiographs than it is to determine maturity using a radiograph of the hand and wrist. When decision-making in the patient with scoliosis, the iliac apophysis is a better measurement of maturity as it relates to remaining spine growth.—P.P. Griffin, M.D.

Costoplasty in Adolescent Idiopathic Scoliosis: Objective Results in 55 Patients

Barrett DS, MacLean JGB, Bettany J, Ransford AO, Edgar MA (Royal Natl Orthopaedic Hosp, Stanmore, England)
J Bone Joint Surg (Br) 75-B:881–885, 1993   129-94-1-22

Introduction.—The unsightly rib prominence often seen in adolescent idiopathic scoliosis may be unchanged by surgery, resulting in patient dissatisfaction and disappointment. Costoplasty, designed to reduce rib prominence in such patients, may be performed as a preliminary procedure, at the time of primary surgery for scoliosis, or as a secondary procedure offered after skeletal maturity. Rib prominence was assessed after simple short-segment costoplasty without internal or external fixation or muscle transfer. Results of costoplasty at the time of primary surgery were compared with results of secondary operations in mature patients.

Patients and Methods.—Thirty-five patients (average age, 14.3 years) had costoplasty during the operation of primary Harrington rod instrumentation and segmental Luque wiring. Twenty mature patients had costoplasty as a secondary procedure, performed at an average age of 24.4 years. All patients had preoperative and postoperative assessments of rib prominence and pulmonary function. The extent of rib prominence was marked on the skin preoperatively while the patient was in a forward-bending position. After the rib was exposed, its prominent costotransverse joints and transverse processes were trimmed. Removed rib segments were used as bone grafts for the spinal fusion. The final review of outcome was at a minimum of 2 years after operation.

Results.—Costoplasty was carried out on an average of 5 ribs for each patient. Both groups of patients showed a significant decrease in the volume of the rib prominence, the maximum skin surface angle, and the Bunnell angle. The reduction of prominence was proportionately greater in the patients who had a primary combined procedure. All patients experienced reformation of the rib within 3.6 months and none had decreased respiratory function. Complications included 8 instances of pneumothorax, which did not prolong hospitalization, and 3 cases of prominence of the scapula.

Conclusion.—Both immature and mature patients can benefit from costoplasty, and the correction achieved does not appear to reduce with time. Two types of rib deformity were distinguished on the basis of whether the rib prominence is placed medially or laterally. Attention to these 2 types of rib prominence aids in planning a successful procedure. Costoplasty should be possible in most patients with idiopathic scoliosis and rib prominence.

▶ Costoplasty has a place in the reduction of rib prominence that is not significantly reduced by the newer techniques for correction of scoliosis curves. Costoplasty is exceptionally successful in patients who have had early correction and fusion and in whom an increased rib hump develops secondary to the crankshaft phenomenon.—P.P. Griffin, M.D.

Long-Term Results of Boston Brace Treatment on Vertebral Rotation in Idiopathic Scoliosis
Willers U, Normelli H, Aaro S, Svensson O, Hedlund R (Huddinge Univ, Sweden; Linkping Univ, Huddinge, Sweden)
Spine 18:432–435, 1993   129-94-1–23

Introduction.—The Boston brace is a popular conservative treatment for idiopathic scoliosis that, because of its better cosmetic appearance, may improve treatment compliance. Treatment of scoliosis has generally emphasized restoration of the coronal plane deformity, although it has been suggested that vertebral rotation may be a better reflection of the severity of disease. The long-term effect of the Boston brace on the 3-dimensional deformity was examined in patients with idiopathic scoliosis.

Methods.—The patients were 30 girls and 3 boys with idiopathic scoliosis (mean age, 14 years) who were treated using a Boston brace without a superstructure. Analysis of the long-term results was based on 25 patients who wore the brace for at least 12 months. The mean Cobb angle was 31 degrees and the mean duration of treatment was 3 years. Patients were followed for a mean of 5 years after the end of treatment. The results were assessed by CT measurement of vertebral rotation, rib hump index, sagittal diameter of the thoracic cage, and translation of the apical vertebra in the coronal plane.

Results.—At a mean follow-up of 8½ years, there were no significant changes in Cobb angle, vertebral rotation, rib hump index, or translation of the apical vertebra. The rib hump was significantly increased in patients with the apex below T12, but this was thought to be of minor cosmetic importance. There was a significant decrease in the sagittal diameter of the thoracic cage.

Conclusion.—Boston bracing does not appear to improve vertebral rotation, translation, rib hump, or Cobb angle in patients with idiopathic scoliosis. Whether bracing prevents progression of the deformity was not determined. The observed reduction in sagittal diameter may be relevant to cosmesis and pulmonary function.

▶ This study of a small number of patients showed no improvement in the several measurable parameters studied. However, there was no increase in the curve or the rotation. The decrease in the sagittal diameter of the thorax is probably a part of the natural history in untreated patients. See my comment after the Goldberg et al. study (Abstract 129-94-1-24).—P.P. Griffin, M.D.

A Statistical Comparison Between Natural History of Idiopathic Scoliosis and Brace Treatment in Skeletally Immature Adolescent Girls
Goldberg CJ, Dowling FE, Hall JE, Emans JB (Our Lady's Hosp for Sick Children, Dublin; Harvard Med School, Boston)
Spine 18:902–908, 1993   129-94-1-24

Background.—Orthoses are widely used to treat late-onset idiopathic scoliosis. Many reports of brace results have appeared in the literature, but few have compared these results with the natural history of the disorder. Brace treatment and the natural history of idiopathic scoliosis were compared in skeletally immature girls.

Methods and Findings.—The study subjects were 32 adolescent girls braced for late-onset idiopathic scoliosis at a Boston hospital and 32 un-

TABLE 1.—Data on Braced Patients

Patient No.	Age (yr) Brace	Age (yr) Weaned	Cobb (°) Brace	Cobb (°) Wean	Change	Site	Menarche*	Status
Braced patients								
1	13.5	15.5	25	40	+15	T	0	
2	13.3	16.3	25	10	-15	L	-	
3	12.2	13.9	25	25	0	D	+	
4	12.1	14.3	25	20	-5	TL	0	
5	14.2	15.2	20	11	-9	L	+	
6	13.4	15.7	23	25	+2	D	-	
7	12.5	15.2	22	15	-7	L	0	
8	14.8	15.7	20	15	-5	T	+	
9	14.3	16.8	20	50	+30	TL	-	Surgery
10	14.0	17.0	20	21	+1	T	-	
11	13.9	15.3	25	21	-4	T	+	
12	13.3	16.3	20	16	-4	D	0	
13	13.0	14.4	20	20	0	T	0	
14	12.9	13.9	20	25	+5	TL	-	
15	12.6	13.8	20	20	0	TL	0	
16	12.4	14.0	20	30	+10	T	-	
17	12.4	14.4	20	17	-3	T	-	
18	12.3	15.3	20	22	+2	D	-	
19	13.2	15.6	19	15	-4	D	0	
20	12.2	13.6	17	20	+3	T	-	
21	12.3	16.3	15	18	+3	L	-	
22	13.0	14.7	30	30	0	TL	+	
23	13.0	15.7	15	14	-1	T	+	
24	14.0	16.1	16	13	-3	T	+	
25	12.4	15.2	16	26	+10	T	-	
26	12.7	15.2	31	32	+1	TL	+	
27	12.2	13.5	31	42	+11	T	0	Surgery
28	12.8	14.9	30	34	+4	T	+	
29	12.3	15.1	26	25	-1	TL	-	
30	14.9	16.6	25	30	+5	L	+	
31	13.7	16.7	25	38	+13	D	0	Surgery late
32	13.6	15.9	25	24	-1	TL	+	

Abbreviations: T, thoracic; L, lumbar; D, dorsal; TL, thoracolumbar.
** Minus sign indicates patient was premenarche at diagnosis; plus sign indicates postmenarche; zero indicates menarchal status at diagnosis is unknown.*
(Courtesy of Goldberg CJ, Dowling FE, Hall JE, et al: *Spine* 18:902–908, 1993.)

treated girls at a Dublin hospital. The groups were matched for curve size and site and age at diagnosis. All subjects were classified as Risser 0 when late-onset idiopathic scoliosis was initially diagnosed. No significant differences were found between groups on any parameter of curve progression (Tables 1 and 2).

Conclusion.—The lack of significant differences between groups in this study casts doubt on the efficacy of bracing in the treatment of late-onset idiopathic scoliosis. Withholding treatment in a randomized, prospective trial may no longer be ethically problematic.

TABLE 2.—Data on Untreated Controls

	Age (yr)		Cobb (°)					
	Diagnosed	Last	Diagnosis	Last				
Untreated control patients								
1	13.5	15.3	18	26	+8	T	-	
2	12.9	16.6	20	34	+14	L	-	
3	12.8	14.6	17	16	-1	L	+	
4	12.6	14.8	20	8	-12	TL	+	
5	14.2	15.9	15	19	4	L	+	
6	13.4	15.5	19	28	+9	TL	-	
7	12.5	14.2	18	24	+6	L	-	
8	14.3	16.2	16	22	+6	T	-	
9	14.5	16.2	24	24	0	TL	-	
10	13.9	15.9	22	20	-2	T	-	
11	14.0	17.2	35	30	-5	T	+	
12	13.1	14.6	19	8	-11	T	-	
13	12.3	15.3	18	20	+2	T	-	
14	12.9	17.5	17	25	+8	T	-	
15	12.1	16.6	17	40	+23	TL	-	Surgery
16	12.5	15.5	20	45	+20	T	-	Surgery
17	13.4	15.0	20	25	+5	T	+	
18	12.9	14.9	18	20	+2	T	-	
19	13.3	16.6	19	47	+28	T	-	Surgery
20	11.9	14.4	17	40	+23	T	-	Surgery
21	12.3	14.7	15	31	+16	TL	-	
22	13.2	16.1	35	38	+3	D	-	
23	12.5	14.4	15	8	-7	TL	-	
24	14.4	15.5	18	18	0	TL	+	
25	12.3	14.6	16	15	-1	L	-	
26	13.4	15.7	27	27	0	T	-	
27	11.9	16.2	24	38	+14	T	-	
28	13.1	13.5	25	38	+13	T	-	Surgery
29	11.9	17.4	21	44	+23	T	-	
30	14.5	16.4	24	15	-9	TL	-	
31	13.8	15.6	25	28	+3	D	+	
32	14.2	15.3	25	25	0	TL	+	

Abbreviations: T, thoracic; *L*, lumbar; *D*, dorsal; *TL*, thoracolumbar.

Note: In the last column, a *minus sign* indicates patient was premenarche at diagnosis; a *plus sign* indicates postmenarche.

(Courtesy of Goldberg CJ, Dowling FE, Hall JE, et al: *Spine* 18:902–908, 1993.)

▶ The results in this paper suggest that bracing has no significant effect on the natural history of scoliosis. However, there were flaws in this project. It was retrospective; patients in the control group were not followed to maturity as were those in the brace group; and the method of selection of patients for the control group was not unbiased. We should not discontinue brace treatment for adolescent scoliosis. At the 1993 meeting of the Scoliosis Research Society, the results of a multicenter prospective study comparing the efficacy of bracing, electrical stimulation, and observation came out strongly in favor of bracing. More prospective long-term studies are needed to evaluate brace treatment of late-onset scoliosis.—P.P. Griffin, M.D.

Anterior Correction of Idiopathic Scoliosis Using TSRH Instrumentation

Turi M, Johnston CE II, Richards BS (Dallas; Texas Scottish Rite Hosp for Children, Dallas)
Spine 18:417–422, 1993   129-94-1-25

Background.—The use of anterior instrumentation and fusion to correct thoracolumbar and lumbar scoliosis is an established technique. In the Texas Scottish Rite Hospital (TSRH) Spinal Instrumentation System, hooks, screws, and Crosslinks are attached to smooth rods to allow correction and fixation of spinal deformities or instabilities, either anteriorly or posteriorly. The results of anterior correction of idiopathic scoliosis using TSRH instrumentation were reported.

Methods and Findings.—The first 14 patients with idiopathic lumbar scoliosis treated with the TSRH system were reviewed. The mean frontal curve correction was 76%, with a 5-degree loss of correction during an average follow-up of 17.6 months. Spinal balance was improved by a mean of 1.8 cm toward the center sacral line. Apical vertebral rotation was corrected by a mean of 49%. Instrumentational kyphosis was minimal. The total L1–S1 lordosis decreased by a mean of 1 degree. There was no measured compensatory hyperlordosis caudal to the instrumented segment. All disk spaces were fused by 8 months, as seen on radiography. No neurologic, septic, or implant complications occurred (Fig 1–5).

Conclusion.—The contoured solid rod used in this system provides the same frontal and rotatory correction as in previous systems. Instrumentational kyphosis is minimized. The stiffness of the construct enables rapid, reliable fusion. The construct may also obviate the need for postoperative immobilization.

▶ The TSRH anterior instruments have improved the results of instrumentation in the anterior correction of scoliosis. Using this system, forces are more evenly distributed because the rotation is decreased as the compression is applied. This, in addition to the rigidity of the system, should result in fewer failures of instrumentation and a lower-rated pseudoarthrosis.—P.P. Griffin, M.D.

Persistent Synchondrosis of the Second Cervical Vertebra Simulating a Hangman's Fracture in a Child: Report of a Case

Smith JT, Skinner SR, Shonnard NH (Univ of California, San Francisco)
J Bone Joint Surg (Am) 75-A:1228–1230, 1993   129-94-1-26

Purpose.—The rare fracture of the cervical spine in a child tends to involve the cephalic portion of the cervical spine. The hangman's fracture, or traumatic spondylolisthesis of the cervical spine, may occur in

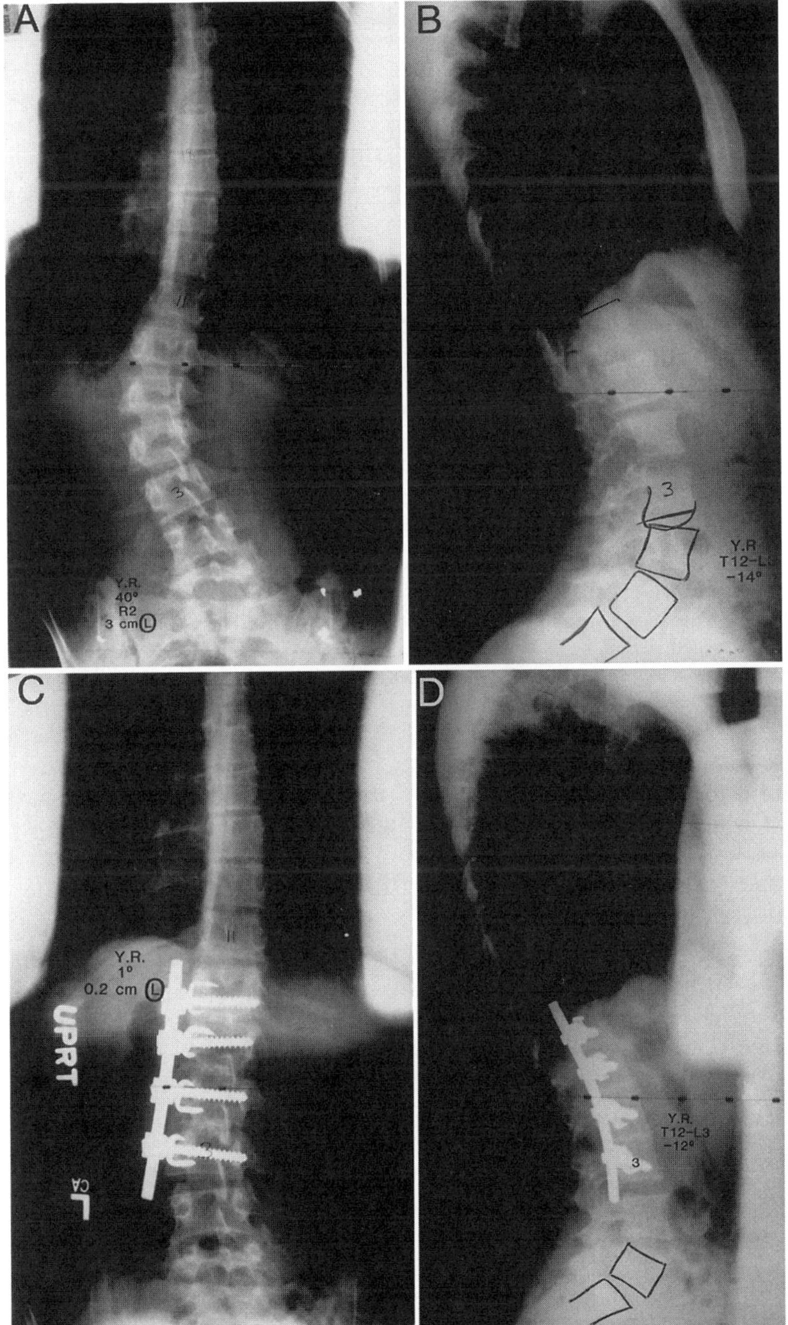

Fig 1–5.—A, preoperative anteroposterior radiograph of a 14-year-old girl with a left lumbar deformity. There is a 3-cm lateral trunk shift to the left. **B,** preoperative lateral radiograph. **C,** postoperative anteroposterior radiograph, 4 months after surgery, showing essentially complete correction of preoperative measured curve and trunk shift. **D,** lateral radiograph, 4 months after operation. There has been a negligible change in the sagittal contour. There is solid arthrodesis of each disk space. No postoperative immobilization was used. (Courtesy of Turi M, Johnston CE II, Richards BS: *Spine* 18:417–422, 1993.)

31

children; it usually causes no neurologic deficit and unites without operative treatment. Traumatic lesions of the cervical spine in children must be differentiated from pseudosubluxation, laminar defects, and synchondrosis. The problems of evaluating the cervical spine were illustrated in a child with neck injury.

Case Report.—Boy, 18 months, fell from a height of 2.5 m, landing in a shrub. Emergency department evaluation showed no sign of neurologic deficit, but the lateral cervical spine radiograph appeared to show an acute fracture of the posterior arch of the second cervical vertebra. The diagnosis was supported by the CT finding of a bilateral cleft of the posterior arch. Treatment was with neck immobilization in a halo vest. The patient fell again while playing 1 month later, and some of the halo pins penetrated the calvarium. There were no signs of healing on radiographs, so the pins were replaced at new sites. A few months later, cellulitis developed on the side of the face from a pin site infection, and the patient was referred for further treatment.

A review of the initial imaging studies gave the impression that the defects represented a synchondrosis of the posterior arch of the second cervical vertebra, where the pedicles met the body of the axis. There were no signs of instability on lateral radiographs of the cervical spine. There was no change in the imaging appearance of the lesion until 5 years after the injury, when some ossification of the synchondrosis was noted.

Discussion.—In children, it may be difficult to distinguish fractures of the arch of the axis from a synchondrosis. The inability to obtain a detailed history contributes to the problem of making a definitive diagnosis. Differentiation of traumatic from congenital spondylolysis may require radiographs, CT, and sometimes MRI.

▶ The persistent synchondrosis of the second cervical vertebra has the appearance of hangman's fracture. Flexion and extension lateral radiographs may not clearly distinguish the two. Magnetic resonance imaging may be needed to make the diagnosis. However, in general, hangman's fracture will have persistent pain, whereas the synchondrosis will be painless.—P.P. Griffin, M.D.

Cervical Spine Subluxation Associated With Congenital Muscular Torticollis and Craniofacial Asymmetry

Slate RK, Posnick JC, Armstrong DC, Buncic JR (Univ of Toronto; Georgetown Univ, Washington, DC)
Plast Reconstr Surg 91:1187–1197, 1993
129-94-1–27

Background.—Craniofacial asymmetry with neck rotation and head tilt can result from congenital torticollis. Cervical spine rotatory subluxation may also produce head and neck postural problems. The relationship between craniofacial asymmetry, congenital muscular torticollis, and cervical spine subluxation was examined.

Patients and Findings.—Thirty children seen in a craniofacial program between 1987 and 1990 were assessed. Twenty-six had craniofacial asymmetry and muscular torticollis without true suture synostosis on head and neck CT scans. These children had positional skull molding with flattening of the contralateral occipitoparietal region and ipsilateral fronto-orbital region. Thirteen of these 26 children also had C1–C2 subluxation. In 12 patients, C1 was rotated forward of C2 on the side contralateral to the muscular torticollis. None of the children with subluxation had neurologic deficits or needed spinal stabilization. Ophthalmologic assessment revealed amblyopia in 4 children and horizontal strabismus in 1. Both of these conditions were thought to be coincidental. There was no evidence of nystagmus in any child. Seven of the 26 children needed surgery for tightness of the neck muscles; the rest responded to physiotherapy. Cranio-orbital reshaping was needed in only 2 children to correct upper facial asymmetry.

Conclusion.—Congenital muscular torticollis is common and can be successfully treated with early physiotherapy for sternocleidomastoid muscle tightness. Craniofacial asymmetry will then improve. A small number of these patients will have a true suture synostosis and need cranial vault and orbital surgery.

▶ The sternocleidomastoid muscle tightness in most patients with torticollis improves without therapy by 1 year of age. Those who do not improve need the muscle lengthened. The recognition by CT that C1 was subluxed on C2 was an interesting finding. All of the subluxations resolved when the muscle tightness was corrected. Further investigation is needed to determine the significance of these findings.—P.P. Griffin, M.D.

General

Hip Abnormalities in Children With Charcot-Marie-Tooth Disease

Walker JL, Nelson KR, Heavilon JA, Stevens DB, Lubicky JP, Ogden JA, VandenBrink KA (Shriners Hosps for Crippled Children, Lexington, Ky; Moore Orthopaedic Clinic, Columbia, SC; Shriners Hosps for Crippled Children, Chicago; et al)
J Pediatr Orthop 14:54–59, 1994   129-94-1–28

Introduction.—In 1985, Kumar et al. reported 5 girls with hip dysplasia associated with Charcot-Marie-Tooth disease (CMT). A retrospective review of the medical records of patients with CMT at 3 centers was done to define the incidence of hip dysplasia in CMT.

Patients.—One hundred patients met both clinical and electrodiagnostic criteria for CMT. Of those, 74 had available radiographs showing the most mature hips. Most radiographs were obtained as a screening procedure for a possible spinal anomaly causing foot deformity; only 6 patients had hip complaints.

Findings.—Six patients had hip dysplasia, constituting 6% of patients with documented CMT and 8.1% of those with available radiographs. All patients with hip dysplasia had hereditary motor and sensory neuropathy type I (HMSN-I), and only 3 had symptoms. There were 5 girls and 1 boy, but the female predominance might have resulted from the sampling of more immature radiographs in males. Another 21 patients had minor hip abnormalities, most frequently increased neck shaft angles. These abnormalities were noted in both HMSN-I and HSMN-II Charcot-Marie-Tooth disease.

Implications.—A high index of suspicion is needed for the diagnosis of hip dysplasia in CMT. Most dysplasia is asymptomatic and detected only on screening radiographs. Because treatment of hip dysplasia in children with CMT depends on the severity of symptoms, earlier diagnosis with screening radiographs in the absence of symptoms may not be expected to change the management of the child's dysplasia.

Latex Allergy in Children With Myelodysplasia: A Survey of Shriners Hospitals

Meeropol E, Frost J, Pugh L, Roberts J, Ogden JA (Shriners Hosps for Crippled Children, Springfield, Mass; Shriners Hosps for Crippled Children, Tampa, Fla)
J Pediatr Orthop 13:1–4, 1993   129-94-1–29

Background.—Families and caregivers have reported latex allergies in children with myelodysplasia. The incidence of latex sensitivity in patients with myelodysplasia was determined in a survey at the Shriners Hospitals for Crippled Children.

Methods and Findings.—A total of 2,952 children at 16 hospitals were surveyed. The mean percentage of children with myelodysplasia and a history of latex allergy was 5%, with a range of 0% to 22%. Significant anaphylactic reaction occurred in 22 patients. Five hospitals had policies and procedures for latex allergy in place or in progress.

Recommendations.—Every child with myelodysplasia should be screened carefully for latex allergy at every outpatient visit and hospital admission. Data on latex allergy need to be documented in the patient's medical record. Children with a clinical history of such allergy should be designated as latex allergic, and all children with myelodysplasia should be considered on latex alert. A latex-free environment in both the hospital and community should be created. Children with a history of latex allergy should be assessed individually by an anesthesiologist for preoperative prophylaxis. All families of children with myelodysplasia should be given printed and verbal information about latex allergy, including the recommended precautions. Health care providers caring for children with myelodysplasia need to be made aware of the potential of latex allergy and should continue to investigate its incidence, prevention, and treatment.

▶ The recommendations made based on this survey of children with myelodysplasia are sound. All physicians and others who care for these children should be aware and react appropriately.—P.P. Griffin, M.D.

Neuromuscular Approach to the Motor Deficits of Cerebral Palsy: A Pilot Study

Pape KE, Kirsch SE, Galil A, Boulton JE, White MA, Chipman M (Univ of Toronto; Ben-Gurion Univ, Beer-Sheva, Israel; Mount Sinai Hosp, Toronto)
J Pediatr Orthop 13:628–633, 1993   129-94-1-30

Introduction.—Various methods have been tried to influence spasticity in cerebral palsy, including casting, massage, splinting, nerve blocks, and electrical stimulation (ES). Both animal and human studies demonstrate that a wide variety of electrical wave forms and current intensities result in muscle growth and strength and change in muscle fiber type. Whether ES could reduce spasticity for the long term was investigated.

Patients and Methods.—Young children with mild ambulatory cerebral palsy were selected for the study. The 2 boys and 4 girls ranged in age from 3 to 6 years. All had normal cognition and had taken part in ongoing therapy programs for several years. Motor delay in the children was confirmed by Psychomotor Developmental Index scores. The children underwent overnight low-intensity transcutaneous ES to the leg muscles. Six months of treatment were followed by 6 months off treatment. Electrical stimulation was then instituted for a second 6-month treatment period. The children continued with their usual physical therapy during the ES study.

Results.—Six months of ES treatment brought about a statistically significant improvement in the gross motor, locomotor, and receipt/propulsion skills scores of the Peabody Developmental Motor Scales. Daytime spasticity was decreased and balance improved. Except for locomotor scores, there was a uniform decline in scores after the 6 months without ES treatment. Further significant improvements were observed after ES was reinstituted.

Conclusion.—Overnight ES may be a useful addition to standard rehabilitation methods in some patients with cerebral palsy, particularly in children who are mildly affected. The therapy is noninvasive, easy to learn, and does not increase the caregiver's burden. Two years after the second period of ES was discontinued, 4 of the 5 patients who were compliant with ES therapy showed no deterioration.

▶ The use of ES to strengthen muscles is not new, but its use in patients with cerebral palsy has not been previously reported. It may have a place in the selected patient. Electrical stimulation plus exercises with biofeedback techniques could be the prescribed treatment of the future.—P.P. Griffin, M.D.

Subtalar Arthrodesis for Stabilization of Valgus Hindfoot in Patients With Cerebral Palsy
Alman BA, Craig CL, Zimbler S (Tufts Univ, Boston; Harvard Med School, Boston)
J Pediatr Orthop 13:634–641, 1993   129-94-1–31

Introduction.—Reported results of extra-articular subtalar arthrodesis for correction of valgus hindfoot in patients with cerebral palsy have varied greatly. Because different techniques are used in the procedure, sorting out the variables that lead to a successful outcome is difficult. Long-term results in patients who were treated by 2 surgeons using identical surgical techniques were evaluated.

Patients and Methods.—Subtalar arthrodesis was performed on 53 feet (29 patients) by 2 orthopedic surgeons between 1971 and 1986. All patients had spastic cerebral palsy and progressive valgus deformity despite bracing. The age of the patients at operation ranged from 4 to 12 years; the average follow-up was 8.9 years. The operative technique was a modification of that reported by Grice, using a lateral approach to the sinus tarsi. Patients were kept non–weight-bearing in a long leg cast until the threaded wires were removed. A short leg cast was then used for 4 weeks, followed by an ankle-foot orthosis for 6 more months. Each patient had standing anteroposterior and lateral radiographs of the foot and ankle before surgery, after final cast removal, and at most recent follow-up. Talar head uncovering was the method used to evaluate hindfoot valgus.

Results.—Two patients were lost to follow-up at 2 and 3 years after arthrodesis. Preoperatively, the percentage of talar uncovering showed a range of 33% to 68% (average, 55%). The range was 0% to 10% (average, 4%) immediately after arthrodesis and 0% to 66% (average, 5%) at most recent follow-up. Alignment of the tibial plafond averaged 4 degrees of valgus before operation, with no change in this angle immediately after operation. At most recent follow-up, tibial plafond alignment averaged 6 degrees of valgus. Sixteen patients had a good result and could discontinue bracing, 8 had a satisfactory result, and 5 operations were failures. Those 5 patients, all with spastic quadriplegia, had progressive hindfoot or ankle deformity at most recent follow-up. There was a significant difference in failure rate between quadriplegic patients and those less severely affected.

Conclusion.—Subtalar arthrodesis is a major treatment option in skeletally immature patients with cerebral palsy and valgus hindfoot. For best results and long-term correction, patients selected for this procedure should be less severely affected. Factors that may lead to a negative outcome include valgus alignment of the tibial plafond and an unpredictable neurologic picture.

▶ The results reported here are similar to mine. Subtalar arthrodesis (the Grice procedure) plus fixation with talocalcaneal screws or Kirschner wire gives excellent early results. Late failures are usually caused by progressive varus when there is overcorrection at surgery or progressive abduction and valgus when there is excessive peroneal tightness and spasticity. Overcorrection should be avoided and peroneal strength decreased by lengthening in selected patients.—P.P. Griffin, M.D.

Posterior Dislocation of the Humeral Head in Infancy Associated With Obstetrical Paralysis: A Case Report
Troum S, Floyd WE III, Waters PM (Med Ctr of Central Georgia, Macon; Macon Orthopaedic and Hand Ctr, Ga; Children's Orthopaedic Surgery Found, Boston)
J Bone Joint Surg (Am) 75-A:1370–1375, 1993   129-94-1–32

Background.—Posterior humeral head dislocation in infants is rare. It is most often associated with brachial plexus palsy from birth trauma.

Case Report.—Girl, 6 months, had limited abduction and external rotation of the left shoulder, with a 20-degree flexion contracture of the elbow and inability to bring the palm to face upward when the forearm was passively supinated maximally and the shoulder was passively flexed. The infant had a history of left Erb paralysis, high birth-weight, and difficult delivery. She was otherwise healthy. Anteroposterior radiographic views showed hypoplasia of the left glenoid and delayed ossification of the humeral head. True lateral and axillary radiographs of the left shoulder showed a posterior dislocation of the humeral head. Computed tomographic scanning and MRI confirmed this finding.

Electromyographic results were consistent with the left Erb palsy. The patient had partial reinnervation of the fifth and sixth cervical levels. When she was 9 months of age, open reduction was done. Immobilization was applied for 1 month postoperatively, at which time range-of-motion exercises were begun. Twenty-six months after surgery, the patient was able to actively abduct the shoulder to 100 degrees. Active forward flexion to 120 degrees and active external rotation to 50 degrees were possible. Internal rotation to the point where the hand touched the sacrum was also observed. The infant was able to pronate and supinate the forearm fully, although she still had a 10-degree flexion contracture of the elbow. An ossified humeral head and concentric glenohumeral joint were evident on radiographs.

Conclusion.—In this report, 2 infants with posterior dislocation of the humeral head associated with obstetric paralysis were treated successfully. Treatment consisted of a combined anterior and posterior approach with posterior capsulorrhaphy. This procedure allowed for the release of the contracted anterior part of the capsule and subscapularis tendon and for a capsulorrhaphy of the redundant posterior part of the capsule to maximize stability after reduction.

▶ Although the details of 1 case are described in this abstract, the author has had experience with 2, both successfully treated by open reduction. Humeral head dislocation after brachial plexus palsy in an infant is almost always posterior. The clinical expression of this condition is severe limitation of shoulder external rotation. Open reduction in the older child is difficult and improvement in function is less likely than in the infant.—P.P. Griffin, M.D.

Surgical Treatment of the Duplicated Thumb
Seidman GD, Wenner SM (Boston Univ)
J Pediatr Orthop 13:660–662, 1993   129-94-1–33

Introduction.—Duplicated thumb occurs in .08 cases per 1,000 live births, with manifestations ranging from bifid phalanx to complete duplication, including the metacarpal. The surgical options include ablation, fusion of the duplicated segments (the Bilhaut-Cloquet procedure), or reconstruction of the retained digit with tissues transferred from the ablated thumb. The results of ablation were compared with those of ablation plus radial collateral ligament reconstruction in 15 patients with duplicated thumbs.

Patients.—The patients, with a total of 18 duplicated thumbs, were operated on at a single hospital during a 65-year period. There were 10 boys and 5 girls (average age, 20 months at operation). There were 1 Wassel type VI, 2 type V, 8 type IV, 4 type III, and 3 type II thumbs; 14 were on the right hand. The first 12 patients were managed with ablation alone, with excision of the radial digit. The next 6 were managed by ablation with radial collateral ligament reconstruction. The patients were followed for an average of 5½ years.

Outcomes.—For the Wassel type IV thumbs, the mean metacarpophalangeal joint angulation of the ulnar thumb improved from 21 to 10 degrees and mean interphalangeal joint angulation from 15 to 10 degrees. Although unmeasured, range of motion was satisfactory. Five further operations were required in 4 thumbs in 3 patients. All of these patients were initially managed by ablation alone. Indications for reoperation included joint instability, contracture, angulation of the digit, and bony prominence. No further operations were needed and no residual deformity or instability has developed in any of the patients who had initial ligament reconstruction.

Conclusion.—Ablation with radial collateral ligament reconstruction may be superior to ablation alone for patients with the rare deformity of duplicated thumb. The radial digit is excised and, in most cases, a periosteal sleeve is used for ligament reconstruction. The joint is fixed using Kirschner wires, with cast immobilization until the wires are removed 4–6 weeks postoperatively.

▶ The angulated unstable joint of the retained digit may have a progressive deformity. Radial collateral reconstruction is an important part of the surgical procedure.—P.P. Griffin, M.D.

Use of Bone Scan in Management of Patients With Peripheral Gangrene Due to Fulminant Meningococcemia

Hamdy RC, Babyn PS, Krajbich JI (Univ of Toronto)
J Pediatr Orthop 13:447–451, 1993   129-94-1-34

Objective.—In 10% of patients with meningococcal disease, the disastrous complication of fulminant meningococcemia will develop, leading to ischemic lesions of any organ system, including the skeleton. In about

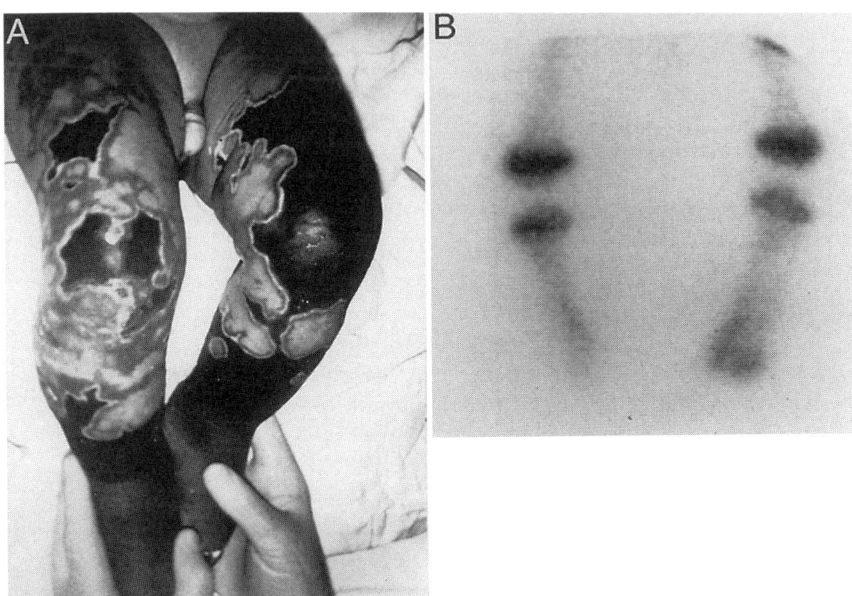

Fig 1–6.—A, patchy, irregular gangrene of both lower extremities in 1 patient 3 weeks after admission. **B,** bone scan of the same patient 39 days after admission showing level of uptake in the lower limbs. (Courtesy of Hamdy RC, Babyn PS, Krajbich JI: *J Pediatr Orthop* 13:447–451, 1993.)

10% of patients with this complication, gangrene of the extremities will develop, probably as a result of disseminated intravascular coagulation and vasculitis. Such gangrene does not follow any uniform pattern, which may make it difficult to assess the proper level of amputation. Experience with technetium bone scintigraphy in 4 children with fulminant meningococcemia and peripheral gangrene was reported.

Patients.—The patients, drawn from a series of 53 patients with fulminant meningococcemia, all required amputation for extensive gangrene of the extremities. All had a progressive, patchy, irregular gangrene within the first 2 hospital days. During the next 3 weeks, the level of gangrene appeared to become demarcated in 12 limbs but could not be clinically determined in the remaining 4. All patients underwent bone scanning 2–5 weeks after the onset of illness. All scans were performed by standard technique, with special attention to blood pool and flow phases.

Outcomes.—All extremities examined in all patients showed variable absent uptake in the distal portion of the limbs (Fig 1–6). All patients had delayed amputation of all 4 limbs. In 13 limbs, the level of amputation was based primarily on the bone scan level; 84% of these amputations were successful. The bone scan confirmed the clinical impression in 5 limbs with a clinically demarcated level of gangrene and showed a more distal level than the clinical estimate in 5 more cases. Bone scanning was useful in deciding on the level of amputation in 4 limbs with no clearly demarcated level of gangrene. Bone scan findings were ignored in 1 limb, which required revision amputation to the level initially suggested by the bone scan.

Conclusion.—Bone scanning appears to be a useful adjunct in determining the appropriate level of amputation in patients with fulminant meningococcemia and extensive peripheral gangrene. It is most useful in patchy gangrenous areas in which there may be islands of viable tissue. Bone scanning should be done soon after the onset of gangrene to allow for an early decision on the level of amputation and for avoidance of unnecessary skin grafts.

▶ The demarcation dictating the level of amputation required in patients with fulminant meningococcemia may take several weeks. This study showed the effectiveness of bone scanning to determine the necessary level of amputation of the terminal tissue of the extremity.—P.P. Griffin, M.D.

One-Bone Forearm As a Salvage Procedure for Recalcitrant Forearm Deformity in Hereditary Multiple Exostoses
Rodgers WB, Hall JE (Boston Children's Hosp)
J Pediatr Orthop 13:587–591, 1993   129-94-1–35

Background.—Multiple hereditary exostoses are metaphyseal protrusions of cartilage-capped bone. They cause significant forearm deformities in 60% of patients, usually as the result of distal ulnar disease. Surgical treatment by excision of exostoses and ulnar lengthening is usually successful; when surgery fails, however, a salvage operation may be necessary to restore function. Creation of the "one-bone forearm" for 2 patients with recurrent multiple hereditary exostoses was reported.

Case Report.—Boy, 4 years, had bony deformities of the hands, hips, and shoulders. He had palpable exostoses of the distal radius and ulna, with full elbow motion and 30 degrees of pronation, 45 degrees of supination, and 10 degrees of ulnar deviation of the hand. The child did not return for further evaluation until nearly 6 years later; he had only 30 degrees of forearm rotation and was unable to deviate his wrist radially. He had a radial articular angle (RAA) of 65 degrees, a carpal slip (CS) of 75 degrees, and a negative ulnar variance of 27 mm, with the left forearm 4 cm shorter than the right.

Excision of the distal ulna and exostoses was performed, along with dome osteotomy of the distal radius to bring the carpus out of ulnar deviation. After 1 year, a painful dislocation of the radial head with a new exostosis developed. The patient lacked 5 degrees of elbow rotation and had a 10-degree arc of forearm rotation; RAA was 30 degrees and CS was negligible. Radioulnar fusion, fixed with threaded Steinmann pins, was performed when the child was 12 years of age. At follow-up 14 years later, the patient reported no pain and had full elbow motion, with 45 degrees of wrist dorsiflexion, 75 degrees of palmar flexion, and a 50-degree arc of radial and ulnar deviation. Although the left forearm is still 2 cm shorter than the right, the patient works as a heavy equipment operator.

Discussion.—Radioulnar fusion—the so-called "one-bone forearm" —is a useful treatment alternative for the rare patient with refractory forearm exostoses. This operation can produce a long-term functional and pain-free extremity.

▶ The 2 cases described in this article show a successful procedure to improve function in the deformed forearm so frequently seen in multiple exostoses. Early excision of exostoses that interfere with forearm rotation and lengthening of the shortened ulna usually will prevent the need for the described procedure.—P.P. Griffin, M.D.

2 Shoulder, Arm, and Elbow

Introduction

This year, some significant information has been added regarding clinical pathology and treatment of the shoulder, arm, and elbow. Radiographic assessment techniques are becoming much better understood. Magnetic resonance imaging is very sensitive, but a number of changes can be seen that also occur in normal individuals and probably cannot clearly be considered pathologic to the extent that aggressive treatment is needed. Using contrast with MRI improves the outline of the glenoid labrum. Whether this is going to be very important in a clinical sense is difficult to know. It is probably not as important as one might think. The role of ultrasonography is becoming more clear, and perhaps it will be a useful screening tool. It usually identifies normal tendons or tendons with larger amounts of tearing; it has a difficult time distinguishing between scar or degenerative changes within the tendon substance and small amounts of tearing. When one is assessing total shoulder arthroplasty, one can achieve much more precise knowledge regarding the interfaces by using fluoroscopic positioning. There is no need to accept inferior images in the analysis of problematic shoulder arthroplasties.

A number of issues have been presented relative to fracture care. A study of fractures of the lateral end of the clavicle indicates that conservative treatment may well be acceptable, but it also points out that nonunion is fairly common (Abstract 129-94-2-5). For the first time, there has been a clear description of the fact that results can be excellent after internal fixation for intra-articular glenoid fractures (Abstract 129-94-2-6). Quite acceptable treatment results have also been outlined for open reduction and fixation of 2- and 3-part fractures and, interestingly, for internal fixation of 4-part fractures (Abstracts 129-94-2-7 and 129-94-2-8). When there is an associated dislocation, the chances of problems after treatment are much greater, and perhaps prostheses will be more strongly considered for this patient group.

Shoulder instability is a very active topic. The pathology of acute shoulder dislocations is delineated in an arthroscopic study (Abstract 129-94-2-11). The capsuloligamentous anatomy is being carefully studied (Abstract 129-94-2-15), and the role of bone torsion has again been questioned as having some importance (Abstract 129-94-2-16). Subdivisions of dislocations—including dislocations in the older age group and chronic anterior dislocations—have been further studied. Concerning treatment, 3 studies have reminded us that internal fixation as a part of surgical repair for instability is problematic (Abstracts 129-94-2-17 through 129-94-2-19). Results may not be as good as one would wish, and the need for subsequent removal of the internal fixation is real. This reader would again have reinforced to him that if one can do repair of shoulder instability without the need for metallic fixation, probably the patients will be better served.

Some interesting information has come to light relative to rotator cuff pathology. Remember the os acromiale, because it has some importance (Abstract 129-94-2-25). In terms of the impingement syndrome, if there is a scar in the bursa, the chances of treatment success are higher than if there is not. Both degenerative changes within the rotator cuff tendon and impingement play a role in the clinical setting. A nice study has reviewed the fact that in the absence of rotator cuff tearing, conservative treatment for rotator cuff disease is perhaps as effective—or almost as effective—as decompressive treatment might be (Abstract 129-94-2-28). Physiotherapy is also helpful, but the placebo limbs did not recover as well as the treatment groups. Arthroscopic decompression is not as effective in treating rotator cuff tears as the usual tendon suturing. Reoperations for failed rotator cuff repair may be effective, as suggested by Abstract 129-94-2-30, which is very hopeful, as past studies have been very pessimistic. Also, the use of a humeral head prosthesis in selected patients with cuff tear arthritis might prove useful, although the results are not nearly so consistent as when prostheses are used for other diagnostic categories.

Shoulder arthrodesis has been revisited. The results may depend on the diagnostic grouping for which the procedure is performed. The use of a plate is technically very effective, and the movement limitations have been clearly defined in a nice study (Abstract 129-94-2-35) outlining motion deficiencies, both for glenohumeral and scapulothoracic arthrodeses.

When a radial head fracture is not accompanied by associated injuries, the results will be much better; when associated injuries are present, the radial head should be preserved if at all possible. When considering tennis elbow, a simple release may be quite effective and may be statistically as effective as any alternate, more complex procedure (Abstract 129-94-2-40).

Degenerative disease of the elbow has been outlined (Abstract 129-94-2-38), and, surprisingly, to stage the disease one might focus more attention on the radiocapitellar articulation rather than the ulnohumeral articulation. Use of an unconstrained prosthesis for total elbow arthroplasty has been quite effective in the rheumatoid patient group (Abstract 129-94-2-39).

As one can glean from the above, a large amount of information has become available this year in this anatomical region. We must be thankful to the authors for conceiving of these studies and for developing the material as they have done. Progress in this area is substantial and continuing.

Robert H. Cofield, M.D.

Shoulder Imaging

The Normal Shoulder: Common Variations That Simulate Pathologic Conditions at MR Imaging

Liou JTS, Wilson AJ, Totty WG, Brown JJ (Washington Univ, St Louis, Mo)
Radiology 186:435–441, 1993   129-94-2-1

Purpose.—Magnetic resonance imaging has been useful in the depiction of full-thickness rotator cuff tears. Focal or diffuse increased signal intensity of T1-weighted and proton density images may represent tendon abnormalities, which are usually managed conservatively; thus, surgical correlation is lacking. Although the MR appearance of the glenohu-

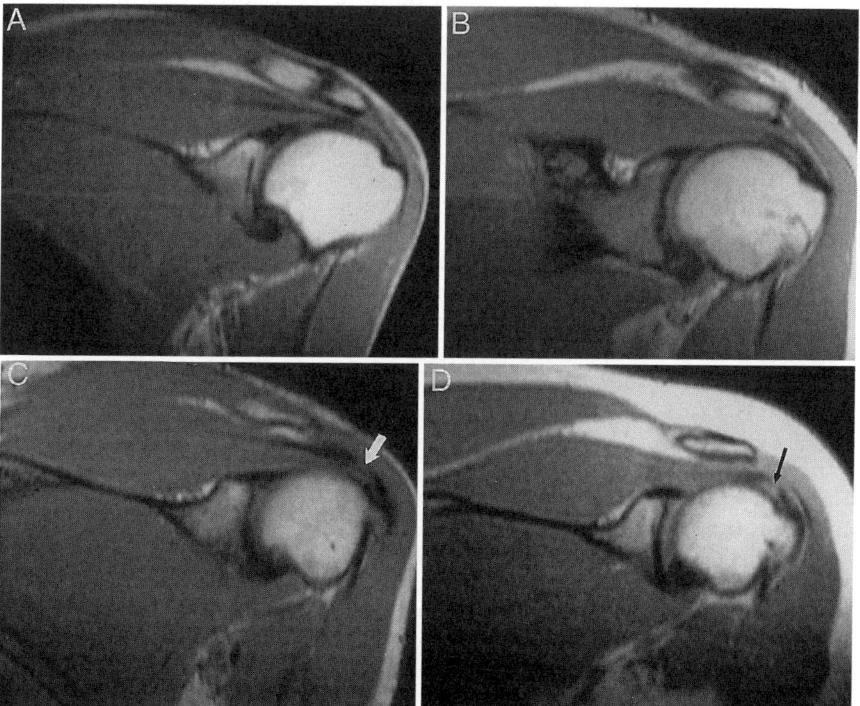

Fig 2–1.—Examples of different patterns of the supraspinatus tendon on proton density oblique coronal images. **A,** type 1, through the central tendon. **B,** type 3, through a short tendon slip. C and **D,** type 5, showing focal increased signal intensity in the distal tendon (*arrow*). (Courtesy of Liou JTS, Wilson AJ, Totty WG, et al: *Radiology* 186:435–441, 1993.)

meral joint in the symptomatic shoulder is well characterized, the normal shoulder has been little studied.

Methods and Results.—Three experienced radiologists analyzed the MR appearance of the supraspinatus and anterior capsular mechanism in 60 asymptomatic shoulders, with special attention to findings that simulate pathologic conditions. Examples of the tendon patterns are shown in Figure 2–1. In most cases, the supraspinatus tendon showed intermediate signal intensity on T1-weighted and proton density spin-echo images. On proton density images, 95% of the shoulders had focal signal intensity within the distal tendon. Ninety-five percent of the shoulders had focal obliteration of the subacromial-subdeltoid fat stripe, and 48% had acromioclavicular joint arthrosis. The shape of the anterior glenoid labrum–glenohumeral ligament (GHL) complex varied considerably, with the appearance of the labrum ranging from triangular, round, or crescentic to absent. The middle and inferior GHLs were close to the upper half of the anterior labrum, with the cleavage plane between the ligaments and labrum sometimes mimicking a tear.

Conclusion.—One should be aware of the varying MR appearance of the normal shoulder to avoid overdiagnosis. The finding of intermediate signal intensity in the supraspinatus tendon, probably explained by tendon anatomy and/or the magic angle phenomenon, is so common that it is unlikely to have any clinical relevance. The anterior capsular mechanism may also vary widely in appearance. The normal anatomy of the labrum-GHL complex appears to be sometimes misinterpreted as labral tears.

▶ This useful study indicates that variations in signal intensity within the supraspinatus tendon are quite common and are not necessarily pathologic. This may diminish the usefulness of MRI in the evaluation of rotator cuff disease; however, one should remember that if the tendon has a homogeneous image, one is unlikely to consider that an abnormal rotator cuff tendon may be the source of the symptoms. Therefore, I think that, in this area as in many other regions of MRI, the study is very sensitive but it is not so specific.—R.H. Cofield, M.D.

Saline Magnetic Resonance Arthrography in the Evaluation of Glenohumeral Instability
Tirman PFJ, Stauffer AE, Crues JV III, Turner RM, Nottage WM, Schobert WE, Rubin BD, Janzen DL, Linares RC (Cottage Community Magnetic Resonance Ctr, Santa Barbara, Calif; Digital and Radiological Imaging, Mission Viejo, Calif; Sports Medicine and Reconstructive Specialists, Laguna Hills, Calif; et al)
Arthroscopy 9:550–559, 1993   129-94-2–2

Introduction.—The results of MRI in the evaluation of glenoid labral tears have been as good or better than those of CT arthrography. The

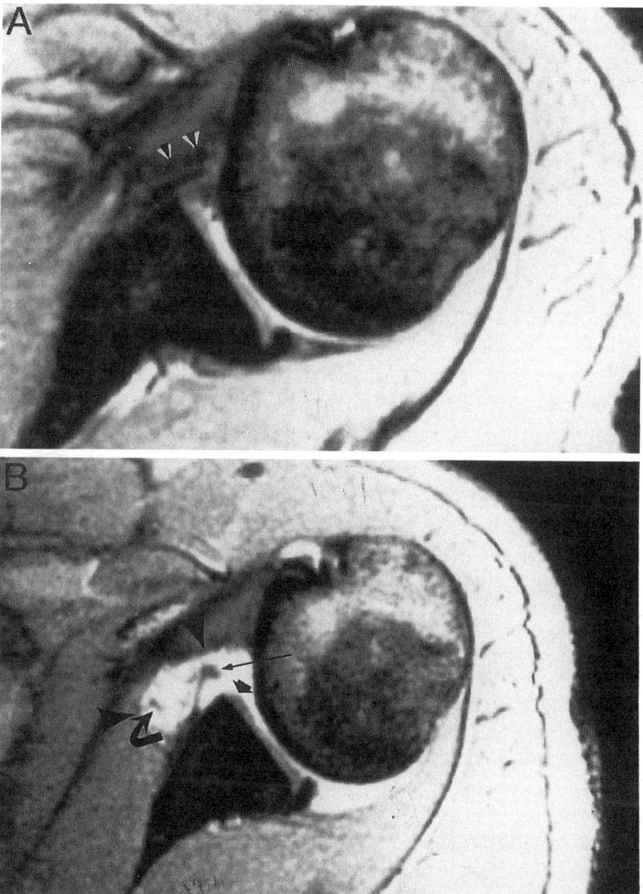

Fig 2–2.—Improved definition of labral and capsular structures after the introduction of intra-articular saline. **A,** axial gradient recalled echo 700/18/30. The routine study demonstrates the lack of a clear definition between the anterior labrum and the joint capsule. The region of the capsulolabral interface is represented as an inhomogeneous, predominantly decreased signal region (*arrowheads*). **B,** after the introduction of saline, the anterior structures are shown to better advantage. Note the torn, detached, anteriorly displaced labrum (*long arrow*). Debris within the joint probably represents the damaged middle glenohumeral ligament (*curved arrow*). Ballooning of the anterior capsule is seen (*arrowhead*). The intact hyaline articular cartilage (*short arrow*) appears as a medium-intensity structure adjacent to the predominantly decreased signal intensity bony glenoid. (Courtesy of Tirman PFJ, Stauffer AE, Crues JV III, et al: *Arthroscopy* 9:550–559, 1993.)

advantages of MRI include multiplanar capability, improved soft tissue contrast, and lack of ionizing radiation. The accuracy of MR arthrography in detecting glenoid labral tears and Hill-Sachs deformities and its value in predicting glenohumeral instability were established.

Patients and Methods.—Sixty-five patients who underwent MR shoulder arthrography were included in the study. The patients' age range was 15–63 years. Thirty-five had a nonspecific history of shoulder pain; 12

were referred for recurrent dislocation, 11 for suspected instability, and 7 to rule out impingement. Forty-eight of the 65 patients underwent examination under anesthesia (EUA). The MR studies were prospectively interpreted by experienced MR radiologists and retrospectively evaluated by an MRI radiologist without prior knowledge of the history for potential imaging indicators of shoulder instability.

Results.—In cases in which a lack of joint fluid on the unenhanced images resulted in a lack of definition between the capsule and the labrum (Fig 2–2), MR saline arthrography offered improved definition of capsular anatomy and contours of the cartilaginous labrum. No correlation was observed between capsular indicators and EUA-documented instability. There was a statistically significant correlation, however, between the presence of a Bankart cartilaginous deformity and Hill-Sachs fractures with EUA-documented instability. Labral tears were detected with a sensitivity of 89% and a specificity of 98%; corresponding values for Hill-Sachs fracture detection were 69% and 87%, respectively.

Conclusion.—The shoulder joint is inherently unstable, and the pain associated with instability can mimic a number of other conditions. Magnetic resonance arthrography is superior to CT arthrography in evaluating the rotator cuff, subtle bone injuries, superior labral and biceps tendon injuries, and many other shoulder abnormalities that can masquerade as or be associated with instability. When unenhanced MRI is inconclusive, MR saline arthrography can be of value in evaluating the anterior labrum. Magnetic resonance arthrography may be the most effective initial diagnostic imaging examination in the young athlete with suspected instability.

▶ We all recognize that MRI is not perfect in the evaluation of the glenoid labrum. (Of course, imaging does not diagnose instability but identifies pathologic lesions associated with instability.) When one wishes to assess the labrum on MRI, fluid in the joint will help, as confirmed by this study. Of course, a Hill-Sachs lesion will be visualizable with or without the presence of fluid.—R.H. Cofield, M.D.

Sonography of the Shoulder in Patients With Tears of the Rotator Cuff: Accuracy and Value for Selecting Surgical Options
Wiener SN, Seitz WH Jr (Mt Sinai Med Ctr, Cleveland, Ohio)
AJR 160:103–107, 1993   129-94-2-3

Introduction.—The choice of treatment for patients with tears of the rotator cuff depends on the presence and magnitude of the pathologic changes. Sonography is useful in detecting tears and classifying them according to size. The accuracy of preoperative sonography and the effect of the findings on subsequent surgical management were studied.

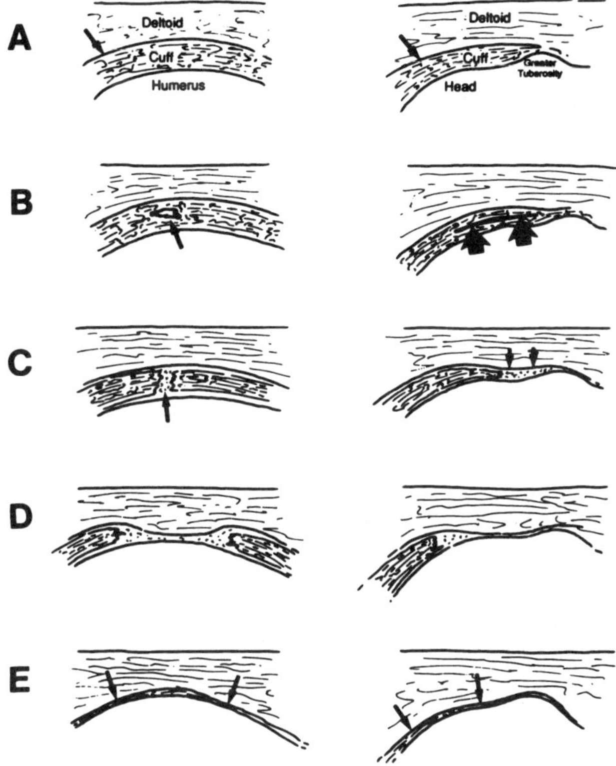

Fig 2–3.—A–E, Drawings show sonographic appearance of rotator cuff integrity in axial (*left*) and sagittal (*right*) planes. **A,** normal rotator cuff with preserved anterior echogenic arc (*arrow*) of subdeltoid fascia and peritendinous fat. **B,** partial-thickness tear appearing as intratendinous hypoechoic (*thin arrow*) or dominant echogenic (*thick arrows*) focus. **C,** small full-thickness tear appearing as hypoechoic area of cuff discontinuity (*long arrow*) and loss of anterior arc and cuff substance at junction of cuff with greater tuberosity (*short arrows*). **D,** large full-thickness tear. **E,** massive tear. Rotator cuff is not visualized. Subdeltoid fascia (*arrows*) "approximates" the humeral head. (Courtesy of Wiener SN, Seitz WH Jr: *AJR* 160:103–107, 1993.)

Patients and Methods.—Between the years 1985 and 1991, 800 patients were referred for shoulder sonography for suspected tears of the rotator cuff; 225 ultimately required surgery. The mean patient age was 59 years; 106 were men and 119 were women. Shoulders were examined anteriorly and laterally in both the axial and sagittal planes with the patient's arm in neutral and internally rotated positions. Preoperative sonographic findings were classified into intact, partial tear, small full-thickness tear, large full-thickness tear, and massive tear groups (Fig 2–3). Surgical treatment was generally based on the sonographic classification.

Results.—Sonography identified an intact rotator cuff in 71 patients and either a partial- or full-thickness tear in 154. Surgical findings confirmed sonographic findings in 92% of the patients. Surgery confirmed 89% of rotator cuffs designated as normal and 93% of those determined to have partial- or full-thickness tears. Eleven patients had more extensive injuries and 8 had less extensive injuries than predicted.

Conclusion.—Some previous reports of less favorable results of shoulder sonography have discouraged the use of this imaging method for suspected rotator cuff injury. The findings of this study, however, show a high correlation between the sonographic classification and surgical evidence. Sonography in this setting is rapid, simple to perform, low in cost, and accurate.

▶ No test is perfect. Sonography seems to readily identify patients with larger rotator cuff tears and to clearly define normal tendons. This, indeed, supports the authors' contention that sonography may be a very useful screening tool because it is so easy to perform and it is inexpensive. When the sonogram is confusing, with interstitial echo changes or, seemingly, the presence of a small rotator cuff tear, a more expensive study or an invasive study could subsequently be performed. As others have suggested, though, when one wishes to do only one test to evaluate the rotator cuff, sonography may not be the one test to do.—R.H. Cofield, M.D.

Fluoroscopically Positioned Radiographs of Total Shoulder Arthroplasty

Kelleher IM, Cofield RH, Becker DA, Beabout JW (Mayo Clinic and Found, Rochester, Minn)
J Shoulder Elbow Surg 1:306–311, 1992   129-94-2-4

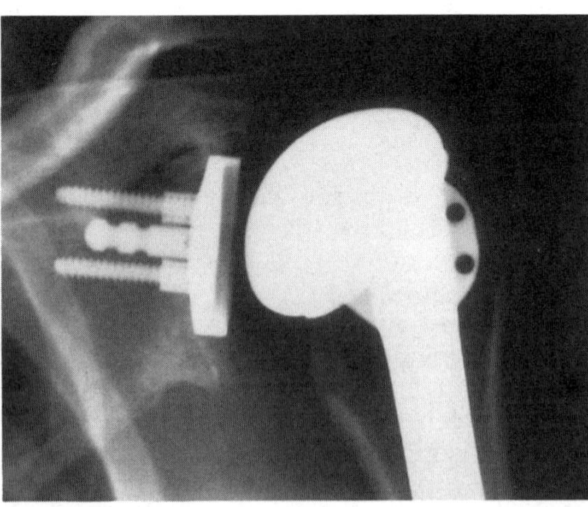

Fig 2–4.—Fluoroscopically positioned Cofield ingrowth shows total shoulder alignment and component-bone interface. (Courtesy of Kelleher IM, Cofield RH, Becker DA, et al: *J Shoulder Elbow Surg* 1:306–311, 1992.)

Background.—Sequential radiographic assessment of the changes at the interface between the arthroplasty component and the adjacent bone can have prognostic value, but standardization of radiographic images is difficult. A fluoroscopically positioned radiographic technique was developed, reviewed, and compared with standard films in detecting the component-bone interface or component cement-bone interface changes in total shoulder arthroplasty.

Methods.—Standard radiographic projections and 2 fluoroscopically positioned localized views were obtained from 87 patients with 100 total shoulder arthroplasties. The radiographs were evaluated and compared for acceptability, with the film considered as acceptable if the components were aligned so that the actual interface between the component and the bone or between the cement and the bone was clearly seen (Fig 2–4). The radiographs were also compared for the presence or absence of radiolucent zones and for differences between size and location of radiolucent zones at the component-to-bone or component cement-to-bone interface.

Results.—Fifty-six standard radiographs (56%) were unacceptable because of obliquity of the x-ray beam projection, compared with only 3 fluoroscopically positioned localized radiographs. In addition, 19 unacceptable standard radiographs had radiolucent zones visible on comparable fluoroscopic views. Forty-four sets were acceptable for evaluation. The changes at the component or component cement-to-bone interfaces were viewed similarly in the standard and localized views in 27 sets, were better in standard views in 1, and were better in localized views in 16. Overall, 68 of 100 total shoulder arthroplasties had clinically useful information that was identified on fluoroscopic views but not on standard radiographic views.

Conclusion.—Fluoroscopic positioning is superior to standard radiographs in detecting implant-bone interface changes in the shoulder. Although fluoroscopy will increase the radiation dose and the cost of total shoulder films, significant additional information is obtained with localized views. Supplementation of plain shoulder radiographs of total shoulder arthroplasties with fluoroscopically positioned localized views is recommended at baseline, during follow-up visits, and in patients with symptoms.

▶ The shoulder is well recognized as a difficult area to image. The scapula is obliquely positioned on the chest wall, and consistent radiographs are difficult to obtain. This positioning difficulty is magnified when a radiopaque implant is used. This study demonstrates the clear advantage of fluoroscopic positioning for radiographs after total shoulder arthroplasty. The interfaces can be clearly and consistently visualized by this method. By relying only on plain films, between one half and two thirds of patients will not receive images that will allow the interpretation of interface changes.—R.H. Cofield, M.D.

Shoulder and Arm Fractures

The Natural Course of Lateral Clavicle Fracture: 15 (11–21) Year Follow-Up of 110 Cases

Nordqvist A, Petersson C, Redlund-Johnell I (Lund Univ, Malmö, Sweden)
Acta Orthop Scand 64:87–91, 1993   129-94-2-5

Objective.—The Neer classification of fractures of the distal clavicular end includes the following: type I, stable fractures that unite promptly without operation; type II, fractures with disruption of the coracoclavicular ligament from the medial clavicular fragment, for which reduction and internal fixation is generally recommended; and type III, fractures leading to acromioclavicular arthrosis or osteolysis, requiring late resection of the clavicular end (Fig 2–5). The natural history of fracture of the lateral end of the clavicle in 110 patients was reported.

Patients.—The patients were 77 males and 33 females. The median age at injury was 36 years, including 17 patients less than 15 years of age. There were 73 Neer type I, 23 type II, and 14 type III fractures. Treatment was with short-term figure-of-8 or sling immobilization and early mobilization exercises in every case. At an average of 15 years after injury, all patients underwent an interview and clinical examination, and 89 were examined radiographically.

Outcomes.—Although there were no cases of severe shoulder disability, 15 patients had moderate persistent symptoms, mainly slight pain on motion. The other 95 were asymptomatic. All patients were able to return to their previous occupation, although 1 altered his level of sports participation. Thirty-three patients had a hump over the lateral clavicle, which was moderately tender on palpation in 11 patients. Radiographic healing was observed in 79 of 89 patients; 26 had lateral clavicular deformity and exuberant bone formation. Healing with deformation was more common in type II fractures. Nonunion was also more common in type II fractures and in older patients. Eight of 10 nonunions were asymptomatic.

Conclusion.—The results of nonoperatively treated lateral clavicular fracture suggest that short-term sling immobilization is an appropriate treatment for these injuries. Deformity was unusual and severe disability was nonexistent. In the uncommon cases of symptomatic arthrosis or clavicular osteolysis, resection of the lateral end of the clavicle may be appropriate.

▶ It is important to heed the authors' overall conclusions. However, one must recall that of those patients with type II fractures, 22% went on to nonunion. One can apply one's own judgment to decide whether conservative treatment of these fractures is justifiable with a significant complication of that frequency. Certainly, in many other areas of fracture care, that percent-

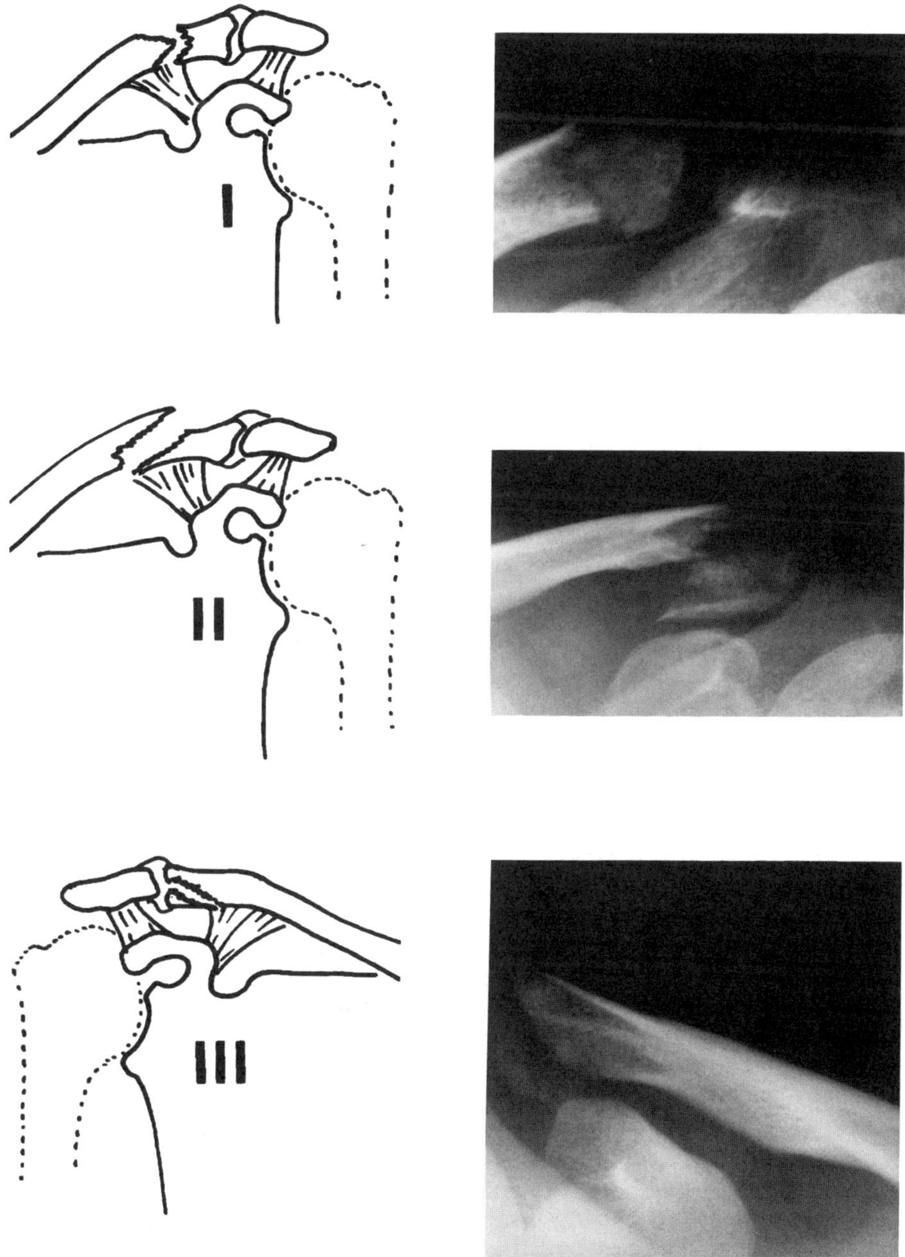

Fig 2–5.—The Neer classification of fractures of the lateral end of the clavicle. **I,** type I fracture of the left clavicle of a 32-year-old man. **II,** type II fracture of the left clavicle of a 42-year-old man. **III,** type III fracture of the right clavicle of an 18-year-old man. (Courtesy of Nordqvist A, Petersson C, Redlund-Johnell I: *Acta Orthop Scand* 64:87–91, 1993.)

age would not imply that the treatment is necessarily satisfactory.—R.H. Cofield, M.D.

Open Reduction and Internal Fixation of Displaced Intra-Articular Fractures of the Glenoid Fossa
Kavanagh BF, Bradway JK, Cofield RH (Mayo Clinic and Found, Rochester, Minn)
J Bone Joint Surg (Am) 75-A:479–484, 1993   129-94-2–6

Introduction.—Although most fractures of the scapula can be treated with nonoperative methods, some patients who desire to remain physically active will require open reduction and internal fixation for optimal results. The outcome and complications of treating displaced intra-articular fractures of the glenoid fossa with open reduction and internal fixation were reviewed.

Patients and Methods.—Ten of 41 patients seen with a glenoid fracture between January 1980 and December 1987 had injuries that included a displaced intra-articular fracture. The range of displacement of the major fracture fragments for these 10 patients was 4–8 mm. All 10 were managed with open reduction and internal fixation, and 9 were available for clinical and radiographic examination at an average of 4 years after operation. The average age of the 7 men and 2 women was 35 years. The time from injury to operative intervention for the scapular fracture ranged from 1 to 38 days. All but 1 patient had a posterior approach (Fig 2–6); the anterior approach was used in that case. A cast was worn for 6–8 weeks and was followed by a program of gentle range-of-motion exercises. More vigorous stretching exercises were started at 2–3 months after cast removal, and isotonic strengthening began at 4–6 months after cast removal.

Results.—All patients expressed satisfaction with the results at the most recent follow-up examination. None reported pain with daily use of the extremity. There were no infections or malunions. Radiographs revealed no displacement of the articular surfaces and no evidence of migration or loosening of the screws or plates. The only complication was heterotopic ossification in 1 patient.

Conclusion.—Operative treatment is rarely considered necessary for patients with scapular fractures. In selected cases of displaced fractures of the glenoid fossa, however, open reduction and internal fixation are needed to restore shoulder function. The outcome in this series of patients confirms the value and safety of this operative technique. The anterior approach used in 1 of the 10 cases was exceptionally difficult and is not recommended.

▶ The surprising outcome of this study was the consistently excellent results after internal fixation of these displaced intra-articular fractures. However, it

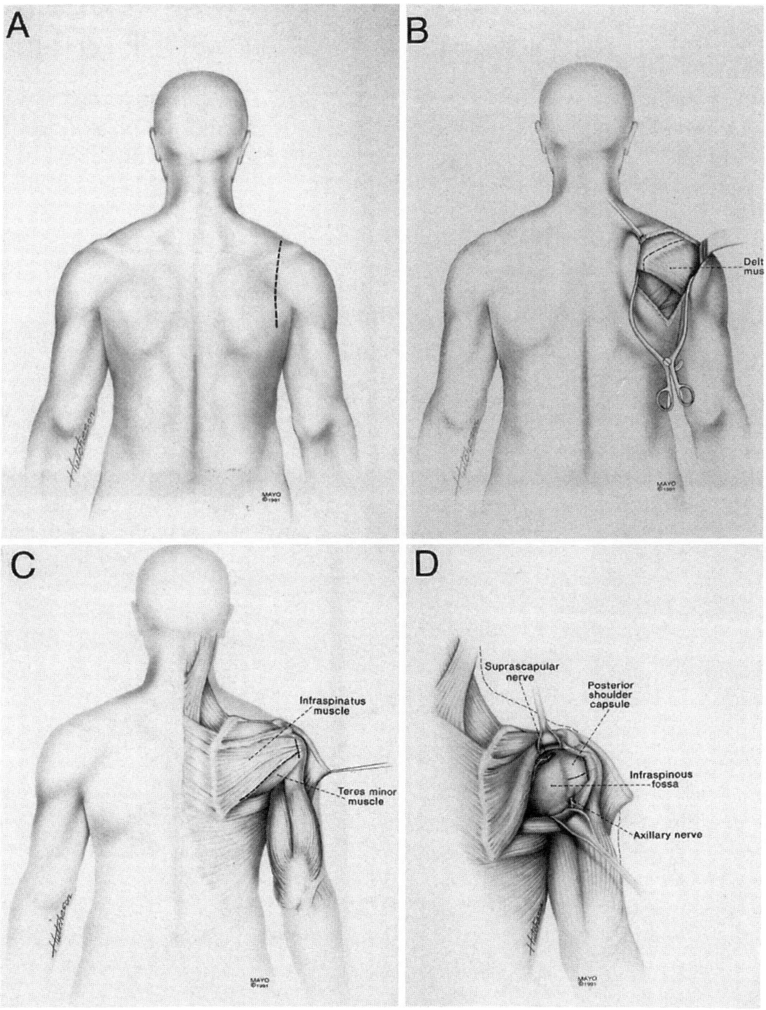

Fig 2–6.—Drawings illustrating the operative procedure. **A,** vertical skin incision is preferred for exposure of fractures involving the intra-articular portion of the glenoid. Incision begins just proximal to the junction of the lateral one third and medial two thirds of the spine of the scapula and extends downward and slightly medially for 15 cm. **B,** the deltoid is released from the spine of the scapula by incision of the fascia between the trapezius and the deltoid muscles and by elevation of the fascia of the deltoid attachment from the spine of the scapula. Often the most medial aspect of the deltoid is divided, which eliminates the need to extend the dissection medially. **C,** the distal border of the infraspinatus muscle is defined, and the interval between the infraspinatus muscle and the teres minor muscles is developed. For a number of these fractures an adjunctive vertical incision through the tendons of the infraspinatus and teres minor muscles augments the exposure of the infraspinous fossa and lessens the need for strong retraction of the muscles. **D,** with elevation of the infraspinatus muscle proximally and the teres minor muscle distally, the infraspinous fossa is exposed. The intra-articular component of the fracture can be identified by capsular incision. The illustrated T-shaped incision is preferable. The suprascapular nerve should be identified as it exits through the spinoglenoid notch and courses along the undersurface of the infraspinatus muscle. The axillary nerve should be palpated and protected. (Courtesy of Kavanagh BF, Bradway JK, Cofield RH: *J Bone Joint Surg (Am)* 75-A:479–484, 1993.)

was necessary to carefully protect the soft tissues during the early healing phase and to institute a progressive rehabilitation program that typically extended between 6 months and 1 year. Certainly, if it is deemed satisfactory to treat a glenoid fracture nonoperatively, recovery will be much quicker; however, when significant displacement exists, it seems that open reduction, internal fixation, postoperative protection, and progressive rehabilitation will lead to an excellent result.—R.H. Cofield, M.D.

Open Reduction and Internal Fixation of Two- and Three-Part Displaced Surgical Neck Fractures of the Proximal Humerus

Cuomo F, Flatow EL, Maday MG, Miller SR, McIlveen SJ, Bigliani LU (Columbia-Presbyterian Med Ctr, NY)
J Shoulder Elbow Surg 1:287–295, 1992   129-94-2–7

Introduction.—Minimal fixation techniques have been advocated for the surgical management of unstable, displaced fractures of the proximal humerus. Between 1981 and 1989, 26 patients underwent open reduc-

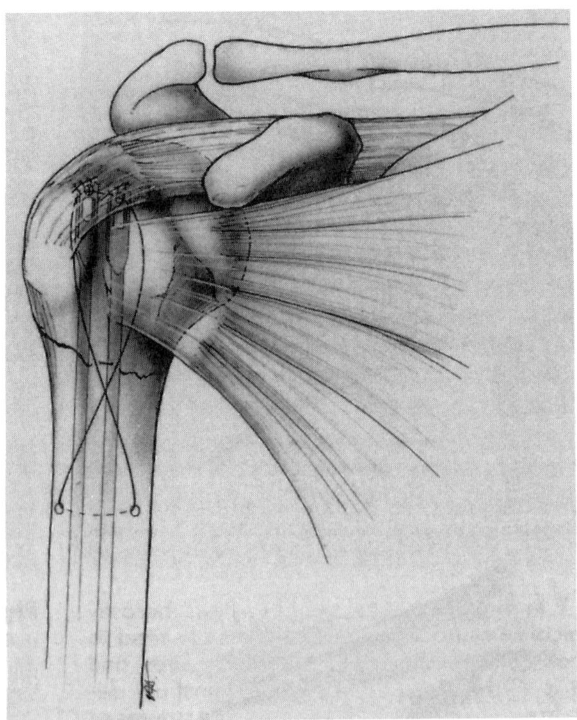

Fig 2–7.—Nails are introduced through small (1 cm) longitudinal incisions in rotator cuff insertion. Suture or wire is brought through proximal holes and under the intervening cuff tendon. (Courtesy of Cuomo F, Flatow EL, Maday MG, et al: *J Shoulder Elbow Surg* 1:287–295, 1992.)

tion and internal fixation of 2-part and 3-part displaced surgical neck fractures of the proximal humerus. There were 14 two-part surgical neck fractures, 7 three-part displaced greater tuberosity and surgical neck fractures, and 1 three-part displaced lesser tuberosity and surgical neck fracture. The average follow-up was 3.3 years (range, 1.1–8.9 years).

Technique.—Fixation is accomplished with heavy nonabsorbable suture or wire that incorporates the rotator cuff tendons, tuberosities, and shaft. For comminuted surgical neck fractures, humeral Enders nails are incorporated into a tension-band construct to provide longitudinal stability. The Enders nail is modified with an additional hole above the eyelet allowing insertion of the nail deeper into the head with its proximal tip well below the surface of the cuff tendons (Fig 2–7). The suture or wire is passed deep to the tendon.

Outcome.—There were 18 good or excellent results (82%), 3 satisfactory results (14%), and 1 unsatisfactory result (5%). All 8 3-part fractures and 10 of 14 2-part fractures (71%) had good or excellent results. All fractures healed, and no infections or nonunions occurred.

Conclusion.—The use of limited internal fixation in displaced fractures of the proximal humerus without the use of plates and screws provides fracture stability and a high percentage of acceptable results. The use of suture or wire fixation requires less extensive exposure and soft tissue stripping with better preservation of head vascularity; it allows incorporation of the rotator cuff tendon, which is generally stronger than the soft bone, into the fixation. In addition, when sutures or wire are combined with intramedullary rods in a figure-of-8, tension-band fashion, one obtains extremely solid fixation, which allows early mobilization and rehabilitation.

▶ This article reinforces the classic approach to care of fractures of the proximal humerus. Open reduction is accomplished, and the fragments are held together with a suture repair or a suture repair combined with longitudinal pins. This affords enough stability to allow passive motion, with active motion started after bone and tendon healing. The results described suggest that one should seriously consider adopting this approach to the care of displaced proximal humeral fractures—2- and 3-part.—R.H. Cofield, M.D.

Four-Part Displaced Proximal Humeral Fractures: Operative Treatment Using Kirschner Wires and a Tension Band
Darder A, Darder A Jr, Sanchis V, Gastaldi E, Gomar F (Hosp Clínico Universitario, Valencia, Spain)
J Orthop Trauma 7:497–505, 1993   129-94-2-8

Introduction.—There is currently no consensus regarding the management of 3-part and 4-part proximal humeral fractures. Displaced 4-part fractures and fracture-dislocations are at high risk of avascular necrosis.

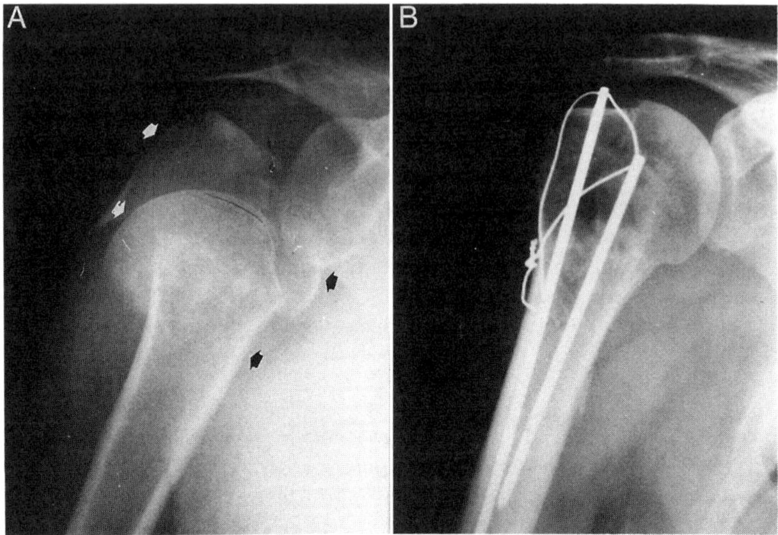

Fig 2–8.—A, a 56-year-old man fell on his right arm and sustained a 4-part proximal humeral fracture (*arrows*). **B,** 3 weeks after operation, the radiographs show an acceptable reduction of the head fragment and tuberosities. (Courtesy of Darder A, Darder A Jr, Sanchis V, et al: *J Orthop Trauma* 7:497–505, 1993.)

Treatment of such fractures with open reduction and internal fixation was discussed, and a method of fixation using 2 modified Kirschner (K) wires and tension-band wiring was described.

Patients and Methods.—Thirty-five patients with 4-part displaced proximal humeral fractures were treated from December 1977 through February 1990; 33 were available for follow-up. The mean patient age was 59 years. Seven had fracture-dislocations and 26 had displaced fractures. Surgery was performed at an average of 6 days after the injury. The surgical technique was as atraumatic as possible and sought to restore normal anatomy of the proximal humerus with a minimal fixation system. Two modified K wires, introduced through the tuberosities and reinforced by tension-band wiring, formed the fixation device. Outcome was evaluated according to Neer's criteria.

Results.—The average length of follow-up was 7 years. All fractures healed in 5–9 weeks. Results were judged excellent or satisfactory in 64% of patients, nonsatisfactory in 30%, and failures in 6%. Most patients (82%) were free of shoulder pain. Only 2 of the 9 patients with avascular necrosis reported mild or occasional pain. Thirty-one patients returned to their usual jobs and other activities and 2 had to change to less strenuous work. Twenty-five of the reductions achieved during surgery were judged acceptable (Fig 2–8). Avascular necrosis developed in 6 of the 8 patients with nonacceptable reductions. The tension-band wiring ruptured in 1 patient.

Conclusion.—Four-part displaced proximal humeral fractures occur infrequently and are generally seen in older patients with osteoporosis (Fig 2–8). Nonsurgical treatment often produces poor results. Open reduction and internal fixation is recommended for these fractures, using the system of osteosynthesis described. Avascular necrosis, the most common complication, is associated with fracture-dislocations and unacceptable reduction.

▶ One could always argue that not all of the patients described in this article truly had 4-part fracture displacement. At the time of follow-up, osteonecrosis had developed in slightly more than one quarter of the patients. In many, this developed in association with fracture-dislocations, highlighting the increased severity of that injury. It also occurred when reduction was unacceptable.

Thus, the important message of this paper is that, when performing open reduction for such fractures, the quality of the reduction is important. It also emphasizes that one might wish to err toward the side of using open reduction and fixation rather than using a prosthesis in many fractures that are borderline in terms of fragment displacement. In fact, one might easily argue that all of these fractures should be fixed except for those with associated dislocation. That, of course, will not be universally true, but it may represent a good guideline.—R.H. Cofield, M.D.

Acute Prosthetic Replacement for Severe Fractures of the Proximal Humerus

Hawkins RJ, Switlyk P (Univ of Western Ontario, London, Canada)
Clin Orthop 289:156–160, 1993   129-94-2–9

Background.—Four-part proximal humerus fractures are difficult to treat successfully. Most American surgeons treat them by immediate prosthetic replacement and rotator cuff reconstruction. A series of patients treated acutely with prosthetic replacement for severe fracture of the proximal humerus was described.

Patients.—From 1979 to 1986, 19 patients with 20 severe proximal humeral fractures were treated at 1 university. Each fracture was managed within 2 weeks of injury. The average patient age was 64 years. Follow-up evaluation was performed at an average of 40 months.

Results.—Overall, 90% of shoulders had little or no pain after treatment. A fair-to-good functional rating was obtained in 75% of shoulders. The patients were personally satisfied with the results in 80% of cases. The average active forward elevation was 72 degrees, the average active external rotation was 16 degrees, and the average passive external rotation was 38 degrees. The average University of California at Los Angeles Shoulder Rating was 24 out of 35, which was considered fair. Complications included 1 case of axillary nerve palsy, 1 case of prosthetic dislocation, 1 case of a loose humeral component, and 1 case of a broken metal wire with painful bursal accumulation. Postoperative rehabilitation was important for regaining function, although pain relief could be obtained without rehabilitation.

Conclusion.—In this patient series, treatment of severe proximal humerus fracture with prosthetic replacement had a variable outcome. Functional results were related to the degree of union of the rotator cuff and tuberosities to the humeral shaft. Techniques to enhance this include the use of cement, secure fixation without wires, and bone grafts under the tuberosities. Functional results were enhanced by prolonged rehabilitation, although good pain relief was obtained without it.

▶ This article describes a severe injury and a rather dramatic treatment for it. The pain relief is acceptable, but the return of active motion and strength are highly variable because of variability in healing of the musculotendinous attachments of the rotator cuff. The findings in this article reinforce the suggestions made in the preceding article (Abstract 129-94-2–8). When there is a borderline situation, it may be preferable to treat the patient with internal fixation. When using a prosthesis, the most critical part of the procedure is secure repair of the rotator cuff attachments and then careful aftercare directed at protecting these attachments; if the attachments do not heal, the best result one can obtain is fair. Unfortunately, many patients who have these fractures are not able to participate in rehabilitation as fully as one might desire. This also leads to a compromise in outcome.—R.H. Cofield, M.D.

Surgical Treatment of Humeral Shaft Fractures: The Basel Experience
Heim D, Herkert F, Hess P, Regazzoni P (Univ Hosp, Basel, Switzerland)
J Trauma 35:226–232, 1993   129-94-2–10

Introduction.—Conservative treatment of humeral shaft fractures has been favored by some over open reduction and internal fixation. Nevertheless, most surgeons accept severe open fractures, fractures in patients with multiple trauma, and fractures with delayed union as indications for surgical treatment. Researchers report their experience of 127 patients with fractures of the humeral shaft treated by osteosynthesis using the AO technique and implants.

Patients and Methods.—The patients were treated from 1980 through 1988. The average patient age was 51.1 years. Forty-one patients had 1 or more fractures in addition to that of the humeral shaft or other concomitant injuries. Seventy-one surgical procedures were done primarily. Patients were treated using 4.5-mm dynamic compression plates. The average hospital stay for the 86 patients with only humeral shaft fractures was 14.4 days.

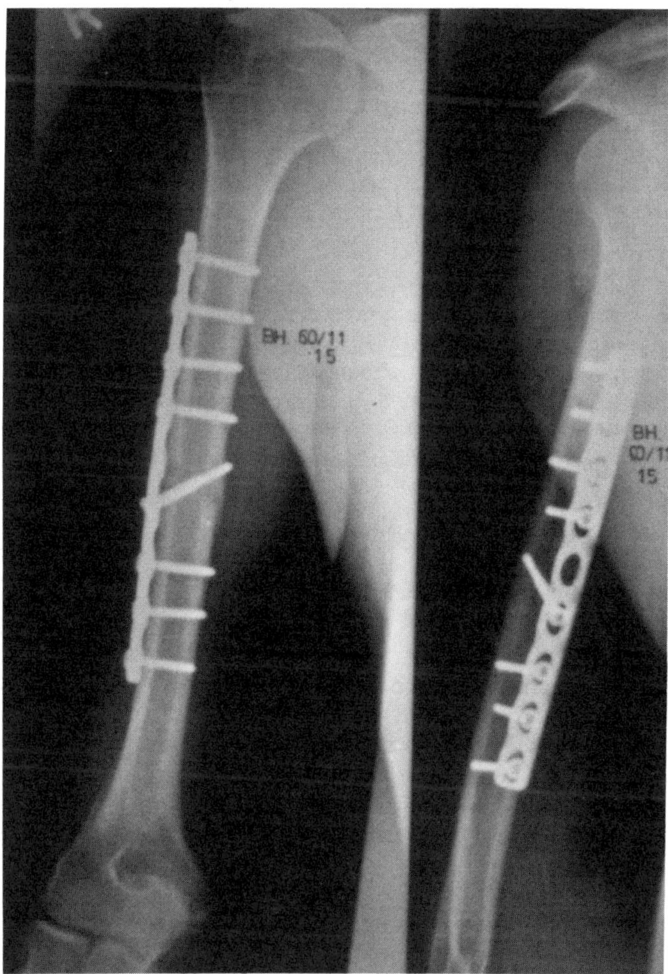

Fig 2–9.—Narrow 4.5-mm limited-contact dynamic compression plate used in a 22-year-old patient with a transverse fracture of the humeral shaft. Osteosynthesis is shown in the anterolateral position at beginning of treatment (**left**) and at 15 weeks (**right**). (Courtesy of Heim D, Herkert F, Hess P, et al: *J Trauma* 35:226–232, 1993.)

Results.—There were 13 postoperative complications in 12 patients. Five cases of early failure of internal fixation were the result of insufficient technique. A pseudoarthrosis developed in 2 patients and 4 had an early infection. There was 1 case of chronic infection and 2 of postoperative radial nerve palsies. Nineteen patients died during the first year, 4 were lost to follow-up, and 2 refused to participate in follow-up. At 1 year of follow-up, all fractures in the remaining 102 patients had healed radiologically. Eighty-nine patients had achieved full functional recovery. The most common causes of limited range of motion were an ipsilateral fracture of the forearm and an old fracture of a neighboring joint. Employed patients with only humeral shaft fractures returned to work in an average of 14.5 weeks.

Conclusion.—In selected patients, a correct plate fixation of the humeral shaft offers an advantageous alternative to conservative treatment with comparable functional outcome at 1 year. Good results can be obtained with narrow 4.5-mm plates (Fig 2–9); broad plates are no longer needed. The authors' implant of choice is now the narrow 4.5-mm limited contact dynamic compression plate, preferably of 9 or 10 holes.

▶ This manuscript carries a simple message: Conservative treatment of humeral shaft fractures is favored; however, if internal fixation is needed, use of a plate and screws is effective. The technique must be meticulous. One must take care to protect the radial nerve, and an occasional patient will be subject to infection.—R.H. Cofield, M.D.

Shoulder Instability

Intraarticular Pathology in Acute, First-Time Anterior Shoulder Dislocation: An Arthroscopic Study
Norlin R (Univ Hosp Linköping, Sweden)
Arthroscopy 9:546–549, 1993   129-94-2-11

Objective.—Intra-articular soft tissue damage in 24 patients with first-time, acute shoulder dislocation is discussed. It was hypothesized that different patterns of injury to the glenohumeral joint might imply a different risk for recurrence, thus affecting the choice of conservative or surgical treatment.

Patients and Methods.—The median age of the patients was 22 years. Eighteen dislocations had occurred during athletic activities. In 15 patients, the dominant arm was involved. All shoulders were reduced and standard radiographs were obtained. Arthroscopy was performed with informed consent 1–3 days after the dislocation. Before the procedure was started, an evaluation under anesthesia was performed in both shoulders.

Results.—All anterior dislocators were unstable anteriorly. There was slight inferior instability in 2 patients. Arthroscopy showed a hemarthrosis of the shoulder with subsequent generalized synovitis in all patients. Anteroinferior damage to the labrum and ligaments was apparent, and the labrum was detached from the glenoid together with the middle glenohumeral ligament and the upper part of the inferior glenohumeral ligament (a Bankart lesion). Hill-Sachs lesions, present in all patients, were chondral in 18 patients and penetrated the cartilage down to the subchondral bone in 6 patients.

Conclusion.—In this series of patients, all shoulders were unstable anteriorly and showed both Bankart and Hill-Sachs lesions. The uniformity of arthroscopic findings limits this procedure's ability to predict future development of recurrent instability. Because the recurrence rate in shoulder dislocation shows a strong negative correlation with age at first dislocation, youth may be an indication for early stabilization. Another possible reason for aggressive therapy is a high level of activity.

▶ This interesting study describes what appears to be rather homogeneous damage in the shoulder joint associated with acute anterior dislocation. One would wish the description of the pathology to be in somewhat more detail. There could be an interesting follow-up of this patient group describing their outcome. It may, in fact, come to pass that the outcome is much more heterogeneous than the pathology and may be dependent on describable variables.—R.H. Cofield, M.D.

Early Complications After Anterior Dislocation of the Shoulder in Patients Over 40 Years: An Ultrasonographic and Electromyographic Study
Toolanen G, Hildingsson C, Hedlund T, Knibestöl M, Öberg L (Univ Hosp, Umeå, Sweden)
Acta Orthop Scand 64:549–552, 1993   129-94-2-12

Objective.—Complications of anterior shoulder dislocation were examined in 65 patients older than age 40 years; the mean patient age was 64 years. Patients with an associated tuberosity fracture were not included.

Methods.—Patients initially underwent closed reduction and had the arm immobilized in a sling. Physiotherapy began 2–3 weeks after injury. Electromyography was performed 6 weeks after injury. Most of the patients also had real-time ultrasonographic assessment of both shoulders 1 month after injury.

Findings.—Electromyography gave evidence of a nerve lesion in 36 of 55 patients, most frequently involving the axillary nerve. Thirty-five patients had denervation of the deltoid muscle, which in 9 patients was marked or total. Sonography revealed a rotator cuff lesion in 24 patients, 12 of whom had a total rupture. Thirteen patients had both nerve and cuff lesions. Twenty-seven of 57 patients had persistent symptoms at follow-up. All but 4 of these patients had cuff and/or nerve lesions, as did 18 of the 30 asymptomatic patients.

Conclusion.—Patients older than age 40 years who incur an anterior shoulder dislocation frequently have lesions of a nerve or the rotator cuff or both and, therefore, should be followed closely after injury. Difficulty in abduction of the arm is an especially important warning sign.

Chronic Anterior Dislocation of the Shoulder

Flatow EL, Miller SR, Neer CS II (Columbia-Presbyterian Med Ctr, NY)
J Shoulder Elbow Surg 2:2–10, 1993   129-94-2-13

Objective.—The treatment of chronic, unreduced anterior dislocations of the shoulder was dismal before the arthroplasty era; a series of these cases was reviewed.

Patients.—Eleven women and 6 men, aged 36–88 years, with chronic, unreduced anterior dislocations of the shoulder were treated. The average duration of dislocation was 2.3 years (range, 8 weeks to 8 years).

Treatment.—Because of health problems or motivational difficulties, 7 patients were treated without surgery despite severe functional deficits. Ten were treated surgically. One patient with preserved joint surfaces underwent open reduction and bone grafting of a large anterior glenoid fracture. The other 9 patients with destroyed articular surfaces underwent unconstrained replacement arthroplasty from an anterior, deltopectoral approach. Humeral retroversion was increased for stability. The soft tissues were reattached, and rehabilitation was modified with gradual introduction of motion similar to rehabilitation after repair of recurrent dislocations. Anterior glenoid bone loss was common and required bone grafting to support the glenoid component in 4 shoulders. Two large, chronic rotator cuff tears were repaired.

Outcome.—Nine patients were followed for an average of 3.9 years (range, 2–6 years). Four had excellent results, 4 were satisfactory, and 1 was unsatisfactory. Seven patients had no significant pain and none reported functional limitations.

Implications.—The availability of replacement arthroplasty has greatly improved the results of surgical reconstruction of chronic anterior dislocation of the shoulder. Although the reconstruction is complex, the surgical results are clearly superior to nonsurgical treatment.

► This seems to be a rare lesion in the absence of a massive rotator cuff tear. This series is interesting in that only 2 large rotator cuff tears were repaired. Perhaps this explains the overall excellent and satisfactory results achieved. This article is useful in supplying some of the details surrounding repair for this uncommon condition, as the arthroplasty technique is modified somewhat, as is the rehabilitation. However, with these modifications, the outcome can be quite acceptable. Please beware that a number of patients with this problem have a large chronic rotator cuff tear and, if this is found to be present, surgery may offer much less than might otherwise be possible.—R.H. Cofield, M.D.

The Structure and Function of the Coracohumeral Ligament: An Anatomic and Microscopic Study
Cooper DE, O'Brien SJ, Arnoczky SP, Warren RF (Cornell Univ, New York)
J Shoulder Elbow Surg 2:70–77, 1993   129-94-2–14

Objective.—To more precisely define the gross and microscopic anatomy of the normal coracohumeral ligament (CHL), 12 fresh-frozen shoulders from cadavers from 30 to 70 years of age were dissected.

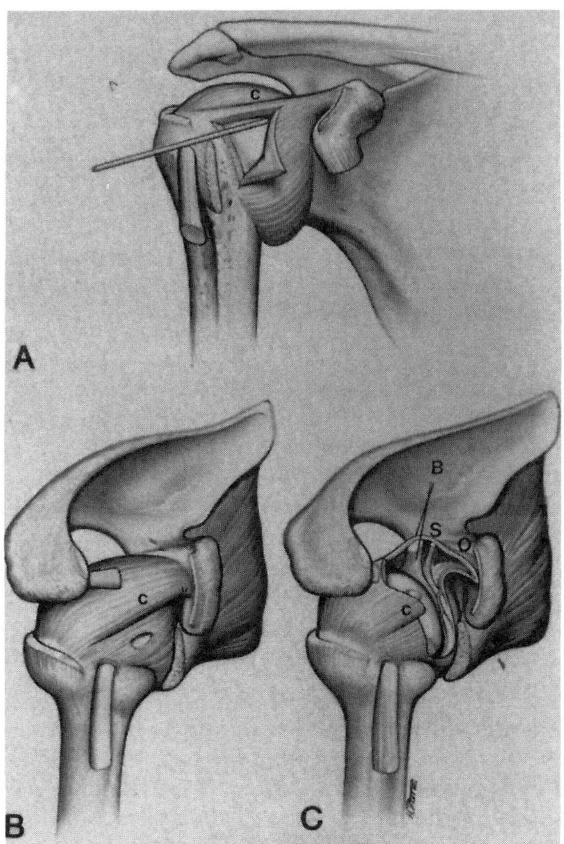

Fig 2–10.—Diagram of coracohumeral ligament anatomy. Coracoacromial ligament has been removed. **A,** drawing of the shoulder capsule after removal of the coracoacromial ligament and rotator cuff. Incision in the elevated ridge of folded CHL allows passage of probe to base of coracoid. **B,** illustration of an intact CHL (*c*). Folded capsular configuration is not evident by external inspection alone. **C,** sagittal plane block of the capsule has been removed. Inverted v-shaped origin (O) of coracohumeral ligament (*c*) is evident, as are biceps tendon (B) insertion and the superior glenohumeral ligament (S) just anterior to it. (Courtesy of Cooper DE, O'Brien SJ, Arnoczky SP, et al: *J Shoulder Elbow Surg* 2:70–77, 1993.)

Observations.—The CHL assumed 1 of 3 structural patterns. In 9 of the 12 dissections, it was merely a fold in the anterosuperior glenohumeral capsule that appeared prominent because of inferior translation of the head of the humerus (Fig 2–10). Microscopy failed to demonstrate discrete collagen bundles in these patients. The insertion of the CHL exhibited variable fiber orientation.

In 2 shoulders, a similar pattern was seen but the capsular fold failed to extend all the way to the anterior aspect of the CHL, leaving the structure with a thin anterior edge. In only 1 of the 12 shoulders were discrete collagenous fiber bundles present, suggesting a ligamentous structure.

Conclusion.—Most often, the CHL is a thin, folded, capsular structure that bears little resemblance to a true ligament.

▶ When shoulders become stiff, there is a propensity for scarring to form around the base of the coracoid and extend into the rotator cuff interval area. If surgical releases are necessary in this condition or if patients have rotator cuff tears involving the supraspinatus tendon, we have been taught that the release of the CHL is a useful adjunct; however, these authors nicely describe the CHL as merely a fold of capsule that is seldom a substantial ligamentous structure. This does not reduce in importance the desirability of releases around the base of the coracoid, but one must bear in mind that this tissue probably does not represent substantial pathology of the CHL per se. On the other hand, the CHL as described is unlikely to play much of a role in the maintenance of shoulder stability. It is merely a fold in the capsule.—R.H. Cofield, M.D.

Dynamic Capsuloligamentous Anatomy of the Glenohumeral Joint
Warner JJP, Caborn DNM, Berger R, Fu FH, Seel M (Univ of Pittsburgh, Pa)
J Shoulder Elbow Surg 2:115–133, 1993   129-94-2–15

Objective and Methods.—To define the relationships among the glenohumeral ligaments during shoulder rotation, 6 shoulders from fresh cadavers from 51 to 66 years of age were dissected and examined. A specially designed dynamic shoulder simulator, which may serve as either an isometric or isotonic model, was used. The superior and middle glenohumeral ligaments and the anterior and posterior bands of the inferior glenohumeral ligament complex were labeled arthroscopically with metallic beads. Rotational torques were applied with the shoulder in 0, 45, and 90 degrees of abduction.

Observations.—The superior and middle glenohumeral ligaments were maximally lengthened in 0 and 45 degrees of abduction and external rotation. Internal rotation in the abducted position caused these structures to shorten and become more vertical. In external rotation, they assumed a nearly horizontal course above the humeral head and be-

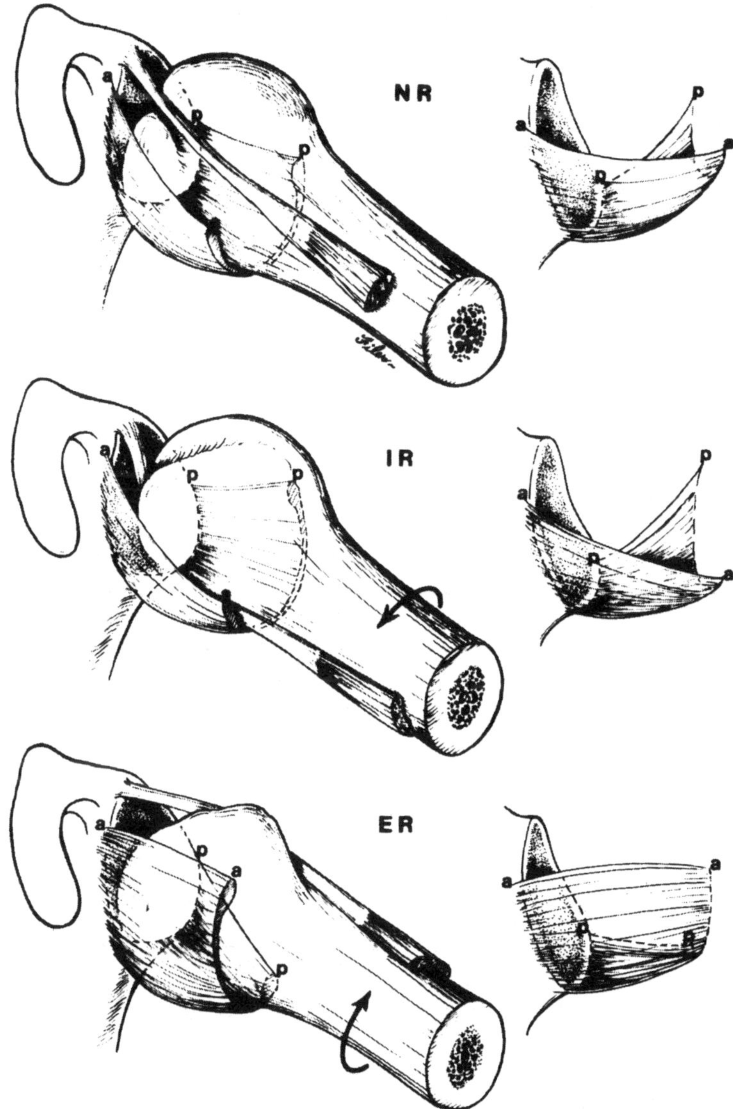

Fig 2–11.—Orientation changes of the inferior glenohumeral ligament complex at 90 degrees of abduction during rotation. In neutral rotation (NR), there is a cruciate arrangement of anterior (*a-a*) and posterior (*p-p*) bands. Internal rotation (IR) causes the anterior band to course underneath the humeral head while the posterior band then courses more superiorly. External rotation (ER) causes the anterior band to course superiorly while the posterior band courses underneath the humeral head. (Courtesy of Warner JJP, Caborn DNM, Berger R, et al: *J Shoulder Elbow Surg* 2:115–133, 1993.)

came longer. The components of the inferior glenohumeral ligament complex remained in a cruciate orientation in all abducted positions in the anteroposterior plane, except at 90 degrees of abduction and external rotation where they were oriented in a parallel manner.

Functional Implications.—The superior and middle glenohumeral ligaments would seem to complement the inferior ligaments, the former tightening in adduction and the latter in abduction. In this way, a large range of glenohumeral joint motion is possible. The cruciate arrangement of the inferior glenohumeral ligament complex allows each component to augment the other in stabilizing the humeral head on the glenoid during rotation (Fig 2–11). Operations for instability that tighten or shift the joint capsule must take these relationships into consideration so that the joint will not be overly constrained and motion limited as a result.

▶ The capsuloligamentous anatomy of the shoulder joint is becoming much better understood as a result of this study and other similar ones. Focusing on the shoulder capsule is very useful clinically in patients with unstable shoulders. Tightening the capsuloligamentous structures in the face of instability is a direct method for improving joint stability; however, the optimal method for doing this is probably yet to be described. Understanding anatomy and pathology and formulating appropriate repair methods are the next steps in synthesizing this information. That has not happened to date.—R.H. Cofield, M.D.

Recurrent Anterior Glenohumeral Joint Dislocation and Torsion of the Humerus
Dias JJ, Mody BS, Finlay DBL, Richardson RA (Leicester Royal Infirmary, England)
Injury 24:329–332, 1993   129-94-2–16

Objective.—The factors that might lead to recurrent dislocation of some glenohumeral joints were examined. Humeral torsion and glenoid version were investigated in 19 patients with recurrent anterior glenohumeral joint dislocation and 23 controls.

Patients and Methods.—The 16 male and 3 female patients (mean age, 27 years) all underwent CT of the shoulder. Two CT sections, 1 taken just below the coracoid process and the other about 2.5 cm proximal to the interepicondylar line, were used to determine glenoid version and humeral torsion. The glenoid was considered to be in neutral version if it was perpendicular to the plane of the scapula, anteverted if it was facing forward, and retroverted if it was facing backward. Humeral torsion was determined by observing the 2 CT sections with their axes superimposed. The angular difference between the proximal and distal axes indicated the magnitude of humeral torsion. Similar sections were obtained

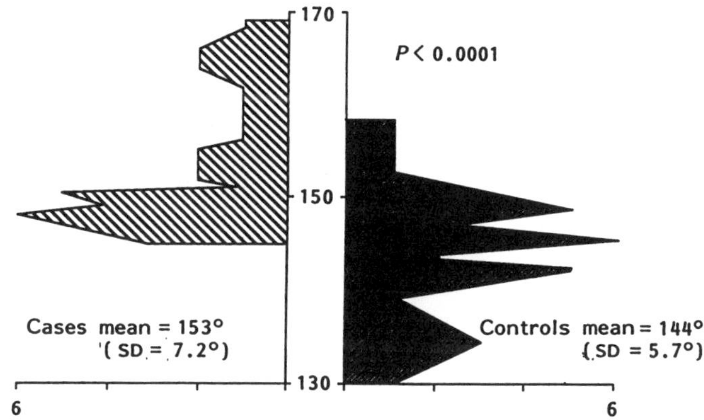

Fig 2–12.—Humeral torsion in patients with recurrent dislocation of the glenohumeral joint and in 23 controls. Humeral torsion was greater in patients than in controls. (Courtesy of Dias JJ, Mody BS, Finlay DBL, et al: *Injury* 24:329–332, 1993.)

in 23 patients with a mean age of 41 years who were undergoing CT scanning of the chest for other reasons.

Results.—Glenoid version and humeral torsion did not differ significantly between the right and left sides of controls or between the involved and contralateral sides of patients. The mean glenoid version was similar in patients (92 degrees) and controls (91 degrees). The humeral torsion, however, was significantly greater in patients (mean, 153 degrees) than in controls (mean, 144 degrees) (Fig 2–12).

Conclusion.—Patients with recurrent anterior glenohumeral joint dislocation appear to have greater torsion (less retroversion) than normal, by a mean of about 9 degrees. In some of the patients in this study, humeral torsion was at the upper limit of the torsion in shoulders of controls. This torsion was markedly increased in a small number of patients with recurrent dislocation. A rotation osteotomy of the proximal humerus to decrease torsion might be considered in these patients.

▶ Although patients with recurrent anterior dislocation had greater torsion (less retroversion) than normal, it is important to recognize that there was considerable overlap between the normal subjects and those with recurrent dislocation (as displayed in the figure). It is difficult to develop a clear mandate that rotational osteotomy of the proximal humerus should be considered.—R.H. Cofield, M.D.

Long-Term Results of Staple Capsulorrhaphy for Anterior Instability of the Shoulder

O'Driscoll SW, Evans DC (Mayo Clinic and Found, Rochester, Minn; Don Mills, Ont, Canada)
J Bone Joint Surg (Am) 75-A:249–258, 1993   129-94-2-17

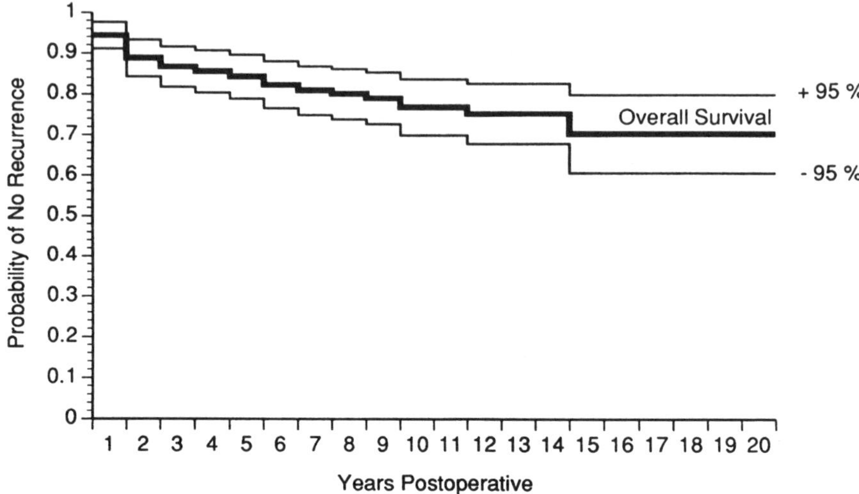

Fig 2–13.—Kaplan-Meier survival curve (*heavy line*) for the 204 shoulders, showing the probability that the shoulder would be stable after staple capsulorrhaphy: the upper and lower lines represent the 95% confidence intervals. The end point is an episode of instability after the operation, defined as either a dislocation that led to reduction or a subluxation that was clearly evident from the history provided by the patient. Two thirds of the end points were dislocations and one third were subluxations. In approximately one half of the shoulders, there was only 1 such episode; in the other half, there were at least 2 recurrent episodes of instability. The frequency of recurrent instability was logarithmically related to the duration of the follow-up period (*P* < .001). (Courtesy of O'Driscoll SW, Evans DC: *J Bone Joint Surg (Am)* 75-A:249–258, 1993.)

Objective.—The short-term results after open staple capsulorrhaphy of the shoulder are very encouraging, with a 90% to 97% rate of success and very few complications. The long-term results and complications of staple capsulorrhaphy of the shoulder were ascertained in a retrospective study.

Patients.—Between 1967 and 1986, 192 patients underwent 204 open staple capsulorrhaphy for recurrent anterior instability of the shoulder, including 88% with recurrent dislocations and 12% with recurrent subluxations. Stapling was combined with a Putti-Platt procedure in one third of the shoulders; a muscle-splitting approach was used in the others. The mean duration of follow-up was 10 years (range, 2–22 years).

Outcome.—Postoperative instability, either as dislocations or subluxations, occurred in 22% of patients, with more than half of these shoulders experiencing recurrent episodes. Half of the failures occurred in the first 2 years, and the frequency of recurrence of instability increased logarithmically with the duration of follow-up, with a 30% failure rate by 20 years (Fig 2–13). Postoperative instability occurred significantly more often in shoulders that had stapling alone (29%), compared with those in which a modified Putti-Platt procedure had been added (8%). Loosening or migration of a staple, or penetration of the articular cartilage by a staple occurred in 12% of shoulders, and the staple was removed in 9%.

The rate of loosening or migration of barbed staples did not differ significantly from that of nonbarbed staples, but incorrect placement of staples was associated with a higher rate of recurrent instability. Pain, physical restrictions, and osteoarthrosis occurred more frequently in patients who had complications associated with a staple. The shoulders that had a complication associated with a staple had greater reduction in average ranges of internal and external rotation, compared with the other shoulders.

In 84% of shoulders, the patients believed that the operation had been worthwhile. However, 51% of shoulders had pain and 50% were different enough from normal to affect the quality of life. In 6% of the shoulders, problems with the shoulder that had not been present preoperatively caused patients to change occupations.

Conclusion.—Staple capsulorrhaphy for anterior instability of the shoulder is associated with unacceptably high rates of serious or potentially serious complications associated with the staple and of recurrent instability. Hence, this procedure is not recommended for anterior instability of the shoulder, even when it is augmented by a Putti-Platt procedure.

▶ It has been consistently recognized that the use of metallic devices about the shoulder is fraught with danger. This study nicely documents that with long-term follow-up, stapling for instability also is not very effective—or at least seemingly so. Will absorbable tacks or staples fare any better? It makes one wonder.—R.H. Cofield, M.D.

Arthroscopic Staple Capsulorrhaphy: A Long-Term Follow-Up
Lane JG, Sachs RA, Riehl B (Kaiser Permanente, San Diego, Calif)
Arthroscopy 9:190–194, 1993   129-94-2–18

Background.—Limitation of motion is a common problem after reconstructive procedures for recurrent anterior shoulder instability. Fifty-four consecutive shoulders that underwent arthroscopic staple capsulorrhaphy were studied, and the long-term results were assessed in terms of stability, function, and range of motion.

Method.—Fifty-four patients underwent arthroscopic staple capsulorrhaphy between 1984 and 1989. All had traumatic instability with a Bankart lesion and had failed conservative treatment. The procedure included arthroscopic evaluation and abrasion of the anterior neck of the glenoid to stimulate a bleeding response. The ligamentous and capsular repair staple was then introduced through the anterior portal, and the tines of the staple were manipulated to snag the middle and inferior glenohumeral ligaments. The tissue and staple were then advanced to the anterior neck of the glenoid below the level of the joint surface, where the tines were embedded in bone. The arm was then immobilized for 3 weeks. Follow-up was carried out at 39 months, when patients were questioned about intensity and performance level before injury and at the time of follow-up.

Results.—The incidence of postoperative problems was high. Thirty-three percent of the patients had recurrent anterior instability. Ten underwent further surgery. Twenty-six percent of the patients had loose staples. Three of the 8 loose staples caused slight discomfort and 1 had migrated into the brachial plexus. Some staples were found in unexpected areas, such as the subacromial space and the area between the rib cage and the body of the scapula. Patients had an average loss of 5 degrees in external rotation with the arm abducted at 90 degrees, and the average loss in internal rotation was 1 spinal segment. Of the 14 patients who had participated in overhead throwing sports, 6 reached preinjury activity; the others were afraid or unable to return.

Conclusion.—Arthroscopic staple capsulorrhaphy is a demanding procedure, with many potential complications. The rates of recurrence and staple problems are high. However, potential benefits include well-maintained range of motion and functional levels. Because of the risk of staple loosening and migration, consideration should be given to the routine removal of staples or long-term radiographic follow-up.

▶ In this study, certain conclusions were reached. One might also conclude that another type of operative procedure would be better—particularly an operative procedure that would avoid insertion of metal and the subsequent need to remove it. Although movement seemed to be well maintained in those who did not have problems, so many patients had problems that one must conclude that the operation is somewhat inconsistent in its outcome. There are other operations that are much more consistent, and most surgeons would opt to use techniques that avoid a number of the problems reported here.—R.H. Cofield, M.D.

Long-Term Followup of the Modified Bristow Procedure
Banas MP, Dalldorf PG, Sebastianelli WJ, DeHaven KE (Univ of Rochester, NY)
Am J Sports Med 21:666–671, 1993   129-94-2–19

Background.—The modified Bristow procedure has been popular for the past 20 years. However, its use as a primary treatment for anterior glenohumeral instability is increasingly being discouraged. The long-term outcome of the modified Bristow procedure was reported.

Patients.—Between 1975 and 1987, 78 patients underwent 86 modified Bristow procedures for anterior shoulder instability. Complete follow-up data were available for 71 patients with 79 treated shoulders (92%). Eight patients had bilateral procedures. The patients ranged in age from 16 to 42 years at the time of operation. Follow-up ranged from

2 to 13.7 years. Indications were recurrent subluxation in 35 shoulders and recurrent dislocation in 44 shoulders. The average time between the initial injury and operation was 35 months.

Results.—Three patients sustained traumatic postoperative redislocations that required revision surgery. Eight other patients (10%) required secondary operations for screw removal because of persistent shoulder pain at an average of 27 months after primary operation. At the follow-up examination, none of the patients had sensory deficits in the extremity operated on. Postoperative subjective shoulder function averaged 86% of the preinjury level. The results were rated as excellent or very good by 66 patients (88%), good by 6 patients (9%), and poor by 2 patients (3%). The Rowe scale for shoulder reconstruction recorded the results as good or excellent in 40 shoulders (85%), fair in 4 (9%), and poor in 3 (6%). All throwing athletes were able to return to throwing, although 54% of those with dominant shoulder involvement reported a decrease in throwing velocity.

Conclusion.—The modified Bristow procedure provides excellent long-term stability, satisfactory shoulder function, and minimal loss of internal and external rotation.

▶ This well-formatted report demonstrates the benefits of the Bristow procedure and also its detriments. I think no one questions that the Bristow procedure may lead to an excellent result, and, indeed, these authors have documented that that is possible. However, of the 79 shoulders treated, 11 required a reoperation. Most of these reoperations occurred because of problems with the internal fixation. This is also something that many surgeons have recognized—that the need for reoperation when using this procedure is much higher than that experienced with techniques that do not use metallic internal fixation. Perhaps that is a primary reason why the Bristow procedure has lost some favor in North America. Certainly, that is true for me.—R.H. Cofield, M.D.

The Inferior Capsular-Shift Procedure for Multidirectional Instability of the Shoulder

Cooper RA, Brems JJ (Cleveland Clinic Found, Ohio)
J Bone Joint Surg (Am) 74-A:1516–1521, 1992   129-94-2-20

Introduction.—Between 1984 and 1990, 38 patients (43 shoulders) underwent an inferior capsular-shift procedure for disabling multidirectional instability of the shoulder that did not respond to nonsurgical management. All patients had severe pain, disabling instability with activities of daily living, or persistent paresthesias during the involved activities. All patients had been followed up for at least 2 years (mean, 39 months).

Outcome.—The range of motion of the shoulders was well maintained, with a mean forward elevation of 172 degrees, external rotation of 77 degrees, and internal rotation up to the level of the eighth thoracic vertebra. Thirty-nine shoulders (91%) functioned well with no recurrence of symptomatic instability. Four patients (4 shoulders or 11%) had recurrent symptomatic instability less than 2 years after the operation.

Thirty-four patients were subjectively satisfied with the status of the shoulder, and 4 with recurrent instability were not satisfied. Thirty-seven shoulders remained stable through the follow-up, whereas 6 shoulders (including the 4 with recurrent instability) deteriorated with time. Nine patients (9 shoulders) reported episodes of apprehension that were associated with the residual inferior and posterior translations evident on postoperative physical examinations.

Conclusion.—Inferior capsular shift is an acceptable procedure for the treatment of severe, incapacitating, multidirectional instability of the shoulder. Although it does not eliminate all translation of the humeral head, the procedure provides satisfactory objective and subjective results that remain stable with follow-up of 2–6 years.

▶ It is difficult to distinguish those who have multidirectional instability, a pathologic condition, from those who have ligamentous laxity in the shoulder—a variant of normal. As these authors have so nicely described it, they made the diagnosis in 251 patients during the time that 43 shoulders were selected for surgery. The others were treated conservatively and presumably did well. Thus, it is still very difficult to select who should be considered for the surgical procedure described. These authors do report that with patient selection done as carefully as possible, careful surgery, and immaculate aftercare, somewhere between 80% and 90% of shoulders will be improved. In this series, the mean patient age was 25 years, ranging from 17 to 36 years. This seems typical, with patients usually presenting in the latter part of the second decade, in the third decade, and occasionally in the fourth decade of life.

A question one must ask is: What is the natural history of this problem? Does the problem persist into middle age and beyond? There is little evidence that that is true. As with the many other patients seen by these authors, one wonders how many of the patients who had the surgery would have improved with time alone. I suspect the number would approach 80% and above. It seems clear, however, that the surgery has hastened this natural recovery process. The surgery has not been shown to cause harm and has benefited a significant number of patients.—R.H. Cofield, M.D.

Arthroscopic Suture Repair of Superior Labral Detachment Lesions of the Shoulder

Field LD, Savoie FH III (Mississippi Sports Medicine & Orthopaedic Ctr, Jackson)
Am J Sports Med 21:783–790, 1993   129-94-2–21

Patients.—Twenty consecutive patients underwent arthroscopic suture repair of anterior and posterior superior labral (SLAP) lesions of the shoulder that involved the attachment of the biceps to the glenoid labrum (Snyder types II and IV). The patients, 16 men and 4 women, had an average age of 39 years. They were symptomatic for 13 months, on average, before repair, and they were followed for an average of 21 months. The most common antecedent was a compression force to the shoulder, most often resulting from a fall on the outstretched and abducted arm. Most of the patients had nonspecific posterior shoulder pain. Eight patients also had a partial rotator cuff tear, and 5 had an impingement syndrome.

Technique.—After arthroscopy has confirmed a type II or type IV SLAP lesion, a superior inflow portal and anterior instrument portal are established. The frayed superior labral tissue is débrided, and, in type IV cases, the bucket-handle tear and small tears of the biceps tendon are excised. The superior glenoid neck is abraded to bleeding bone, and 4–7 sutures of 2-0 polydioxanone are placed in the labrum-biceps tendon complex using a suture punch. One or 2 anchor stitches are placed in the biceps tendon itself. A hole is then drilled through the glenoid neck about 3–5 mm medial to the articular surface of the glenoid, exiting

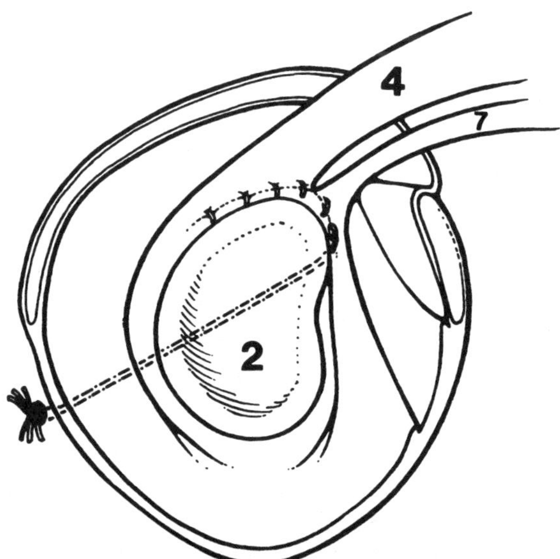

Fig 2–14.—The repaired labral ligamentous complex shows sutures in position, effecting excellent, tight closure of the superior labrum-biceps tendon complex to the superior glenoid: biceps tendon (4), glenoid (2), and superior glenohumeral ligament (7). (Courtesy of Field LD, Savoie FH III: *Am J Sports Med* 21:783–790, 1993.)

in the infraspinous fossa of the posterior scapula. Sutures are passed through this hole and tied over the infraspinatus muscle fascia (Fig 2–14). A shoulder immobilizer is used for 1–2 weeks postoperatively, and an arm sling is used for another 3–4 weeks before starting a progressive rehabilitation program.

Results.—Pain scores improved significantly after repair, as did functional scores. The Rowe scale indicated good or excellent results in all patients. No patient had discomfort from the subcutaneous sutures. All 6 patients involved in throwing sports returned to activity with no loss of velocity. Recreational athletes and patients with work-related injuries also resumed their activities. One patient had adhesive capsulitis that responded well to manipulation under general anesthesia.

Conclusion.—Arthroscopic suturing is a reliable and relatively simple means of repairing unstable superior labral detachment lesions of the shoulder.

▶ This arthroscopically diagnosed lesion is more common than one might have anticipated. In patients with significant shoulder symptoms, this method of repair seems quite reasonable. It is not unduly difficult and does not involve internal fixation, which might require removal or cause other subsequent problems. This article, in essence, shows that this technique can be effective in the treatment of these lesions.—R.H. Cofield, M.D.

Arthroscopic Repair of Superior Glenoid Labral Detachment (the SLAP Lesion)
Resch H, Golser K, Thoeni H, Sperner G (Univ Hosp of Innsbruck, Austria)
J Shoulder Elbow Surg 2:147–155, 1993   129-94-2–22

Background.—Abnormalities of the glenoid labrum at the superior pole of the glenoid range from degenerative changes to complete detachment of the glenoid labrum, including destabilization of the origin of the long biceps tendon. Detachment of the long head of the biceps tendon from the superior glenoid pole alters the functioning of the shoulder joint, especially in overhead activities. Snyder et al. have described this lesion as superior labrum, anterior and posterior (SLAP). Two surgical techniques, similar in principle, for reattachment of the glenoid labrum to the glenoid were reported.

Methods.—The screw fixation technique was used in 6 patients. The glenoid labrum was reattached with small cannulated titanium screws just behind the origin of the long biceps tendon. In 5 of the patients, the screws were inserted under arthroscopic control from a cranial direction. Percutaneous probing around the acromion with a Kirschner wire identified the most favorable portal. A transacromial hole was drilled if access via a portal placed anterior or medial to the acromion was not possible. The screws were removed by arthroscopy after 3–5 months.

Absorbable tacks were used instead of screws for reattachment in 8 patients. The mean follow-up for the 14 patients was 18 months.

Results.—Fourteen patients underwent surgical reattachment to treat a complete detachment of the glenoid labrum from the superior pole of the glenoid with destabilization of the attachment of the biceps tendon. At follow-up, 8 patients were completely rehabilitated and had resumed overhead sports, 4 patients were improved, and 2 patients had no improvement. Only 1 of the 4 patients who were treated without reattachment of the labrum has experienced a definite improvement in his symptoms. He had a "bucket-handle" displacement of the labrum and the displaced part was resected. The other 3 had shaving of the free margin of the glenoid labrum only and have shown no significant improvement in their symptoms when performing overhead activities.

Conclusion.—Fourteen patients with SLAP lesions underwent surgery to reattach the glenoid labrum to the superior aspect of the glenoid. Eight patients had excellent results, 4 were improved, and 2 had no improvement. In contrast, there was improvement in only 1 of the 4 patients without reattachment.

▶ This article, like Abstract 129-94-2–21, explores other alternatives for treatment of superior glenoid labral detachments. Direct fixation is used instead of suture repair. The authors show how this can be accomplished. The results are reasonable.—R.H. Cofield, M.D.

Instability of the Shoulder After Arthroplasty

Moeckel BH, Altchek DW, Warren RF, Wickiewicz TL, Dines DM (Middlesex Orthopedics, Middletown, Conn; Hosp for Special Surgery, New York)
J Bone Joint Surg (Am) 75-A:492–497, 1993   129-94-2–23

Background.—Replacement arthroplasty of the shoulder is generally a highly successful procedure with pain relief in 90% to 95% of patients and a range of motion two thirds of normal. Anterior or posterior instability of the shoulder is a rare complication of replacement arthroplasty. The outcome of operative management of instability in 10 patients was assessed.

Method.—A retrospective record review identified 236 patients who underwent a total shoulder replacement in 1 center. Instability developed in 10 patients, all of whom had been treated with an unconstrained prosthesis. Seven patients had anterior instability caused by rupture of the repaired subscapularis tendon. Three patients had posterior instability with multifactorial causes. After repair, the patients were followed clinically and radiographically for at least 2 years.

Operative Treatment.—The 7 patients with anterior instability were treated with mobilization and repair of the tendon, which was successful in 4 patients. A static stabilizer, consisting of an allograft of Achilles tendon, was inserted in the remaining 3 patients with good results. Posterior instability was treated with correction of any soft tissue imbalance and revision of the prosthetic components as necessary.

Results.—All 10 patients had some loss of motion of the shoulder, but there were no other complications or problems related to the allografts.

Conclusion.—During total shoulder replacement, instability can be prevented by proper positioning of the component and balancing of the soft tissues. Postoperative physical therapy must be based on the range of motion achieved in the operating room. Early recognition and treatment of instability is important as repairs become increasingly difficult with time. Treatment of any dislocation or subluxation includes reconstruction of the soft tissue envelope, revision of the prosthetic components, the use of allografts to correct soft tissue deficiencies, or a combination of these techniques.

▶ Instability is the most common complication after shoulder arthroplasty. It is surprising that there are only a few articles on the treatment of this complication. This article nicely outlines the fact that correction of soft tissue problems is essential and that, as an adjunct to this, it may be necessary to revise the components or to use other special reinforcement techniques. Treatment will not always be successful, but for a substantial number of patients there will be significant improvement.

Of note, this article does not address other common problems leading to instability, such as diffuse rotator cuff deficiency in patients with rheumatoid arthritis or iatrogenic lesions involving either component displacement or disruption of supporting soft tissue structures. It is important to recognize that there can be a number of factors contributing to the instability. This is a difficult condition to treat and probably most, if not all, of the associated problems need to be addressed at the time of revision surgery.—R.H. Cofield, M.D.

Rotator Cuff Disease

Suprascapular Neuropathy Restricted to the Infraspinatus Muscle in Volleyball Players

Montagna P, Colonna S (Univ of Bologna, Italy; Univ of Siena, Italy)
Acta Neurol Scand 87:248–250, 1993   129-94-2-24

Introduction.—Isolated neuropathies of the infraspinatus muscle may result from suprascapular nerve lesions at the spinoglenoid notch. Many reported cases have involved sports and muscular effort. Six volleyball players who sustained suprascapular nerve lesions restricted to the infraspinatus muscle were described.

Patients.—The patients were 3 women and 3 men ranging in age from 16 to 32 years. All were active volleyball players competing on amateur to professional levels. All had moderate shoulder pain and weakness after practice, particularly with serving and smashing, and isolated atrophy of the infraspinatus, which was noticed by others. There were no apparent reasons for the onset of symptoms. All patients continued competition despite being warned not to do so. Electromyography demonstrated denervation, loss of motor units with effort, and signs of reinnervation restricted to the infraspinatus on the dominant side only. The supraspinatus was normal in all patients. Five of the patients had increased latency to the infraspinatus with small and polyphasic motor potentials.

Conclusion.—An isolated infraspinatus neuropathy associated with the sport of volleyball is described, presumably resulting from a lesion of the suprascapular nerve at the spinoglenoid notch. This injury may occur when excessive muscular effort of the shoulder is associated with anatomical predisposing factors, such as a tight spinoglenoid ligament.

▶ A variation of suprascapular neuropathy is described. Speculation continues that this is related to an entrapment lesion. That may be true, but it may also be related to repetitive stretching of the nerve as a part of activity. If this is indeed true, consideration of surgery would be substantially lessened. In North America, many would obtain an MRI if this lesion is apparent to assess whether there is an associated lesion, such as a large ganglion adjacent to the suprascapular nerve. If so, many surgeons would probably consider removal of the ganglion and release of the ligament in an effort to improve the patient's condition.

A second feature of this article is that the individuals involved were competitive athletes. They were having difficulties with their shoulders but could still compete. Therefore, more aggressive patient management might not be indicated in a number of individuals with this affliction.—R.H. Cofield, M.D.

Os Acromiale: Anatomy and Surgical Implications

Edelson JG, Zuckerman J, Hershkovitz I (Poriya Hosp, Tiberias, Israel; Hosp for Joint Diseases Orthopaedic Inst, New York; Tel Aviv Univ, Israel)
J Bone Joint Surg (Br) 75-B:551–555, 1993   129-94-2-25

Background.—An os acromiale is the result of an unfused acromial epiphysis. An os acromiale is usually asymptomatic, but it can cause localized degenerative changes, impingement syndromes, and rotator cuff tears. A cadaveric study was carried out to examine the anatomy of os acromiale, and surgical treatment of 7 patients with this anomaly was evaluated.

Methods.—The study material for the anatomical study consisted of 190 well-preserved scapular specimens obtained from 3 archaeologic sites in Israel and 80 specimens obtained from dissecting room cadavers. All scapular specimens came from mature individuals aged 30–60 years at the time of death.

Findings.—Twenty-two of the 270 scapulae (8.2%) had os acromiale. Degenerative changes were observed at the site of nonunion in 12 of the 22 specimens. The degenerative changes were usually on the proximal acromial fragment in the form of a distinctive pattern of osteophytic lipping. The length of the free bone fragments was approximately one third of the overall length of the respective acromions. In 20 specimens, the facet of the acromioclavicular joint was located on the os acromiale.

Patients.—Of 7 patients with shoulder pain, 5 underwent total excision of the acromion and repair of the coincident rotator cuff tears. Because no rotator cuff abnormality was found in the other 2 patients, their os acromial lesions were treated by fusion. After a follow-up of 18–40 months, 6 of the 7 surgically treated patients were satisfied with the outcome. The only treatment failure occurred in a 70-year-old man with an irreparable rotator cuff tear.

▶ This descriptive article further defines os acromiale. It is important to recognize that this variation can be overlooked unless an axillary x-ray study is done as a part of patient evaluation. Certainly, if one is considering surgical treatment, it is wise to be aware that this condition is present before the operation is undertaken.—R.H. Cofield, M.D.

The Subacromial Bursa and the Impingement Syndrome: A Clinical and Histological Study of 30 Cases
Rahme H, Nordgren H, Hamberg H, Westerberg C-E (Central Hosp, Västerås, Sweden; Univ Hosp, Uppsala, Sweden)
Acta Orthop Scand 64:485–488, 1993   129-94-2–26

Introduction.—The impingement syndrome was first described 2 decades ago by Neer who introduced an operation—anterior acromioplasty—designed to treat the syndrome. Few studies have considered the microscopic morphology of the subacromial bursa in patients with a presumed diagnosis of an impingement syndrome. This study sought to determine whether biopsy specimens taken from patients differed morphologically from biopsy specimens from normal shoulders, and whether there was an association between microscopic findings and outcome of surgery.

Patients and Methods.—Operative bursal biopsy specimens were taken from 30 patients whose history was compatible with impingement syndrome. The group had a mean age of 42 years and a mean duration of symptoms of 3 years. Preoperatively and at regular intervals up to 1 year after operation, patients rated their pain on a visual analogue scale and were evaluated by an independent examiner. Bursal specimens were obtained at autopsy from 13 individuals with no known history of shoulder disorders. The biopsy specimens were classified by 2 pathologists on the basis of the absence/presence of fibrosis.

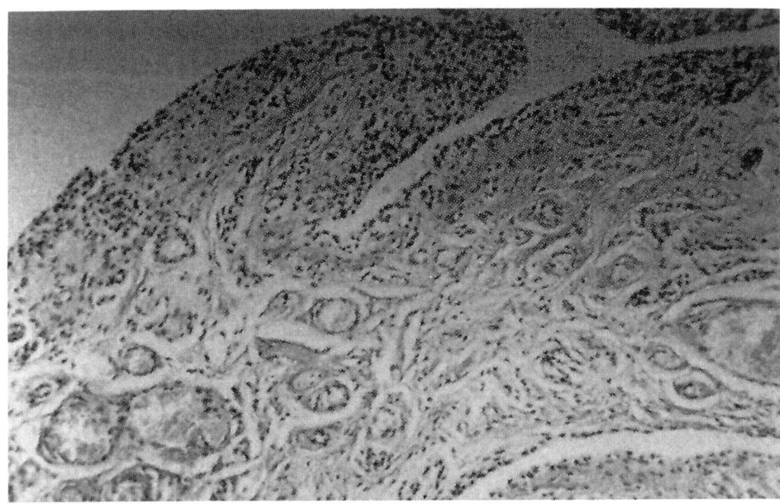

Fig 2–15.—Bursa specimen. Van Gieson stain, original magnification, ×100. Pathologically altered bursa with fibrous thickening of the wall and dilated blood vessels. There is no evident synovial proliferation or any infiltration of inflammatory cells. (Courtesy of Rahme H, Nordgren H, Hamberg H, et al: *Acta Orthop Scand* 64:485–488, 1993.)

Results.—Pathologists agreed regarding the absence/presence of fibrosis 91% of the time and showed complete agreement on the classification of autopsy specimens. Fibrosis appeared to be characteristic of the patients with impingement syndrome (Fig 2–15) and was an occasional finding in the autopsy series. Inflammatory cells were found in 7 of 30 specimens from patients but in none of the autopsy samples. Microscopic findings could not be predicted from preoperative observations. Successful outcome after surgery was associated with the presence of bursal fibrosis.

Conclusion.—Impingement syndrome is diagnosed on the basis of pain at rest, during a standardized provocation maneuver, and after an injection of a local anesthetic. Poor outcome after Neer's operation may result from the fact that mechanical impingement did not exist. The presence of fibrosis might be predictive of a favorable outcome after surgery. At present, however, knowledge of the microscopic appearance of the subacromial bursa cannot be obtained before operation.

▶ These authors nicely reinforce that the result of surgery is improved if pathology can be identified. One associated feature of the impingement problem is scarring within the subacromial bursa. If that is absent, one wonders whether the acromioplasty should be considered. One also asks oneself whether, if that is the only pathologic abnormality present, acromioplasty should be considered; perhaps it should not be undertaken unless more substantive changes, such as either partial or complete rotator cuff disruption, accompany this change.—R.H. Cofield, M.D.

Degenerative Change and Rotator Cuff Tears: An Anatomical Study in 160 Shoulders of 80 Cadavers

Hijioka A, Suzuki K, Nakamura T, Hojo T (Univ of Occupational and Environmental Health, Kitakyusyu, Japan)
Arch Orthop Trauma Surg 112:61–64, 1993   129-94-2–27

Introduction.—The etiology of rotator cuff tearing has recently become a matter of controversy. In 1 study of cadavers, it was concluded that intrinsic tendon degeneration is dominant, but in another the theory of a contribution by friction and rubbing by the subacromial undersurface was supported. Details of a study of 80 cadavers examining the effects of friction and rubbing in the development of rotator cuff tears were reported.

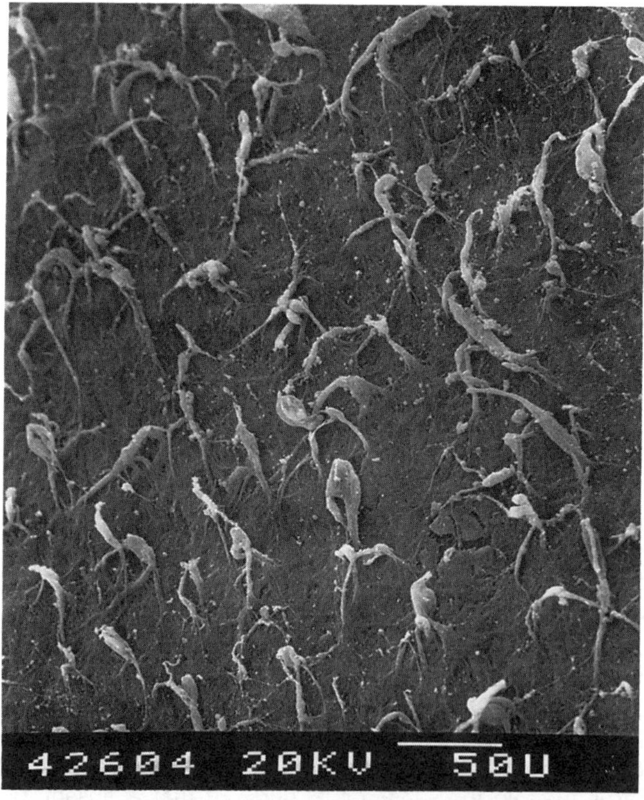

Fig 2–16.—In specimens with grade 1 degeneration, scanning electron microscopy showed regularly arranged wool-like spherical structures on the surface of the supraspinatus tendon. Small spherical structures appeared to be made of fine reticulum fibers. (Courtesy of Hijioka A, Suzuki K, Nakamura T, et al: *Arch Orthop Trauma Surg* 112:61–64, 1993.)

Methods.—Both shoulders of 56 male and 24 female cadavers were dissected. The mean age of the subjects at death was 69.3 years. The surface of the cuff and the undersurface of the acromion were observed macroscopically. Cuff degeneration was classified into 4 grades and the undersurface of the acromion into 3 grades. Scanning electron microscopy was used to examine shoulders in the 8 fresh cadavers.

Results.—Degenerative changes of the supraspinatus tendon were observed in 98 specimens (61%). The size of the tear increased with age, and the number of tendons with degeneration and tearing increased from the fifth to sixth decade of life. There was no sustained increase in incidence from age 60 to 90 years, however, and the percentage with degenerative changes remained at approximately 60%. Ninety-six specimens had degeneration of the subacromial surface, but there was no sustained increase in the incidence of degeneration with age. A significant correlation was observed between the severity of the changes in the rotator cuff and the subacromial surface. In specimens with grade 1 cuff degeneration (loss of the bursa on the cuff), scanning electron microscopy revealed wool-like spherical structures on the surface of the tendon (Fig 2–16). These regularly arranged structures and the rounded ruptured ends of the tendon fibers suggested the effects of friction and rubbing on the rotator cuff.

Conclusion.—The findings suggest that degenerative changes in the rotator cuff appear mainly in the fifth and sixth decades of life. Cuffs that do not begin degeneration in these years may not develop a tear in later years. Whatever the initial cause of degeneration, changes in the cuff may be aggravated by friction and rubbing and may lead to the development of a complete tear.

▶ This study is probably closest to the truth of any that have been published recently. It shows that tendons of the rotator cuff do degenerate with age; it also clearly shows that friction in the subacromial region creates changes in the tendons, augmenting or adding to the degenerative changes that do occur. Both processes are important in the genesis of the clinical syndromes involving rotator cuff pathology.—R.H. Cofield, M.D.

Arthroscopic Surgery Compared With Supervised Exercises in Patients With Rotator Cuff Disease (Stage II Impingement Syndrome)
Brox JI, Staff PH, Ljunggren AE, Brevik JI (Ullevaal Univ, Oslo, Norway)
BMJ 307:899–903, 1993   129-94-2-28

Objective.—A randomized clinical trial was planned to compare the efficacy of arthroscopic surgery, a supervised exercise program, and a placebo treatment using a detuned soft laser in patients with rotator cuff disease (stage II impingement syndrome).

Patients.—A total of 125 patients, aged 18–66 years, who had had shoulder pain for at least 3 months despite physiotherapy, nonsteroidal anti-inflammatory drugs, and steroids were included in the trial. All of them had pain or dysfunction on abduction of the upper extremity and positive results on tests for impingement, but the passive range of glenohumeral motion was normal. Lignocaine was injected into the anterior subacromial space to confirm the diagnosis.

Treatments.—Two experienced surgeons performed subacromial decompression arthroscopically by creating space for the rotator cuff. The procedure entailed bursectomy and resection of the anterior and lateral parts of the acromion and coracoacromial ligament. Exercises were designed to normalize dysfunctional neuromuscular patterns and enhance the nutritional status of collagen in the rotator cuff. Placebo treatments were given twice per week for 6 weeks.

Results.—There were no significant treatment-related differences in the duration of sick leave or the use of analgesics. Patients in both actively treated groups improved significantly more than the placebo patients at 6 months. Overall Neer scores did not differ significantly in the surgery and exercise groups. Men had a better outcome after operative treatment, and women did slightly better after exercises. Pain was reduced to a nearly identical degree in these groups. Surgery proved to be more costly than the supervised exercise program.

Conclusion.—Most patients with rotator cuff disease can be effectively managed by supervised exercises.

▶ This interesting study reinforces the benefits gleaned by conservative, nonoperative treatment for rotator cuff symptomatology in the absence of rotator cuff tearing. Unlike many other studies, a placebo limb was included, and it is useful to see that either surgery or physiotherapy caused improvement and placebo treatment did not. As might be anticipated, treatment costs were at least twice as high in those patients who underwent surgery. As an adjunct to this study, it would be helpful for the authors to resurvey these patients 5 years later to ascertain whether any additional treatment has been necessary among the 3 groups. If the results remain unchanged, the value of physiotherapy would be confirmed, but one wonders whether the nonoperatively treated group might not be more likely to have recurrent symptomatology. It is, of course, impossible to tell at this point.—R.H. Cofield, M.D.

Arthroscopic Treatment of Full-Thickness Rotator Cuff Tears: 2- to 7-Year Follow-Up Study
Ellman H, Kay SP, Wirth M (Univ of California, Los Angeles; Univ of Texas, San Antonio)
Arthroscopy 9:195–200, 1993
129-94-2–29

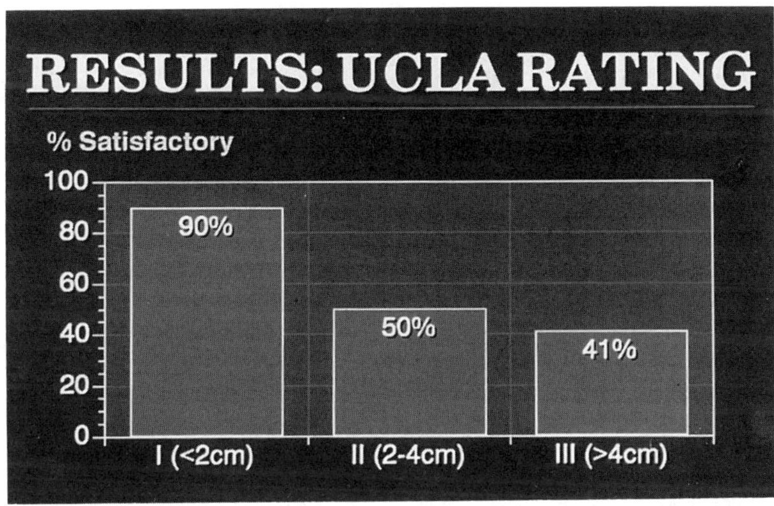

Fig 2–17.—Overall satisfactory results (excellent and good) based on pain, function, range of motion, strength in forward flexion, and patient satisfaction are compared by group. (Courtesy of Ellman H, Kay SP, Wirth M: *Arthroscopy* 9:195–200, 1993.)

Purpose.—Arthroscopic subacromial decompression (ASD) is an effective treatment for shoulder impingement syndrome, but its efficacy for full-thickness rotator cuff tears has not been determined. Whether ASD could be useful in selected patients with shoulder impingement syndrome that has progressed to a full-thickness rotator cuff tear was evaluated.

Methods.—During a 6-year period, 40 patients with full-thickness rotator cuff tears underwent ASD and cuff débridement. Only older, relatively sedentary patients who did not want to undergo major surgery were included in the study. When grouped by rotator cuff tear size as measured during arthroscopic inspection, 10 patients with an average age of 63 years had fixable cuff tears of less than 2 cm; 8 patients with an average age of 66.7 years had fixable but larger cuff tears of 2–4 cm; and 22 patients with an average age of 73.9 years had irreparable cuff tears greater than 4 cm in length. A 35-point University of California at Los Angeles (UCLA) shoulder rating scale was used to assess pain, function, range of motion, strength in forward flexion, and patient satisfaction.

Results.—Arthroscopic subacromial decompression and débridement improved pain and function scores in 90% of the patients with small, fixable cuff tears as reflected by good or excellent scores on the UCLA shoulder rating scale. Furthermore, 90% of these patients were satisfied with the outcome. Only 50% of the patients with larger rotator cuff tears had satisfactory UCLA outcome scores and only 62.5% of these patients were satisfied with the outcome. Only 40.9% of the patients with large, irreparable cuff tears received satisfactory UCLA ratings, but 86.4% of these patients were satisfied with the outcome (Fig 2–17).

Conclusion.—Arthroscopic subacromial decompression with cuff débridement is useful for treating small rotator cuff tears in a carefully selected subset of patients. Open surgical repair remains the most effective approach, even for small cuff tears.

▶ From a common sense point of view, this article hits the spot. For smaller amounts of rotator cuff pathology, arthroscopy may be helpful; for larger amounts of rotator cuff pathology, it is much less useful—probably approaching a placebo level of effectiveness. As with Abstract 129-94-2-28, it would be interesting to know what will happen to these patients in 5 years. It is unlikely that the results for any of the 3 groups will improve over time. Perhaps this form of treatment will not be enduring for any of the patient groups. Of course, that is impossible to know without more long-term information.—R.H. Cofield, M.D.

Reoperation for Failed Rotator Cuff Repair: Analysis of Fifty Cases
Neviaser RJ, Neviaser TJ (George Washington Univ, Washington, DC)
J Shoulder Elbow Surg 1:283–286, 1992   129-94-2-30

Introduction.—Clinical failure occurs in up to 25% of repaired ruptures of the rotator cuff. The prevailing view has been that reoperation for failed repairs is unlikely to increase motion. An analysis was made of 50 cases of reoperation for failed cuff repair to determine whether functional improvement can be achieved.

Patients and Methods.—The patient group included 39 men and 11 women with an average age of 54.5 years at the time of final reoperation. The average number of previous operations was 1.6, and the average interval between the last failed surgery and the final operation was 16.9 months. All patients had night pain and significant pain both at rest and with use. Active forward elevation in the scapular plane averaged 92 degrees before surgery. Degenerative changes in the acromioclavicular joint were observed on preoperative radiographs in all patients. After surgery, the patients were immobilized for 4–6 weeks. All started passive elevation and external rotation (arm at side) within 48 hours after surgery and active rehabilitation was initiated within 4–6 weeks. The mean follow-up was 30 months.

Results.—Twenty-two patients retained their preoperative motion, and 26 had an average increase in elevation of 50 degrees. Two patients lost motion but still had more than 90 degrees. All 6 patients who had less than 90 degrees after surgery had deltoid abnormalities. Pain improved in 46 patients and remained unchanged in 4. The number of patients with more than 150 degrees of elevation was doubled after surgery. The final results did not appear to be related to the size of the tear at reoperation or the number of previous failed procedures. Forty-five patients expressed satisfaction with the results of reoperation. Four of the 5 dissatisfied patients had no change in their pain.

Conclusion.—Successful reoperation for rupture of the rotator cuff depends on having an intact deltoid for improved function and adequate decompression for reduction of pain. The mobilization and closure of all defects with tendon-to-bone junctures and early passive mobility after surgery also contribute to favorable results. Weights and resistive exercises should be avoided in the early postoperative rehabilitation period.

▶ This study offers physicians and patients alike great hope, reinforcing the idea that it may be possible to obtain a good outcome after repeat rotator cuff surgery. About half of the patients in this group had massive tears; seemingly they did reasonably well, although it is difficult to be certain from the way the data are tabulated. One must mention that this is unlike the experience that other people have had. Rerepairing massive rotator cuff tears is often not as effective as one would wish. As implied from the above, this article serves as a useful counterpoint to that viewpoint.—R.H. Cofield, M.D.

Anterior Dislocation of the Shoulder and Rotator Cuff Rupture
Neviaser RJ, Neviaser TJ, Neviaser JS (George Washington Univ, Washington, DC; Fairfax, Va; Loris, SC)
Clin Orthop 291:103–106, 1993   129-94-2–31

Background.—The mechanism of shoulder dislocation may vary for individuals younger than and older than 40 years of age. After age 40, rotator cuff rupture is frequently associated with a primary dislocation. Unfortunately, the rotator cuff rupture is often mistaken for an axillary neuropathy. Thirty-seven patients were treated for rotator cuff ruptures resulting from a documented primary dislocation.

Patients.—The patients, all but 1 older than 40 years of age at the time of their first shoulder dislocation, had a history of inability to elevate the arm after reduction and many were treated for suspected axillary nerve palsy. Eleven patients had recurrent instability almost immediately after reduction. The diagnosis of rotator cuff rupture was made an average of 7.2 months after the dislocation. The patients were all treated with subacromial decompression and rotator cuff repair or reconstruction for associated rotator cuff ruptures. All the patients had ruptured the subscapularis and underlying anterior capsule from the lesser tuberosity. None of the patients had associated Bankart lesions. Repair of the tendon and capsule to the tuberosity was sufficient to close the defect and repair the cuff. Function and stability were restored to all patients.

Conclusion.—Rupture of the rotator cuff should be considered first in the differential diagnosis when a patient with the first shoulder dislocation after age 40 years is unable to elevate the arm after reduction.

▶ This paper carries a clear message that one should consistently consider the possibility of rotator cuff tearing in older patients with shoulder dislocations—or in older patients with shoulder dislocations who have recurrent instability. The results reported are surprisingly good. It has been this reviewer's experience that, on many occasions, the tearing is massive and, even in spite of direct tendon-to-bone repair, recovery of active movement and strength is not assured. As with Abstract 129-94-2–30, this article also offers physicians and patients hope that treatment based on sound orthopedic principles can be effective.—R.H. Cofield, M.D.

Prosthetic Replacement of the Shoulder for the Treatment of Defects in the Rotator Cuff and the Surface of the Glenohumeral Joint

Arntz CT, Jackins S, Matsen FA III (Renton, Wash; Univ of Washington, Seattle)

J Bone Joint Surg (Am) 75-A:485–490, 1993   129-94-2–32

Introduction.—The patient with an irreparable defect of the rotator cuff, together with destruction of the surfaces of the glenohumeral joint, presents a challenge to the orthopedic surgeon. Reconstruction of the glenohumeral joint using the humeral component of the Neer-II prosthesis was described for 19 such patients.

Patients and Methods.—All 19 patients (21 shoulders) had disabling pain but nearly normal or normal function of the deltoid and good passive motion of the shoulder. None had responded to nonsurgical treatment. In all patients, the tissue of the cuff in the shoulder was of such poor quality that not even mobilization or transfer techniques could repair the tear. Eighteen shoulders in 16 patients were available for follow-up for periods ranging from 25 to 122 months. After reconstruction with the humeral prosthesis, the shoulders were moved with assisted exercises within the first few days postoperatively. Patients were hospitalized until they could independently initiate, and complete with assistance, 140 degrees of forward flexion and 40 degrees of external rotation.

Results.—At operation, each shoulder was found to have a massive deficiency of the rotator cuff and destruction of most of the articular humeral cartilage. Fourteen patients had experienced marked or disabling pain before surgery. Postoperatively, 3 shoulders were pain-free, 8 had slight pain, and 4 had pain only after unusual activities. Active forward elevation improved from an average of 66 degrees to an average of 109 degrees. Three patients underwent revision procedures because of persistent, substantial pain. No patient had infection or prosthetic loosening.

Conclusion.—Patients with irreparable tears of the rotator cuff and a loss of the articular surface of the glenohumeral joint, but with excellent function of the deltoid, can be treated successfully by reconstruction with a humeral prosthesis. Pain was reduced or eliminated and function improved in most of these patients. A sufficiently small prosthesis should be selected in order to avoid excessive tightness of the posterior aspect of the capsule.

▶ This is a very difficult patient group. The results as reported are believable. Approximately 8 of 10 patients will have a satisfactory reduction in pain and moderate movement will be maintained or regained. Interestingly, in this patient group, only 1 shoulder of 18 was noted to have postoperative instability. No doubt the authors are very skilled in patient selection and treatment, but probably they were also quite fortunate in this patient sample because, other than obtaining a poor result (insufficient pain relief or failure to regain active movement), the most common problem encountered in this patient group should be recurrent subluxation, or perhaps even dislocation. More than a few patients will be prone to this, and one of the factors in patient selection would be whether enough scar has formed surrounding the joint to confer some stability to the arthroplasty. If a patient has overt instability before surgery, it is unlikely that placing a prosthesis will resolve the problem.—R.H. Cofield, M.D.

Shoulder Arthritis

The Shoulder in Sickle-Cell Disease

David HG, Bridgman SA, Davies SC, Hine AL, Emery RJH (Cardiff Royal Infirmary, Wales; Central Middlesex Hosp, London; St Mary's Hosp, London)
J Bone Joint Surg (Br) 75-B:538–545, 1993   129-94-2–33

Background.—Avascular necrosis (AVN) is a common complication of sickle-cell disease (SCD), which is the most common cause of hip deformity in black children worldwide. Although AVN of the humeral head has been reported, its clinical and functional abnormalities have not been systematically studied. The shoulders of 138 patients with SCD were examined for the presence of AVN.

Patients.—Sixty-four male patients with SCD and 74 female patients with SCD, aged 5–66 years, had their shoulders examined. The examination included a posteroanterior chest radiograph of both shoulders.

Results.—Fifty-three shoulders of 36 patients had a total of 59 AVN lesions on shoulder radiographs. Sixteen patients had bilateral AVN lesions. None of the children younger than 10 years of age had AVN, but 33% of all skeletally mature patients were affected. Half of the patients who averaged 4 or more sickle-cell crises per year had evidence of AVN. Twenty-three of the 36 patients with radiographically proven AVN had impaired function. An additional 42 patients with no radiographic evidence of AVN had abnormal shoulder function. Thus, of 138 patients with SCD, 28.3% had radiographic evidence of AVN and 47% had impaired shoulder function. The incidence of AVN in patients with heterozygous SCD was higher than that in patients with homozygous disease.

Conclusion.—The incidence of AVN of the humeral head in patients with SCD appears to be similar to previously reported rates of femoral head involvement.

▶ The authors clearly describe a high frequency of osteonecrosis of the humeral head in patients with SCD. They mention in the discussion part of the paper that both of the patients who had shoulder replacements had prosthetic loosening. In reviewing the literature on treatment relative to this condition, the authors recognized a high complication rate after treatment, including not only loosening but also infection. It was difficult for the authors to find, as it must be difficult for us to envision, consistently effective treatment methods for this patient group. It is to be hoped that some new information will come to light.—R.H. Cofield, M.D.

Shoulder Arthrodesis

Shoulder Arthrodesis With Plate Fixation: Functional Outcome Analysis
Richards RR, Beaton D, Hudson AR (St Michael's Hosp, Toronto; Univ of Toronto)
J Shoulder Elbow Surg 2:225–239, 1993   129-94-2-34

Introduction.—The experience of a single surgeon using a standardized technique to perform shoulder arthrodesis on 57 consecutive patients between June 1980 and June 1991 was described. The technique used involved both glenohumeral and acromiohumeral arthrodesis with a single 10-hole plate for internal fixation. The position was 30 degrees of abduction, 30 degrees of internal rotation, and 30 degrees of flexion.

Patients.—There were 51 men and 6 women. Of these 57 patients, 46 underwent surgery for brachial plexus injury, 6 for multidirectional shoulder instability, 2 for osteoarthritis, 2 for failed arthroplasties, and 1 for infection. The patients were independently evaluated by a clinician, and function was assessed according to the ability to perform tasks of daily living, subjective satisfaction, and degree of pain.

Results.—Of the 57 shoulders, 54 fused within 10 degrees of the desired position. Secondary bone grafting was required by 3 patients. The complication rate was 14%. Patient satisfaction was highest among those patients undergoing this procedure for brachial plexus injury, osteoarthritis, or failed arthroplasty. The 4 patients with multidirectional shoulder instability continued to complain of instability despite the solid arthrodesis.

Conclusion.—Preoperative diagnosis and workers' compensation status were the major determinants of both perceived benefit and activity of daily living scores after this procedure. Hand function was a major determinant in patients with brachial plexus injury who underwent this procedure. Shoulder arthrodesis is a poor choice for patients with multidirectional instability who have had multiple procedures attempting to stabilize their shoulders. Shoulder arthrodesis is a good therapeutic alternative in carefully selected patients with brachial plexus injuries and good hand function, osteoarthritis, or failed shoulder arthroplasty if the patient has a positive work status.

▶ Shoulder arthrodesis has its advantages and its disadvantages. These authors have introduced us to some nuances in patient selection that are seemingly important determinants of outcome. The material presented has also reinforced that plate fixation for shoulder arthrodesis is quite effective. Seven of the patients (12%) required plate removal because of prominence of the fixation device. Although it is not always possible to do so, it is useful in this setting to advance the deltoid over the plate whenever possible, rendering the plate submuscular rather than subcutaneous.—R.H. Cofield, M.D.

Residual Motion and Function After Glenohumeral or Scapulothoracic Arthrodesis

Harryman DT II, Walker ED, Harris SL, Sidles JA, Jackins SE, Matsen FA III
(Univ of Washington, Seattle)
J Shoulder Elbow Surg 2:275–285, 1993   129-94-2–35

Introduction.—Newly developed spatial kinematic techniques can accurately characterize motion after shoulder fusion and allow this residual movement to be compared with motion of the normal shoulder. This methodology was used in 17 patients who had undergone glenohumeral or scapulothoracic arthrodesis.

Patients and Methods.—Eleven patients (12 shoulders) with a mean age of 46.4 years underwent glenohumeral arthrodesis. Ten had massive rotator cuff insufficiency and 2 experienced recurrent dislocation. Before fusion, the patients had an average of 2.9 operations on the affected shoulder. They were evaluated at an average of 71 months after fusion. The 6 patients who underwent scapulothoracic arthrodesis had a mean age of 32.9 years. They were evaluated at an average of 32 months after the procedure. Eight men with normal shoulders served as controls. All patients underwent standard clinical range-of-motion tests and were assessed for function in various activities of daily living. A spatial position sensor was used to measure residual motion of the unfused articulation.

Results.—The patients who underwent glenohumeral fusion had a poorer functional outcome overall than those with scapulothoracic fusion (Fig 2–18). However, in both groups, nearly all humerothoracic motions were significantly decreased. Although patients with a glenohumeral fusion maintained their scapulothoracic motion at levels comparable to controls, they were limited in their ability to perform activities requiring extremes of internal rotation or elevation. Patients un-

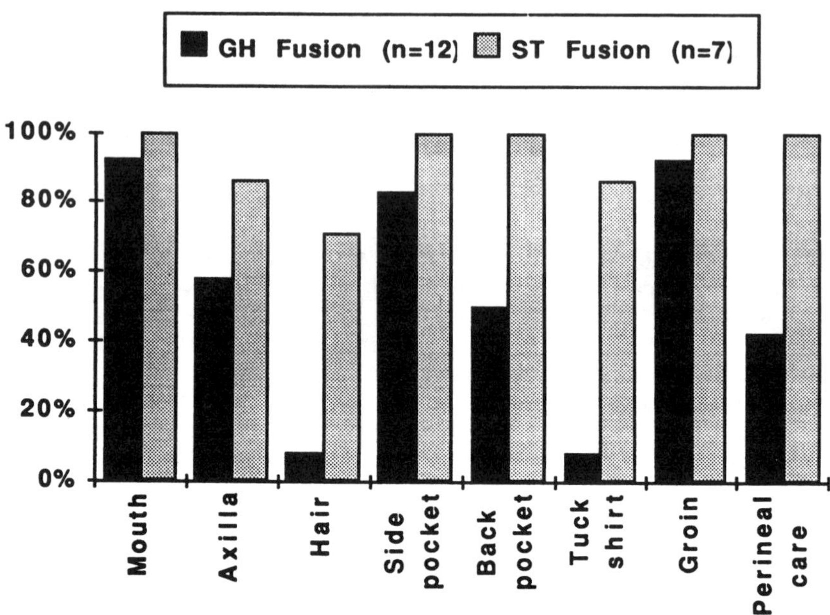

Fig 2–18.—The functional ability of patients with fusions was assessed on the basis of their observed ability to perform 8 personal care activities. Shown is the percentage of extremities that could perform each personal hygiene activity after glenohumeral *(GH)* or scapulothoracic *(ST)* fusion. (Courtesy of Harryman DT II, Walker ED, Harris SL, et al: *J Shoulder Elbow Surg* 2:275–285, 1993.)

dergoing scapulothoracic fusion had relatively good function in the areas of personal care requiring internal rotation. Most patients in both groups reported satisfaction with the outcome of arthrodesis and were relatively free of pain.

Conclusion.—Three-dimensional in vivo measurement of motion allows the functional results of these shoulder procedures to be quantitated. Residual motion was similar to normal motion at the corresponding articulations except for increased scapulothoracic internal rotation after glenohumeral fusion and decreased glenohumeral external rotation and extension after scapulothoracic fusion. Reaching toward the back and above shoulder level are problems after both procedures.

▶ Applied technology again proves very helpful. For decades, people have questioned the functional abilities of individuals after glenohumeral or scapulothoracic fusion. That, of course, is clearly outlined in this study. The scientific method serves us well. Another question has been answered and another issue put to rest.—R.H. Cofield, M.D.

Elbow

Radial Head Fracture Treated by Resection: Long-Term Results
Postacchini F, Morace GB (Cattedra di Chirurgia della Mano, Modena, Italy;

Università "La Sapienza," Rome)
Ital J Orthop Traumatol 18:323–330, 1992   129-94-2-36

Introduction.—The optimal choice of treatment for comminuted or displaced fractures of the radial head remains uncertain. Resection, the most commonly used surgical procedure, may lead to valgus deformity of the elbow and proximal migration of the radius. The long-term outcome in patients who underwent resection of the radial head was evaluated.

Patients and Methods.—Thirty-one patients were evaluated at an average of 17.2 years after surgery. Their average age at the time of injury was 34 years. Based on the presence of other lesions in the same arm and the type of surgical procedure, the patients were divided into 3 groups. The 18 patients in group 1 had isolated radial head fracture and underwent complete resection. Group 2 was made up of 3 patients with marginal fractures of the radial head who were treated by removal of the displaced fragment alone. The 10 patients in group 3 had other lesions and underwent complete resection of the upper end of the radius. Results were rated as excellent, good, fair, or poor using a scoring formula based on pain, muscle force, range of flexion-extension, and range of pronation-supination. Radiographs of the elbow and wrist were made in all patients.

Results.—Results were excellent or good in 72% of group 1 patients. Elbow motion was severely impaired in 1 patient and moderately or slightly impaired in 5. All 3 patients in group 2 had unsatisfactory outcome, with severe or moderate impairment of elbow motion. Results were satisfactory in 60% of group 3 patients. Loss of motion occurred in 4 patients and decrease in muscle force occurred in 3 patients; pain was reported by 3 patients. Of the entire 31 patients, 80% had clinically asymptomatic distal subluxation of the radioulnar joint, and 55% had an increase in the valgus angulation of the elbow. A new radial head had formed in 14 patients, all of whom had normal range of motion.

Conclusion.—Loss of elbow motion was the most common cause of unsatisfactory outcome after resection of radial head fracture. Complete resection in patients with isolated fractures generally yielded satisfactory long-term results. Partial resection and the presence of other osteoarticular lesions in the same arm were associated with poor outcome. The degree of displacement of the fragment should guide the choice of treatment.

▶ These authors have reinforced what many have believed to be true, namely, if there is a simple radial head fracture that cannot be reconstructed, removal is a satisfactory treatment option. If a segment of the radial head is fractured and it is removed, treatment outcome may not be satisfactory. However, perhaps most importantly, if the radial head fracture is associated with other regional injuries, the outcome might well be in question and all efforts should be made to maintain the radial head, if possible.—R.H. Cofield, M.D.

Primary Replacement of the Fractured Radial Head With a Metal Prosthesis
Knight DJ, Rymaszewski LA, Amis AA, Miller JH (Glasgow Royal Infirmary, Scotland; Imperial College of Science, Technology and Medicine, London)
J Bone Joint Surg (Br) 75-B:572–576, 1993   129-94-2–37

Background.—There is no agreement on the best treatment for an unstable elbow injury associated with comminuted radial head fracture. Studies have shown that the functional outcome after radial head replacement with a silicone rubber prosthesis is not better than that after simple head excision. Because silicone rubber is relatively soft and easily compressed under physiologic forces, a Vitallium radial head prosthesis was tested.

Methods.—Using 100 radiographs of normal elbows, Vitallium radial head prostheses were designed with 3 different diameters and 2 thicknesses for each diameter. When tests in cadaveric specimens showed that the metallic implants restored normal elbow mechanics whereas silicone rubber implants did not, the Vitallium implant was tested in the clinical setting.

Patients.—Vitallium radial head prostheses were implanted in 36 patients with comminuted radial head fractures. After a mean follow-up of 4.5 years, 31 patients who then ranged in age from 21 to 83 years were available for evaluation. Ten patients had isolated fractures and 21 had associated dislocations or ulnar fractures.

Outcome.—Of 31 evaluated patients, 24 had little or no elbow pain, 6 had some pain but only with activity, and 1 had pain at rest. None of the patients had infection, prosthetic fracture, or dislocation. Two patients had mild ulnar nerve paresthesia. The implants had been removed in 2 patients because of painful loosening. Anteroposterior and lateral follow-up radiographs showed radiolucent lines around 7 implants, but these did not appear to be progressive. Capitellar erosion or osteoporosis could not be reliably evaluated on these radiographs.

Conclusion.—The Vitallium radial head implant is recommended for use as a spacer to aid elbow stability while the soft tissues heal. Routine replacement in uncomplicated radial head fractures is not advocated.

▶ These authors offer one seemingly reasonable treatment choice for radial head fractures that occur with other injuries in the same area. Interestingly, prostheses were not cemented in place, and very few problems with loosening arose. I suspect that many surgeons in North America would consider the adjunctive use of bone cement if this prosthesis were selected. It is difficult to know how that might influence outcome.—R.H. Cofield, M.D.

An Anatomic Investigation of the Elbow Joint, With Special Reference to Aging of the Articular Cartilage

Murata H, Ikuta Y, Murakami T (Hiroshima Univ, Japan)
J Shoulder Elbow Surg 2:175–181, 1993   129-94-2-38

Objective.—Although osteoarthritic degeneration is common in the radiohumeral joint cartilage, there have been no qualitative and quantitative analyses of the cartilage degeneration occurring in the elbow. Cadaveric findings of the shape of the articular surface of the elbow joint and the location of cartilage degeneration were detailed.

Methods.—A total of 131 elbow joints of 66 cadavers preserved by arterial embalming were examined. The average age at death was 79 years. All specimens were observed macroscopically and classified by degree of degeneration.

Findings.—The radiohumeral joint always had more and greater degenerative changes than the humeroulnar joint (Fig 2–19). In the radiohumeral joint, destruction of the radial head and the crest was more severe than that of the capitulum. The erosion angle, or center of the chondral defect, in the capitulum was located about 45 degrees anterior to the long axis of the humerus. Similarly, the anterior part of the erosion in the crest separating the trochlea from the capitulum was about 48.5 degrees to the long axis of the humerus. Four types of radial head changes were noted, based on the degree and area of cartilage degeneration. No degeneration was found in 18% of joints (type 1); mild degeneration, such as hypertrophy of the ulnar edge of the radial head or a roughened cartilage surface, was found in 28% (type 2); cartilage defects limited to the ulnar side of the radial head were found in 28% (type 3); and cartilage degeneration affecting more than half of the central region of the radial head was found in 25% (type 4).

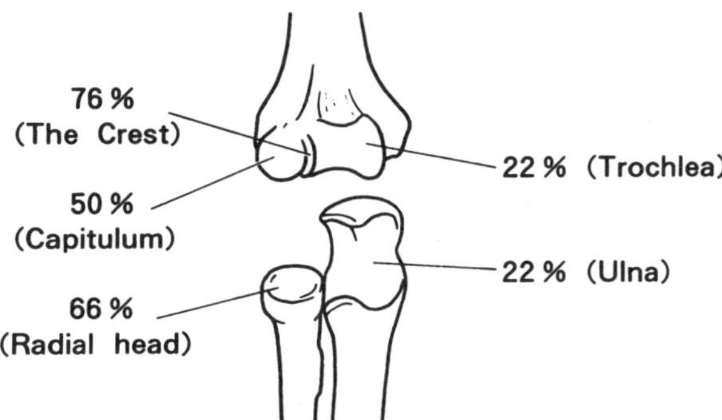

Fig 2–19.—Incidence of degeneration of the elbow joint (50 joints). Degeneration in the radiohumeral joint was always more advanced than in the humeroulnar joint. Furthermore, severe degenerative changes occurred in the radiohumeral joint rather than in the humeroulnar joint. (Courtesy of Murata H, Ikuta Y, Murakami T: *J Shoulder Elbow Surg* 2:175–181, 1993.)

Conclusion.—Autopsy findings suggest that the crest, capitulum, and ulnar side of the radial head are the localized sites of age-related degeneration in the elbow joint. Cartilage degeneration of the radial head shows 4 types of progression, correlating well with the pattern of the radiohumeral and elbow joints. In most cases, the extent of elbow joint osteoarthritis can be classified by the extent of radial head degeneration.

▶ This interesting article supplies new information about degeneration of the elbow joint and focuses on the radiohumeral joint as an indicator of the extent of arthritic involvement. I believe that many individuals have not recognized this in the clinical setting. We will do so in the future, as we all tend to see what we look for.—R.H. Cofield, M.D.

Capitellocondylar Total Elbow Replacement in Rheumatoid Arthritis: Long-Term Results
Ewald FC, Simmons ED Jr, Sullivan JA, Thomas WH, Scott RD, Poss R, Thornhill TS, Sledge CB (Harvard Med School, Boston; Buffalo Gen Hosp, NY; Lane Cove, New South Wales, Australia)
J Bone Joint Surg (Am) 75-A:498–507, 1993   129-94-2–39

Introduction.—Total elbow replacement is a means of relieving pain and restoring functional motion in patients with rheumatoid arthritis or other inflammatory arthritic conditions. Other operative procedures often yield disappointing results in such patients. The long-term outcome in 172 patients who underwent 202 capitellocondylar total elbow replacements was studied.

Patients and Methods.—The patient group included 143 women and 29 men; their average age at the time of the operation was 56 years. Thirty patients had a bilateral replacement. Rheumatoid arthritis was the diagnosis in 91% of the patients, juvenile rheumatoid arthritis occurred in 8%, and post-traumatic osteoarthritis was the diagnosis in 1%. The replacement procedures were performed from July 1974 through June 1987. Until 1978, an all-plastic ulnar component was used (56 elbows). In 1978 and 1979, 26 elbows were replaced by a metal-backed ulnar component through a posterior approach. A metal-backed ulnar component with a modified Kocher approach was used for 120 elbows in the final years of the study. The mean duration of follow-up for the total group was 69 months.

Results.—On a 100-point rating scale, patients had an average preoperative score of 26; the average postoperative score increased to 91 points. Improvement was greatest in the categories of pain relief, functional status, and range of motion (in all planes except extension). These improvements, as well as changes in the roentgenographic appearances, did not deteriorate with time. The most recent follow-up x-ray films demonstrated radiolucency adjacent to 8 humeral components and 19 ulnar components. Preoperative and postoperative evaluations showed

supination to have improved from 45 degrees to 64 degrees and pronation to have improved from 56 degrees to 72 degrees. Revision of the
prosthesis was required in 6 cases because of loosening without infection
or dislocation of the prosthesis. There were 15 wound-related problems,
3 cases of deep infection, 6 cases of ulnar nerve palsy, and 7 dislocations.

Conclusion.—Capitellocondylar total elbow replacement should be
performed before there is extensive loss of the capitellum, the trochlea,
or the trochlear notch of the ulna. With proper indications, careful attention to alignment of the prosthesis, and adequate soft tissue reconstruction, elbow replacement in patients with rheumatoid arthritis can
achieve good function and a lasting result.

▶ It will be hard to improve on these results with any alternate design of elbow arthroplasty. In rheumatoid arthritis and in carefully selected patients, it
is hard to imagine that one would consider another category of prosthesis.
Using this design, one is fearful of postoperative elbow instability. The authors have nicely shown that this can be minimized when attention is directed to the details of patient selection, surgical technique, and postoperative care. Mechanical problems with the device are almost nil, and revision
surgery for any reason is uncommon.—R.H. Cofield, M.D.

**Lateral Extensor Release for Tennis Elbow: A Prospective Long-Term
Follow-Up Study**
Verhaar J, Walenkamp G, Kester A, Van Mameren H, Van Der Linden T (Univ
Hosp Maastricht, The Netherlands; Univ of Limburg, Maastricht, The Nether-
lands)
J Bone Joint Surg (Am) 75-A:1034–1043, 1993   129-94-2-40

Objective.—There are many effective operations available for the
treatment of tennis elbow, including the technically relatively simple lateral release of the common extensor origins. A prospective follow-up
study was performed to assess the long-term outcome after lateral extensor release for tennis elbow.

Patients.—Of 63 patients with tennis elbow who underwent a lateral
extensor release, 57 were followed for a mean of 59 months. Indications
for operation included severe pain that interfered with activities of daily
living and occupation despite at least 6 months of conservative therapy.

Results.—Overall results were rated excellent or good in 37% of the
patients at 6 weeks, in 69% of patients at 1 year, and in 89% at 5 years.
Complete satisfaction with the outcome was reported by 66% of the patients at 1 year and by 91% of the patients at 5 years. There were no recurrences. Analysis of the data did not identify any variables significantly
related to either a good or a poor outcome.

Conclusion.—Lateral extensor release for tennis elbow is a relatively simple operation that should be considered the procedure of choice with which all other operations are to be compared.

▶ The early results are those with which we are familiar. The results reported at 5 years, however, are significantly better, and, as the authors imply, perhaps as good as one can get. I would think that, in North America, many surgeons would prefer to excise the abnormal tissue and rerepair the muscle-tendon attachment, if at all possible. However, we must also be fully aware that this might not improve the result at all, or it might lead to recurrent symptomatology.—R.H. Cofield, M.D.

Call Mosby Document Express at **1 (800) 55-MOSBY** to obtain copies of the original source documents of articles featured or referenced in the YEAR BOOK series.

3 Hip Replacement, Osteoporosis, and Related Issues

Introduction

The literature from the past year records long-term results of total hip replacement and further experience with certain aspects of perioperative care. New work on osteonecrosis suggests that the natural history and prognosis may be determined early in the course of disease, depending on the radiographic and MRI characteristics. Basic research on osteolysis and hip arthroplasty give new insights into the pathogenesis and possible prevention of complications associated with this procedure. Further data from around the world concerning the incidence of osteoporosis and the complications associated with decreased bone mass confirm the importance of a systematic approach to this problem as a major public health issue. Finally, in this era of cost containment, an intuitively attractive, short-term approach is proposed (Abstract 129-94-3–45) that raises provocative questions about the appropriate time frame in which the concept of cost containment ultimately must be addressed.

Robert Poss, M.D.

Results of Total Hip Replacement

The Outcome of Charnley Total Hip Arthroplasty With Cement After a Minimum Twenty-Year Follow-Up: The Results of One Surgeon
Schulte KR, Callaghan JJ, Kelley SS, Johnston RC (Univ of Iowa, Iowa City; Univ of North Carolina, Chapel Hill; Des Moines Orthopaedic Surgeons, Iowa)
J Bone Joint Surg (Am) 75-A:961–975, 1993   129-94-3–1

Introduction.—Between July 1970 and April 1972, 1 surgeon performed 330 total hip arthroplasties using a Charnley hip prosthesis in 262 patients. All patients were disabled because of pain in the hip or a fracture of the hip, and 81% used walking aids. All patients were thoroughly evaluated preoperatively to document functional level.

Patients.—At least 20 years after the index operation, the outcome of 322 arthroplasties was known at the last follow-up evaluation; 5 patients

TABLE 1.—Combined Prevalence of Aseptic Loosening

Determinant of Loosening	All Hips* (N = 319)	Hips in Patients Alive at Least 20 Yrs. after Index Op. (N = 94)
Acetabular component		
Revision	18 (6%)	10 (11%)
Radiographic criteria	25 (8%)	12 (13%)
Total	43 (13%)	22 (23%)
Femoral component		
Revision	8 (3%)	3 (3%)
Radiographic criteria	12 (4%)	4 (4%)
Total	20 (6%)	7 (7%)

* At the time of death or of the most recent follow-up. Eight of the original 330 hips were lost to follow-up and 3 were revised for dislocation, leaving a total of 319 hips.

(Courtesy of Schulte KR, Callaghan JJ, Kelley SS, et al: *J Bone Joint Surg (Am)* 75-A:961–975, 1993.)

(8 hips) were lost to follow-up. Eighty-three patients (98 hips) were still living and 174 had died (224 hips). Radiographs were available for 63 patients (76 hips) who were still alive. For patients who were alive at least 20 years postoperatively, the average age at the time of index arthroplasty was 59 years.

Outcome.—Of the 98 hips in 83 patients still alive at least 20 years after the index arthroplasty, 86% caused no pain and 14% had occasional mild pain. More than half (52%) of the patients walked without support, 19% used a cane part-time, and 24% used aids full-time. Furthermore,

TABLE 2.—Most Recent Outcomes (Number of Hips)

Outcome	Hips for Which the Outcome Was Known at Latest Follow-up Visit (N = 322)	Hips in Patients Alive at Least 20 Yrs. after Index Op. (N = 98)
Original prosthesis retained	291 (90%)	83 (85%)
1 revision	20 (6%) (0, 18, 2*)	9 (9%) (0, 9, 0*)
2 revisions	2 (1%) (0, 2, 0*)	2 (2%) (0, 2, 0*)
3 revisions	2 (1%) (0, 2, 0*)	2 (2%) (2, 0, 0*)
Resect. arthroplasty	7 (2%) (6, 0, 1*)	2 (2%) (1, 0, 1*)

* The reasons for the revisions are in parentheses (the number of hips with loosening associated with infection, the number with aseptic loosening, the number with dislocation).

(Courtesy of Schulte KR, Callaghan JJ, Kelley SS, et al: *J Bone Joint Surg (Am)* 75-A:961–975, 1993.)

84% of patients maintained their own home, 6% lived at home with assistance, and only 10% needed someone for full-time care.

For all 322 hips, 32 (10%) had been revised, including 8 (2%) because of loosening with infection, 21 because of aseptic loosening, and 3 because of dislocation. For patients still alive, 15 (15%) hips were revised because of loosening with infection in 3, aseptic loosening in 11, and dislocation in 1. Aseptic loosening of the acetabular component necessitating revision occurred in 6% (18 hips) of all hips and in 10% (10 hips) of the patients who were still alive. The rate of revision because of aseptic loosening of the femoral component was 2% for all hips and 3% for the living patients. For the acetabular component, the combined prevalence of definite or probable radiographic loosening and aseptic loosening confirmed at revision was 13% for all hips and 23% for patients who survived at least 20 years, whereas 6% of all femoral components and 7% of those in living patients had loosened (Table 1). In addition, 90% of the 322 implants and 85% of the 98 implants in patients who were still alive at least 20 years after the index operation were still in place, and only 2 patients needed a third revision because of aseptic loosening (Table 2). Only patients with an infection of the hip had a resection arthroplasty as the most recent outcome.

Summary.—The Charnley total hip prosthesis has performed well over the long term. The rate of aseptic loosening of the acetabular component is 3 times greater for patients who survived at least 20 years after the index arthroplasty and 2 times greater for all hips for which the outcome is known. Loosening because of infection remains a major problem, accounting for all of the third revisions and for all but 1 of the resection arthroplasties.

▶ This valuable 20-year follow-up of Charnley total hip arthroplasties performed by a single experienced hip surgeon provides the gold standard by which other long-term results must be measured. It is of interest that in this carefully followed study, only 83 of the original 362 patients who had undergone the operation 20 years earlier were still alive. Only 7% of the arthroplasties performed in the original cohort had been revised because of aseptic loosening. Eleven percent of the living patients had required revision because of aseptic loosening. Importantly, at this long-term follow-up, revision because of acetabular loosening was 3 times that of the revision rate for femoral loosening (6% vs. 2%). Ninety percent of patients with the original 322 hips had retained the original implant until the patient died or until the most recent follow-up.—R. Poss, M.D.

Fracture and Loosening of Charnley Femoral Stems: Comparison Between First-Generation and Subsequent Designs

Dall DM, Learmonth ID, Solomon MI, Miles AW, Davenport JM (Hosp of the Good Samaritan, Los Angeles; Princess Alice Orthopaedic Hosp, Cape Town, South Africa)

J Bone Joint Surg (Br) 75-B:259–265, 1993 129-94-3–2

Background.—Early experience with fractures of the Charnley low-friction femoral prosthesis prompted design changes intended to strengthen the component and avoid fatigue fracture. This was achieved mainly by increasing its cross-sectional area. Later stems consequently were stiffer than those used initially. Stem fractures have virtually ceased, but the rate of loosening may have increased at the same time despite improved cementing methods.

Objective.—The results obtained with 264 first-generation Charnley stems, which were followed up for 3–17 years, were compared with those obtained by using 401 second- and later-generation stems. The earlier implants were followed up for a mean of 8.8 years, and the later implants were followed up for a mean of 7.8 years.

Observations.—The likelihood of survival without stem fracture at 10 years was 94.6% for first-generation hips and 99.6% for second-generation hips, a significant difference. The respective results for stem loosening at 10 years were 99.3% and 86.8%. When both complications were considered, the first-generation stems survived significantly better at 10 years than did the second-generation components. Endosteal cavitation was more frequent in first-generation hips, but resorption of the shaft or cortical thinning was slightly more frequent in second-generation hips.

Conclusion.—The increased risk of loosening in later-generation Charnley stems is ascribed to their larger cross-sectional area, which has the effect of increasing flexural stiffness.

▶ Surprisingly, subsequent designs of the Charnley stem produced inferior results when compared with the first-generation design. Whereas the incidence of stem fracture was markedly reduced in later-generation stems, stem loosening increased threefold with second-generation stems. The authors attribute the increased loosening rate in the more contemporary design to a larger cross-sectional area, which produced an increase in flexural stiffness. The authors correctly point out, however, that there are other factors that might influence these results. The subsequent designs had a slightly decreased offset, thus producing an increased joint reactive force. Most intriguing, however, is that the subsequent designs had a matted surface finish compared with the polished finish of the original Charnley stem. Ling and associates reported increased and earlier loosening rates in the Exeter prosthesis when a matted finish was introduced (1).—R. Poss, M.D.

Reference

1.   Fowler JL, et al: *Orthop Clin North Am* 19:477, 1988.

Cemented Total Hip Arthroplasty in Patients Younger Than 50 Years of Age: Ten- to 18-Year Results

Boeree NR, Bannister GC (Winford Orthopaedic Hosp, Bristol, England)
Clin Orthop 287:153–159, 1993   129-94-3-3

Introduction.—Earlier research suggested that total hip arthroplasty (THA) carries an unacceptably high failure rate in young patients, but more recent reports have indicated more favorable results.

Patients and Methods.—The results of cemented THA in 34 patients younger than 50 years of age who survived the procedure in 1973–1979 were reviewed. A total of 49 hips were operated on, 29 with a Charnley prosthesis and 17 with a Howse implant. The average patient age at operation was 38 years, and the average postoperative follow-up was 12 years. The method of grading the roentgenographic appearances is illustrated in Figure 3–1.

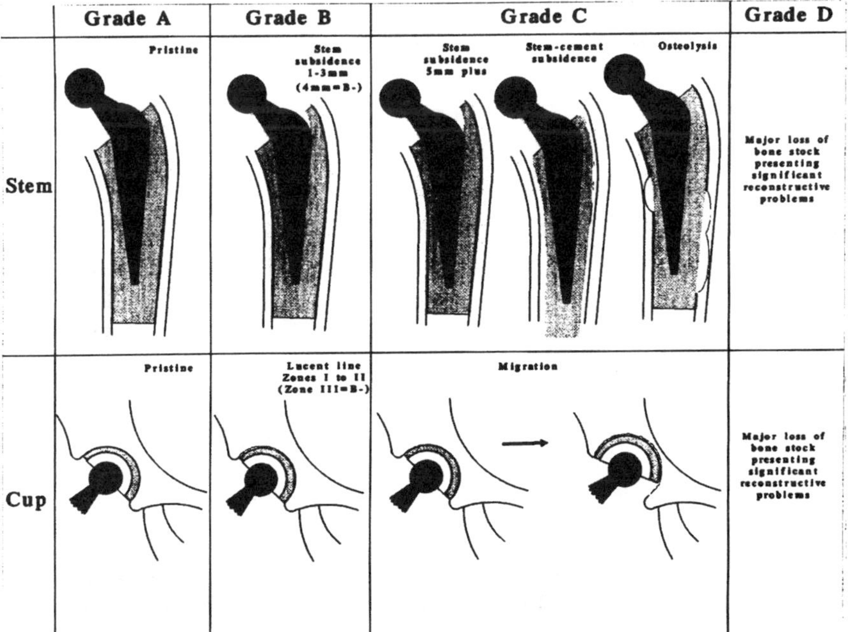

Fig 3–1.—Schematic representation of the grading of roentgenographic appearances according to prognostic significance. (Courtesy of Boeree NR, Bannister GC: *Clin Orthop* 287:153–159, 1993.)

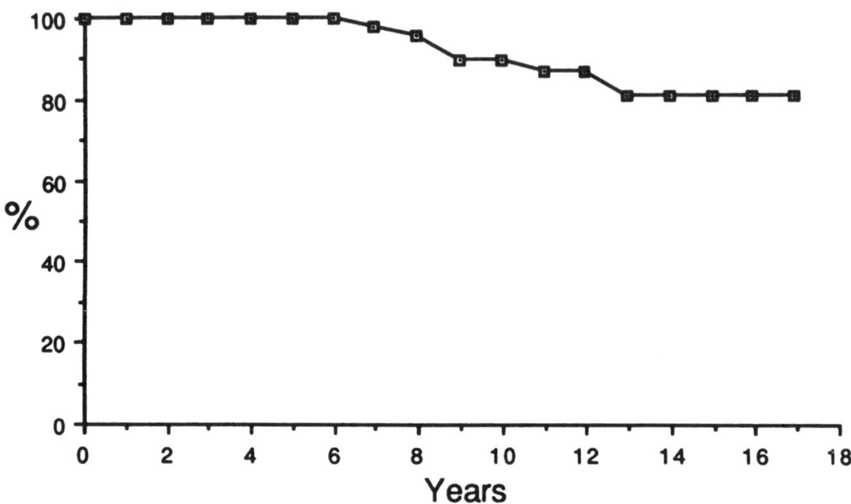

Fig 3–2.—Survivorship curve derived from actuarial table. Survivorship analysis predicts a revision rate of 2% at 7 years, 10% at 10 years, and 12.7% at 12 years. (Courtesy of Boeree NR, Bannister GC: *Clin Orthop* 287:153–159, 1993.)

Results.—Twenty-eight patients had a surviving primary THA at final follow-up; their mean Harris hip score was 93 points. Survival declined gradually with time (Fig 3–2); the average annual risk of failure throughout the follow-up was 1.1%. Seven hips (15%) required revision an aver-

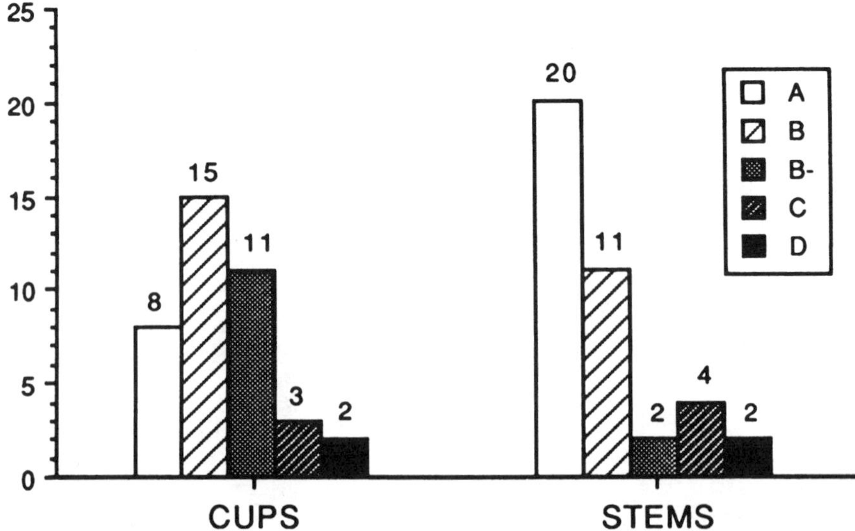

Fig 3–3.—The numbers of femoral and acetabular components in each prognostic grade as determined from the roentgenographic appearances. (Courtesy of Boeree NR, Bannister GC: *Clin Orthop* 287:153–159, 1993.)

age of 9 years after primary surgery, and 3 other hips were scheduled for revision. No failures resulted from sepsis. Hip scores 3 years after revision were as good as for primary arthroplasties. Roentgenographic assessment gave no evidence of failure in 85% of stems and 87% of cups (Fig 3–3).

Conclusion.—Patients younger than 50 years of age appear to benefit from cemented THA as much as those who are older. However, they must be advised not to perform heavy manual work. Regular radiographic review will detect failure before there is significant loss of bone stock.

Long-Term Results of Charnley Low-Friction Arthroplasty in Young Patients

Joshi AB, Porter ML, Trail IA, Hunt LP, Murphy JCM, Hardinge K (Wrightington Hosp, Wigan, England; Royal Preston Hosp, Lancashire, England; Manchester Royal Infirmary, England)
J Bone Joint Surg (Br) 75-B:616–623, 1993   129-94-3–4

Introduction.—The long-term outcome of 218 Charnley low-friction arthroplasties was examined in 141 patients who were aged 40 years or younger at the time of surgery.

Patients.—A total of 103 patients (166 hips) (recall rate, 88%) were followed up for a mean of 16 years (range, 10–24). For the 218 hips operated on, 74 had rheumatoid arthritis, 47 had congenital dysplasia, 41 had ankylosing spondylitis, and 56 had osteoarthritis. Kaplan-Meier survival rates were calculated for all 218 hips.

Results.—At 20 years, the probability of survival of the femoral component was 86% and of the acetabular component was 84%. For both components, the probability of survival was 75%. The diagnosis significantly affected the probability of implant survival: the probability of both components surviving at 20 years was 96% in rheumatoid arthritis, compared with 51% in osteoarthritis. In addition, acetabular components with 2 or more areas of zonal demarcation at 1 year were significantly more likely to loosen than those that did not. For the 103 patients who were followed up for a mean of 16 years, 94% of the implants that had not been revised had little or no pain, 68% had excellent or very good function, and 78% had a full or almost full range of motion. None of the patients had pain at rest or severe pain with limited activity.

Implications.—In young patients, cemented total hip replacement is a good procedure for those with rheumatoid arthritis. However, there is a greater risk of revision for those with osteoarthritis.

▶ These 2 mid-term results (Abstracts 129-94-3–3 and 129-94-3–4) suggest satisfactory longevity for Charnley cemented total hips in younger patients. In the latter study by Joshi et al., patients with rheumatoid arthritis (presumably less active) had a high probability of surviving with both components at 20 years compared with those patients who had a diagnosis of osteoarthritis (presumably more active), whose chance of surviving with both components intact were only 51%.—R. Poss, M.D.

The Porous-Coated Anatomic Total Hip Prosthesis, Inserted Without Cement: Results After Five to Seven Years in a Prospective Study
Heekin RD, Callaghan JJ, Hopkinson WJ, Savory CG, Xenos JS (Walter Reed Army Med Ctr, Washington, DC; Univ of Iowa, Iowa City; Columbus, Ga)
J Bone Joint Surg (Am) 75-A:77–91, 1993   129-94-3–5

Background.—Loosening of first-generation prostheses inserted with cement and cementing methods has prompted attempts to improve prosthetic design, cementing technique, and fixation by biological ingrowth. Long-term follow-up data were reported from a prospective study of arthroplasties performed with a porous-coated anatomical total hip prosthesis.

Methods.—The results of 100 consecutive primary arthroplasties done in 91 patients were analyzed. Patients were followed up for 5–7 years or until their death.

Findings.—The mean sequential hip ratings were maintained between 92 and 93 points during follow-up. After 1 year, 18% of the thighs were painful, although function was not limited. In years 2–5, these rates were 19%, 23%, 26%, and 15%, respectively. Radiography showed that the fixation of the femoral component was by ingrowth of bone in 94% of the hips, by stable fibrous fixation in 1%, and by unstable fibrous fixation in 5%. Six percent of the acetabular components had migrated by 5 years, and 5% of the femoral components had subsided. Two acetabular components were revised within the first 5 years. One revision of a femoral component was pending.

Conclusion.—Two to 7 years after surgery more than 90% of the hips in this series had good or excellent clinical ratings. Seventy-four percent of the 27 hips followed up for 7 years had an excellent rating. Further assessment is needed to establish the long-term durability of the prosthesis-bone interface.

▶ These patients have been followed prospectively and have been the subject of serial reports concerning their progress. In the current update at 5–7 years, radiographic analysis finds that 6% of the acetabular components have migrated and 5% of the femoral components have subsided. Two acetabular components have been revised and one revision of a femoral component is anticipated. Of the 91 original patients, 82 still survive. Continuing follow-up of these surviving patients will provide important information on the outcome of this first-generation cementless prosthesis.—R. Poss, M.D.

Primary Total Hip Reconstruction With a Titanium Fiber-Coated Prosthesis Inserted Without Cement

Martell JM, Pierson RH III, Jacobs JJ, Rosenberg AG, Maley M, Galante JO (Univ of Chicago; Rush-Presbyterian-St Luke's Med Ctr, Chicago)
J Bone Joint Surg (Am) 75-A:554–570, 1993   129-94-3–6

Objective.—The intermediate-term results of primary total hip reconstruction were examined in a prospective series of 110 patients who received a total of 121 cementless Harris-Galante porous titanium fiber-coated prostheses.

Patients.—The average patient age at the time of surgery was 49 years. The primary diagnosis was osteoarthrosis in 58% of the operated hips and avascular necrosis in 30%. Only 5% of the hips had a diagnosis of rheumatoid arthritis. The average postoperative follow-up was about 5½ years.

Results.—The average Harris hip score increased from 55 points preoperatively to 93 points at the most recent follow-up. Excellent results, as reflected by hip scores of 90–100 points, were achieved in 75% of the operated hips, and good results (80–89 points) were achieved in another 12%. Seven percent of the hips had a poor outcome. One patient had the acetabular component revised because of recurrent dislocation. Eleven femoral implants were unstable, and 4 of them have been revised. Nine patients whose implants were stable had cortical erosion about the distal part of the femoral stem. One of them underwent revision because of extensive erosion. Implant survival was 97% at 5 years. Heterotopic ossification developed in 70% of the hips, but no patient had the most marked degree of ossification.

Conclusion.—Clinical success is likely when a cementless Harris-Galante femoral prosthesis fits well. Bony ingrowth does occur after this procedure.

▶ The Harris-Galante porous titanium fiber-coated femoral prosthesis was inserted in 110 patients, and the results were reported at an average follow-up of 67 months. At this early follow-up, 11 femoral implants were unstable and 4 had been revised. Distal osteolysis was present in 9 patients (8%) who had stable implants. The authors had postulated elsewhere that an important barrier to the migration of particulate debris is a circumferential coating of ingrowth material. In this design, the fiber metal pads do not circumferentially provide such a barrier.—R. Poss, M.D.

Hybrid Total Hip Replacement: A 6.5-Year Follow-Up Study

Schmalzried TP, Harris WH (Harbor-Univ of California Los Angeles Med Ctr; Massachusetts Gen Hosp, Boston)
J Bone Joint Surg (Br) 75-B:608–615, 1993   129-94-3–7

Background.—The hybrid total hip replacement, consisting of a cemented femoral component and a cementless acetabular component, has given excellent results at 2-year follow-up. Clinical and radiographic results were examined at a minimum follow-up of 5 years in 97 consecutive primary hip replacements.

Methods.—In the first half of the study, most patients received an HD-2 cobalt-chrome implant with a medial collar as the cemented femoral component and a hemispherical, cobalt-chrome acetabular reconstruction component. In the latter part of the experience, most patients received a Precoat femoral stem and a Harris-Galante porous hemispherical, titanium acetabular component. Most femoral heads were 26 mm in diameter. The patients (average age, 61 years) were followed for a mean of $6\frac{1}{2}$ years.

Results.—At final follow-up, the average Harris hip score was 93, which was slightly better for patients in the latter part of the experience. Ninety-one percent of the hips had excellent results, and 88% had no pain or only slight pain. Only 1 patient with a radiographically loose femoral component complained of thigh pain. Three hips required surgical revision, but only 1 as the result of component loosening. Good collar-medial neck contact was maintained in 88% of the patients. Some loss of calcar bone was common, but new lucencies at the femoral cement-bone interface were rare. There were only 2 cases of femoral osteolysis.

Conclusion.—There were good long-term results with the hybrid total hip replacement. The use of second-generation cementing techniques has improved long-term femoral fixation, and the third-generation techniques have improved fixation even more. The authors have not had to revise any cementless acetabular components for loosening.

▶ At an average follow-up of $6\frac{1}{2}$ years, hybrid total hip replacement (cemented femoral component; uncemented acetabular component) has provided excellent results. In these 97 consecutive primary total hip replacements, one stem has been revised for loosening and no acetabular components have been revised.—R. Poss, M.D.

Revision of the Acetabular Component Without Cement After Total Hip Arthroplasty: Three to Six-Year Follow-Up

Padgett DE, Kull L, Rosenberg A, Sumner DR, Galante JO (Naval Hosp, San Diego, Calif; Rush-Presbyterian-St Luke's Med Ctr, Chicago)
J Bone Joint Surg (Am) 75-A:663–673, 1993   129-94-3–8

Background.—Mechanical loosening of the acetabular component is still a serious problem after total hip arthroplasty. The outcome of surgical revision of the acetabular component has not been consistently good. The results of revising the acetabular component without cement after total hip arthroplasty were reviewed.

Methods.—Between 1983 and 1986 a total of 132 patients underwent 138 acetabular component revisions. The prosthesis used in revision was a hemispherical component coated with porous titanium mesh. It was secured to the pelvis with a variable number of screws. The patients were 75 women and 57 men with a mean age of 52 years at the time of revision surgery. Eighty percent of the hips were treated with bone grafts because of defects in the acetabulum. These grafts were usually a mixture of local autogenous graft and freeze-dried allograft. One hundred twenty-four patients with 129 affected hips were available for follow-up at a mean of 44 months.

Outcomes.—Seven of the hips (5%) were revised again. Four hips were infected, and 3 were unstable. No revisions were done for loosening without infection, and none of the components migrated in the absence of infection. Radiolucent lines were common and usually corresponded to areas involving allograft. All bone grafts united within 12 months. Noncontained medial grafts underwent resorption, consolidation, and remodeling to a sclerotic rim within 24 months. No complications were associated with screw placement.

Conclusion.—These outcomes were superior to the results of revisions of acetabular components with the use of cement, which were associated with failure rates of nearly 10% after a comparable follow-up. The method of maximizing host-bone coverage and packing all defects with cancellous autogenous graft or allograft, or both, was successful for all classes of acetabular defects.

▶ A cementless bone ingrowth hemispherical cup, the maximization of host-bone coverage, and the packing of all defects with cancellous bone autograft or allograft have provided excellent 3- to 6-year results that are superior to those of cemented acetabular revision.—R. Poss, M.D.

High Failure Rate of Bulk Femoral Head Allografts in Total Hip Acetabular Reconstructions at 10 Years

Kwong LM, Jasty M, Harris WH (Massachusetts Gen Hosp, Boston; Harvard Med School, Boston)
J Arthroplasty 8:341–346, 1993   129-94-3-9

Objective.—Short-term results of bulk femoral head allografts in complex acetabular reconstructions for total hip arthroplasty (THA) are excellent, but the long-term performance of these bulk autografts is associated with a high failure rate. To investigate further, a longer follow-up was conducted of bulk femoral head allografts in complex acetabular reconstructions for THA.

Methods.—The radiographic appearance and functional performance of 30 cemented THA acetabular reconstructions in 28 patients were analyzed during a mean follow-up of 10 years (range, 8–13.3 years). Bulk, weight-bearing, femoral head allografts were used to augment severe acetabular bone deficiency. The graft was placed within the acetabulum in 12 hips and against the lateral wing of the ilium in 18. On average, the grafts supported approximately 60% of the acetabular component. Eight were primary THAs, and 22 were revisions of failed cemented THAs. The average patient age at the time of surgery was 51 years.

Outcome.—All grafts united, but failure of acetabular fixation occurred in 47% of the acetabular reconstructions. Four hips had radiographic loosening and the other 10 had a loose acetabular component at reoperation. Loosening occurred in 58% of the sockets with intra-acetabular grafts and in 40% of those bolted to the lateral wing of the ilium. Typically, failure of the reconstruction followed a pattern of graft resorption, graft collapse, and subsequent acetabular component migration on serial radiographs.

Conclusion.—The high 10-year failure rate of bulk femoral head allografts in total hip acetabular reconstructions is in sharp contrast to the high success rates at less than 5 years. Bulk weight-bearing allografts should be limited to use as an extreme salvage procedure in which the only other surgical option is a resection arthroplasty. For reconstructions involving severe acetabular bone deficiency, cementless porous-coated acetabular components are fixed rigidly into the remaining viable host bone using supplemental screws, and nonstructural particulate allografts are used to fill the bony defects.

▶ At a mean follow-up of 10 years, bulk weight-bearing femoral head allografts used to augment severe acetabular bone deficiency failed in 47% of acetabular reconstructions. The failure rate at 10 years is in contrast to the good success rate at 5 years in the same series of patients. The authors, therefore, recommend that alternative methods of acetabular reconstruction be pursued.—R. Poss, M.D.

Perioperative Considerations

Effectiveness of Perioperative Recombinant Human Erythropoietin in Elective Hip Replacement
Laupacis A, for the Canadian Orthopedic Perioperative Erythropoietin Study Group (Ottawa Civic Hosp, Ont, Canada)
Lancet 341:1227–1232, 1993   129-94-3–10

Background.—Because of the risk of viral infection transmission, attempts are made to reduce the transfusion requirements of patients undergoing surgery. Whether recombinant human erythropoietin decreases blood transfusion needs in patients having elective hip arthroplasty was determined.

Methods.—A total of 208 patients were enrolled in the multicenter, double-blind, randomized, placebo-controlled trial. All patients were given daily subcutaneous injections of erythropoietin or placebo beginning 10 days before surgery. Then, 78 patients (group 1) received placebo for 14 days; 77 patients (group 2) were given erythropoietin, 300 units/kg to a maximum of 30,000 units, for 14 days; and 53 patients (group 3) were given placebo on days 10–6 before surgery, with erythropoietin administered for the next 9 days.

Findings.—A primary outcome event, defined as any transfusion or a hemoglobin concentration of less than 80 g/L, occurred in 46% of group 1 patients, 23% of group 2 patients, and 32% of group 3 patients. The mean number of transfusions in groups 1, 2, and 3 were 1.14, .52, and .70, respectively. The respective mean reticulocyte counts the day before the operation were 72, 327, and 170 $\times$ 10⁹/L. Five patients in group 1, 8 in group 2, and 8 in group 3 had deep venous thrombi. Patients with a hemoglobin concentration of less than 135 g/L before randomization benefited most from erythropoietin.

Conclusion.—In these patients undergoing elective hip arthroplasty, erythropoietin given for 14 days perioperatively reduced the need for blood transfusion. This treatment was also well tolerated.

▶ The use of recombinant human erythropoietin in patients undergoing elective orthopedic procedures offers an attractive alternative to autologous blood donation. Reports of its efficacy during the past few years suggest that it may become an increasingly useful blood replacement tool.—R. Poss, M.D.

The Effectiveness of Suction Drainage in Total Hip Arthroplasty
Murphy JP, Scott JE (Westminster Hosp, London)
J R Soc Med 86:388–389, 1993   129-94-3–11

TABLE 1.—Wound Scores

Classification of wound	Drained group	Non-drained group
Satisfactory healing	18	19
Disturbance of healing	1	1
Minor infection	0	0
Moderate infection	1	0
Severe infection	0	0
Mean wound score	4.4	3.6
Total	20	20

Note: No statistically significant difference occurred in scores when analyzed by a Mann-Whitney U test.
(Courtesy of Murphy JP, Scott JE: *J R Soc Med* 86:388–389, 1993.)

TABLE 2.—Blood Loss

Group	TBL (ml)	Perop (ml)	RV* (ml)	RD* (ml)
Drained	1455	420	397	640
Non-drained	1134	530	—	600

*Abbreviations: TBL, total blood loss; Perop, peroperative; RV, redivac: RD, residual.
Note: Total blood loss was statistically significant at .05 level; Peroperative was statistically not significant; residual was not statistically significant at .05 level.
(Courtesy of Murphy JP, Scott JE: J R Soc Med 86:388–389, 1993.)

Introduction.—Most orthopedic surgeons use suction drainage of total hip arthroplasty wounds, with the goal of reducing the size of the wound hematoma and thus the wound infection rate. However, recent retrospective and small prospective studies have demonstrated no benefit associated with suction drainage.

Methods.—This prospective, randomized trial assessed the efficacy of suction drainage in 40 patients undergoing elective total hip arthroplasty. The patients received either 2 redivac drains or no drainage at the end of their surgical procedure. Total blood loss was estimated, and wounds were scored clinically according to the ASEPSIS scoring system on postoperative days 2, 4, 5, 7, and 10.

Results.—One case of wound infection occurred in the drainage group (Table 1). Total blood loss was 321 mL greater in the drainage group, which was a significant difference. Residual blood loss into the thigh was only 40 mL higher in the drainage group (Table 2).

Conclusion.—Suction drainage in patients undergoing total hip arthroplasty increases blood loss with no reduction in wound hematoma size. As such, the practice is unlikely to achieve any reductions in wound infection rates.

▶ In this prospective and randomized trial, suction drainage increased blood loss without reducing wound hematoma size in patients undergoing total hip arthroplasty. These findings agree with recent publications that question the role of routine suction drainage after total hip arthroplasty.—R. Poss, M.D.

Influence of Age on Measurement of Health Status in Patients Undergoing Elective Surgery

Mangione CM, Marcantonio ER, Goldman L, Cook EF, Donaldson MC, Sugar-

baker DJ, Poss R, Lee TH (Harvard Med School, Boston)
J Am Geriatr Soc 41:377–383, 1993   129-94-3–12

Objective.—In an era of increasing emphasis on global measures of health status, there is continuing uncertainty regarding the best such methods, both in general and specific populations. Health status evaluation is particularly important in elderly individuals. Although there are a number of specific evaluations of functional status of elderly individuals, this is only 1 dimension of the patient's perception of quality of life. This cross-sectional cohort study sought to determine the effect of age on the relationship between global health measures and specific health dimensions in elderly individuals.

Methods.—The analysis was based on 745 patients older than age 50 years who were admitted for major elective noncardiac surgery. Of these, 469 were 70 years of age or younger and 276 were older than age 70 years. Preoperative evaluation included a medical history, physical examination, and health status assessments. Measures of global health status were the Medical Outcomes Study Short Form (SF-36) and a verbal measure of global health on a scale of 0–100. The SF-36 was also used to measure specific dimensions of health, including physical, role, and social function; mental health; energy and fatigue; and pain. The patients also completed the Specific Activity Scale, another validated measure of physical functioning.

Findings.—The older patients had lower scores for role function, energy fatigue, and physical function on both the SF-36 and Specific Activity Scale. However, the younger and older patients had a similar perception of their overall health. For the overall cohort, global health status on the SF-36 health perception scale showed the best correlation with the energy and fatigue scale and lesser correlations with the mental health, social function, physical function, and pain scales, in that order. The older patients had a significantly lower correlation of global health perception with pain and with role functioning than the younger patients did.

Conclusion.—Elderly patients and younger adults report similar perceptions of their global health, despite differences in role function, energy and fatigue, and physical function. Thus, global health perception may be related to different factors in the elderly or elderly individuals may have a fundamentally different notion of what global health status they may expect to have. Multidimensional assessment is a key part of the quality-of-life assessment. Particularly in elderly individuals, global measures themselves may not consider key, dimension-specific health impairments.

▶ With the increasing use of global health assessment instruments in outcome studies, this paper points to the differences between younger and older patients' perceptions of global health. The evaluation of quality of life in patients of different ages may require more sensitive multidimensional scales.—R. Poss, M.D.

Routine Use of Adjusted Low-Dose Warfarin to Prevent Venous Thromboembolism After Total Hip Replacement
Paiement GD, Wessinger SJ, Hughes R, Harris WH (San Francisco Gen Hosp; Harvard Med School, Boston)
J Bone Joint Surg (Am) 75-A:893–898, 1993   129-94-3–13

Background.—Earlier studies suggest that prophylactic low-dose warfarin for 12 weeks after total hip replacement, without routine phlebography or sonography, may be safe, effective, and less expensive. The results of a prospective study on the efficacy and safety of routine use of adjusted low-dose warfarin, without sonography or venography, for the prophylaxis of deep-vein thrombosis after total hip replacement were examined.

Treatment.—Between 1986 and 1989, 268 patients aged 40–85 years were given warfarin orally both before and after total hip replacement. The initial dose was usually 10 mg on the night before and 5 mg on the night after the operation. Thereafter, the dose was adjusted to keep the prothrombin time between 1.25 and 1.5 times the control time (10–12 seconds). The partial thromboplastin time was used as an additional determinant of the daily dose of warfarin: if the partial thromboplastin time exceeded 50 seconds, patients were given fresh-frozen plasma and the dose of warfarin was reduced. All patients continued to take low-dose warfarin for 12 weeks after the operation. All patients were followed 6 months after the operation.

Outcome.—None of the patients had phlebography or sonography routinely. None of the patients had fatal pulmonary emboli while hospitalized or after discharge from the hospital. Two patients had nonfatal pulmonary emboli, both during hospitalization. Ten (4%) patients had a major bleeding complication, including 9 wound hematomas and 1 gastrointestinal bleeding, all during hospitalization. There were no major bleeding complications after discharge from the hospital, although 16 patients had minor bleeding episodes that did not require treatment.

Conclusion.—Adjusted low-dose warfarin for 12 weeks is effective in the prevention of fatal pulmonary embolism after total hip replacement. Patients should be constantly monitored using prothrombin and partial thromboplastin times. For all 268 patients, this form of prophylaxis is also cost-effective when compared with performing routine bilateral radiographic phlebography. Between $116,000 to $176,000 was saved by using low-dose warfarin for 12 weeks after the operation in all 268 patients, even when the costs of treatment of all complications that occurred during hospitalization and after discharge were taken into account.

▶ Considerable savings can be realized if preventive measures against thromboembolism include a low-cost medication that can be monitored fairly inexpensively without the requirement of expensive surveillance techniques such as venography or duplex sonography. In this study, warfarin prophylaxis was monitored by prothrombin times, and neither venography nor sonography was done routinely. There were no fatal pulmonary emboli; 2 nonfatal pulmonary emboli were identified during hospitalization. Four percent of the patients had an episode of major bleeding. No major bleeding episode occurred after discharge from the hospital. Warfarin prophylaxis, when carefully monitored and continued for an appropriate time after hospital discharge, is believed to be a safe and cost-effective method of prophylaxis.—R. Poss, M.D.

Ischaemic Complications of Graduated Compression Stockings in the Treatment of Deep Venous Thrombosis

Merrett ND, Hanel KC (St George Hosp, Sydney, New South Wales, Australia)
Postgrad Med J 69:232–234, 1993　　　　　　　　　　　　　　129-94-3-14

Background.—Graduated compression stockings have proven effective in preventing deep venous thrombosis (DVT) in the postoperative state, and they also have been used to treat established thrombosis. Their use has been considered to be relatively free of side effects, but recent research suggests that ischemic complications may be more frequent than has been recognized.

Two Cases.—Two patients who wore graduated compression stockings because of DVT experienced ischemic lesions of the lower extremity. The first patient was a man, 77 years of age, who also was anticoagulated for bilateral DVT extending to the pelvic veins. He spent most of the day sitting and continued using the stockings even though they became painful. Gangrenous areas were noted on both feet after 2 weeks, with mottling of the thigh and calf. Ischemic necrosis developed in the right forefoot and several left toes. The patient died of intracerebral hemorrhage in the hospital. The other patient was a man, aged 39, who had a stroke and was noted to have no pedal or popliteal pulses on the right side. A sympathectomy had been done for right-sided claudication 6 years before; DVT developed on the right side. The patient was anticoagulated and fitted with compression stockings, which were removed 3 days later after an ulcer appeared over the lateral malleolus. When dysphasia lessened, the patient described having had marked discomfort at this site but had been unable to communicate it to nursing staff.

Implications.—Compression stockings may pose a much greater risk of ischemia than has been thought. Great care is needed to ensure that a proper-sized stocking is used, especially if leg swelling is a possibility. The stockings should be removed if any tightness or pain develops.

▶ The authors provide an important reminder of a complication that can occur with the use of graduated compression stockings.—R. Poss, M.D.

Antibiotic Prophylaxis With Two Doses of Cephalosporin in Patients Managed With Internal Fixation for a Fracture of the Hip

Bodoky A, Neff U, Heberer M, Harder F (Univ of Basel, Switzerland)
J Bone Joint Surg (Am) 75-A:61–65, 1993   129-94-3–15

Background.—Two-day antibiotic prophylaxis in surgical repair of proximal femoral fracture may promote the growth of resistant bacteria and increase morbidity for elderly patients. Studies using shorter antibiotic courses have provided mixed results. This randomized, double-blind, prospective study evaluated a 2-dose prophylactic cephalosporin regimen in femoral-neck fracture repair surgery.

Methods.—A total of 239 patients with a fracture of the proximal femur underwent open reduction and internal fixation with a dynamic hip screw. At anesthesia induction and 12 hours later, 124 patients received 2 g of cefotiam; 115 received placebo. An uninvolved third party monitored the postoperative course.

Results.—Major wound infections were significantly more prevalent among placebo-treated patients: 6 vs. only 1 in the antibiotic group. Eighteen minor wound infections occurred: 5 in the antibiotic group and 13 with placebo. Twenty-five systemic infections occurred in 22 antibiotic-treated patients; 33 systemic infections occurred in 31 placebo-treated patients. Predictors for major wound infection were duration of postoperative urinary catheterization, duration of operation, and interval between accident and hospital admission. Predictors for minor wound infection and systemic infection were preoperative serum albumin level and absolute lymphocyte count. No complications occurred secondary to prophylactic antibiotic use.

Conclusion.—Patients at risk for postoperative wound and systemic infections can be identified preoperatively. Nevertheless, because short-term antibiotic prophylaxis is effective, low risk, and cost-effective, all patients undergoing internal fixation for a femoral fracture should receive short-term antibiotic prophylaxis.

▶ A number of factors are associated with the incidence of wound infection after internal fixation for a hip fracture. In a prospective and randomized double-blind study, the use of perioperative antibiotics significantly reduced the incidence of wound infection from 5% to 1%. Associated predictors of major wound infections included the duration of surgery, the duration of postoperative urinary catheterization, the level of serum albumin, and the absolute lymphocyte count as indicators of a patient's nutritional status.—R. Poss, M.D.

Effect of Antiseptics, Ultraviolet Light and Lavage on Airborne Bacteria in a Model Wound

Taylor GJS, Leeming JP, Bannister GC (Southmead Hosp, Bristol, England; Bristol Royal Infirmary, England)
J Bone Joint Surg (Br) 75-B:724–730, 1993   129-94-3–16

Background.—Antibiotics, pulsed lavage, and antiseptics are used to prevent primary infection in joint replacement surgery, but they are not effective in all surgical fields. Ultraviolet C (UVC) light is bactericidal and is used to disinfect theater air. However, it has not been used directly to decontaminate a wound or in combination with pressure lavage or antiseptics. The decontamination effect of UVC, hydrogen peroxide, povidone-iodine, and chlorhexidine was assessed.

Methods.—Irradiated ovine muscle, ovine adipose tissue, and agar plates were inoculated with airborne bacteria. The specimens were coated with blood or plasma and subsequently exposed to UVC or mixed with 3% hydrogen peroxide, 1% and 10% povidone-iodine, and .05% chlorhexidine. Ten inoculated muscle specimens were treated with pulsed jet lavage and UVC, or with syringe and needle lavage with chlorhexidine .05%.

Results.—Ultraviolet C inhibited airborne organism growth on agar; it was less effective on muscle and in the presence of blood. The antiseptics were effective on agar; adding blood or plasma neutralized hydrogen peroxide and povidone-iodine 1%. Antiseptic activity was reduced on tissue samples, but the antiseptics were more effective on adipose tissue than on muscle. Addition of blood or plasma to muscle specimens before disinfection reduced the effectiveness of all antiseptics except chlorhexidine. Ultraviolet C had an additive effect with pulsed jet lavage, significantly reducing colony count. Lavage with chlorhexidine .05% by syringe and needle eliminated colonies on both muscle and adipose tissue. One-minute jet lavage eliminated colonies by 99.8%.

Conclusion.—One-minute jet lavage was the most effective method tested; chlorhexidine was the most effective decontamination agent. The use of chlorhexidine in clean surgical wounds should be investigated; the technique of pressurized chlorhexidine lavage may also be useful in contaminated wounds.

▶ In a laboratory model, agar, muscle, and adipose tissue were contaminated with airborne bacteria and then treated with agents commonly used to sterilize or prep surgical surfaces. Blood or plasma neutralized the cleansing effects of hydrogen peroxide and povidone-iodine 1%. All agents were less effective on tissue specimens when compared with agar, and the most resistive tissue was muscle. Ultraviolet light enhanced the positive effect of pulse jet lavage. In this model, chlorhexidine was the most effective method tested.—R. Poss, M.D.

Functional Recovery of Noncemented Total Hip Arthroplasty
Long WT, Dorr LD, Healy B, Perry J (King–Drew Med Hosp, Los Angeles; Kerlan–Jobe Orthopaedics, Inglewood, Calif; Centinela Hosp, Inglewood, Calif; et al)
Clin Orthop 288:73–77, 1993   129-94-3–17

Background.—In the past 10 years, there have been many technological advances in the design and surface finish of total hip prosthetic components. Clinicians can now choose between cemented fixation and cementless fixation with bone ingrowth. However, little is known about the effect of muscle function and the durability of total hip arthroplasty (THA).

Methods.—Eighteen patients with unilateral hip disease and noncemented THA were examined to investigate the functional recovery in the hip. Clinical follow-up data up to 5 years after surgery were available.

Findings.—Force plate data indicated continued weakness in the affected hip in all patients 2 years after the procedure. Preoperative dynamic electromyograms (EMGs) were abnormal in 8 patients. Two patterns were observed: in 3 patients, stance loss was characterized by absence of activity of the gluteus medius and upper and lower gluteus maximus muscles, whereas 5 patients had continuous activity in the tensor fascia lata, rectus femoris, and adductor longus muscles during the whole gait cycle. All abnormal EMGs normalized after surgery. Four patients with a normal preoperative EMG had abnormal EMG patterns after surgery, with either a prolonged stance or stance loss pattern. All 4 hips were revised.

Conclusion.—Although gait characteristics returned to normal within 2 years in this series, hip weakness persisted, which jeopardizes the implant fixation interface. Thus, patients should avoid activities producing high impact loading of THA. In addition, a prolonged exercise program should be initiated after surgery.

▶ Gait analysis was performed preoperatively and at intervals of 2 years postoperatively on 18 patients who underwent cementless total hip arthroplasty. Gait characteristics returned to normal by 2 years postoperatively, but weakness of the hip persisted. The authors conclude that persisting muscle weakness causes additional high impact loading and recommend that a prolonged muscle strengthening program be used postoperatively.—R. Poss, M.D.

Intraoperative Events

Hypotension During Cemented Arthroplasty: Relationship to Cardiac Output and Fat Embolism

Wheelwright EF, Byrick RJ, Wigglesworth DF, Kay JC, Wong PY, Mullen JB, Waddell JP (Stobhill Hosp, Glasgow, Scotland; Univ of Toronto; The Toronto Hosp; et al)

J Bone Joint Surg (Br) 75-B:715–723, 1993   129-94-3–18

Background.—Acute hypotension during cemented joint replacement is common during cement and prosthesis insertion. The pathophysiology remains unresolved, but particulate fat and marrow pulmonary embolism are suspected causes. The mechanism of hypotension during simulated bilateral cemented arthroplasty (SBCA) and the relationship between hemodynamic changes and lavage were investigated.

Methods.—Twelve mongrel dogs underwent SBCA. In 6, pulsatile intramedullary lavage preceded cement and prosthesis insertion. All pressures and heart rate were monitored continuously. The lungs and heart were removed en bloc postmortem and processed for histologic examination.

Results.—Blood pressure decreased within 3 minutes of SBCA in both groups; however, a significantly greater and longer-lasting decrease was observed in the no-lavage group. Pulmonary artery pressure was significantly greater at all time periods post-SBCA in the no-lavage group. Cardiac output, stroke volume, and vascular resistance all showed significantly greater changes from baseline in the no-lavage group. Postmortem lung tissue from no-lavage dogs contained significantly more pulmonary fat emboli and a higher volume of fat-occluded lung tissue compared with the lavage group. The severity of hypotension, decreased cardiac output, and increase in prostaglandin metabolites correlated with the magnitude of pulmonary fat embolism.

Conclusion.—Significant fat embolism during cement and prosthesis insertion increases peripheral vascular resistance and right ventricular afterload, causing an acute decrease in cardiac output that creates severe hypotension. Lavage reduces the fat embolism and maintains cardiac output, producing less severe and self-limiting hypotension. Preventing the early physiologic effects of pulmonary fat and marrow embolism should be a major focus in cemented arthroplasty.

▶ In a dog model, the hypotension associated with fixation of total hip arthroplasty components was positively correlated to the magnitude of pulmonary fat embolism. Pulsatile lavage prevented much of the fat embolism and resulted in less hypotension and a decrease in cardiac output.—R. Poss, M.D.

Total Hip Replacement, Lower Limb Blood Flow and Venous Thrombogenesis

McNally MA, Mollan RAB (Queen's Univ of Belfast, Northern Ireland)
J Bone Joint Surg (Br) 75-B:640–644, 1993   129-94-3-19

Introduction.—Deep vein thrombosis (DVT) remains a serious problem for patients who have undergone hip surgery. There is renewed interest in the role of venous stasis in the development of this complication, but it is difficult to establish the presence of venous stasis postoperatively. Strain-gauge plethysmography was used to ascertain the effects of total hip arthroplasty on venous hemodynamics days and weeks after the operation. The association between venous flow and DVT was also examined.

Methods.—The study sample comprised 413 consecutive patients undergoing Charnley cemented total hip replacement (mean age, 67.5 years). All underwent venous occlusion strain-gauge plethysmography preoperatively and 412 were assessed at postoperative day 3; 311 also were assessed at day 5 and 186 were assessed at day 7. Two measures of venous function were assessed in both legs: venous capacitance and venous outflow. Two hundred eighty-one patients were also assessed at a review clinic 6 weeks postoperatively.

Results.—Plethysmographic results indicated venography in 76 patients, and DVT was confirmed in 15 operated and 5 nonoperated legs. Both venous capacitance and venous outflow were reduced postoperatively, particularly in the operated leg. Both measures remained significantly below preoperative levels in the operated leg at 6-week follow-up. The occurrence of DVT was significantly correlated with the degree of reduction in venous blood flow. Venous capacitance was reduced postoperatively by 15.7% for legs without DVT vs. 24.8% for those with DVT; reductions in venous outflow were 9% and 35.3%, respectively.

Conclusion.—Venous stasis is an important factor in the development of DVT after total hip replacement. The operation causes a reduction in venous flow, which persists for weeks after operation. The "at-risk" period for development of DVT appears to be at least 6 weeks; the authors are currently assessing this series of patients at 3 months postoperatively to determine when venous flow in the operated leg finally recovers.

▶ A group of patients who underwent total hip arthroplasty through the posterior approach were found to have a reduction in both venous capacitance and venous outflow affecting both legs but greater in the operated leg after total hip arthroplasty. There was a highly significant correlation between the reduction in blood flow and the development of DVT. The authors concluded that venous stasis is a major factor in venous thrombogenesis.—R. Poss, M.D.

Complications: Sepsis

A 43-Year-Old Woman With Right Hip Pain

Yin Y, Gilula L (Beijing Ji Shui Tan Hosp, Peoples Republic of China; Washington Univ, St Louis, Mo)
Orthop Rev 22:943–949, 1993   129-94-3–20

Introduction.—Tuberculous arthritis is uncommon in the United States. It occurs in less than 1% of patients with tuberculosis and can lead to complete destruction of the joint if untreated. An evaluation of clinical features, diagnosis, and treatment of tuberculous arthritis was studied.

Clinical Features.—Tuberculous arthritis is seen as a mild, slowly progressing process, frequently affecting the weight-bearing joints. The most common early symptom is the insidious onset of joint pain and swelling.

Diagnosis.—The diagnosis of tuberculous arthritis is not difficult when classic radiographic features appear in typical locations. Radiologic findings include osteopenia of the involved joint, soft tissue swelling, bone destruction without evidence of bone formation, and sequestrum formation (Figs 3-4 and 3-5). Haziness and widening of the joint space may develop because of effusion in the joint; narrowing of the joint space occurs in later stages (Fig 3-6). The definitive diagnosis is based on identification of *Mycobacterium tuberculosis* and/or granulomas in the synovial fluid and/or synovial membrane. Differential diagnosis includes rheumatoid arthritis, ankylosing spondylitis, calcium pyrophosphate deposition disease, pyogenic infections, osteonecrosis of the femoral head, idiopathic synovial osteochondromatosis, and pigmented villonodular synovitis.

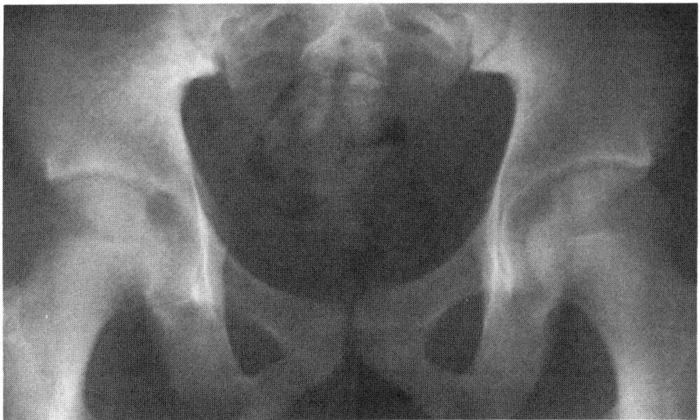

Fig 3–4.—Anteroposterior view of bilateral hip joints. (Courtesy of Yin Y, Gilula L: *Orthop Rev* 22:943-949, 1993.)

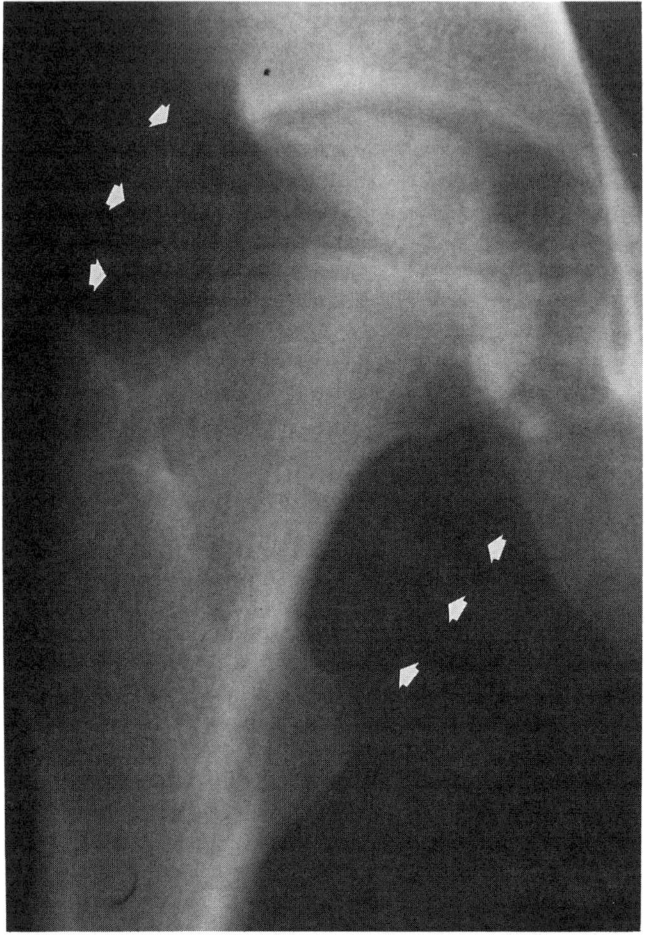

Fig 3–5.—An enlargement of a portion of Fig 3-4 (anteroposterior view of the right hip joint) shows haziness of cortical surface of the hip and widening of the joint space medially. Swelling of the soft tissue surrounding the joint is suggested by bulging of the fat planes around the hip (*arrows*). (Courtesy of Yin Y, Gilula L: *Orthop Rev* 22:943–949, 1993.)

Treatment.—Chemotherapy is almost always effective. Surgery may be needed to relieve pain by evacuating debris or fusion in a severely disorganized joint.

▶ This case report serves as a reminder that tuberculosis must be considered in the differential diagnosis of slowly progressive destructive processes about the hip.—R. Poss, M.D.

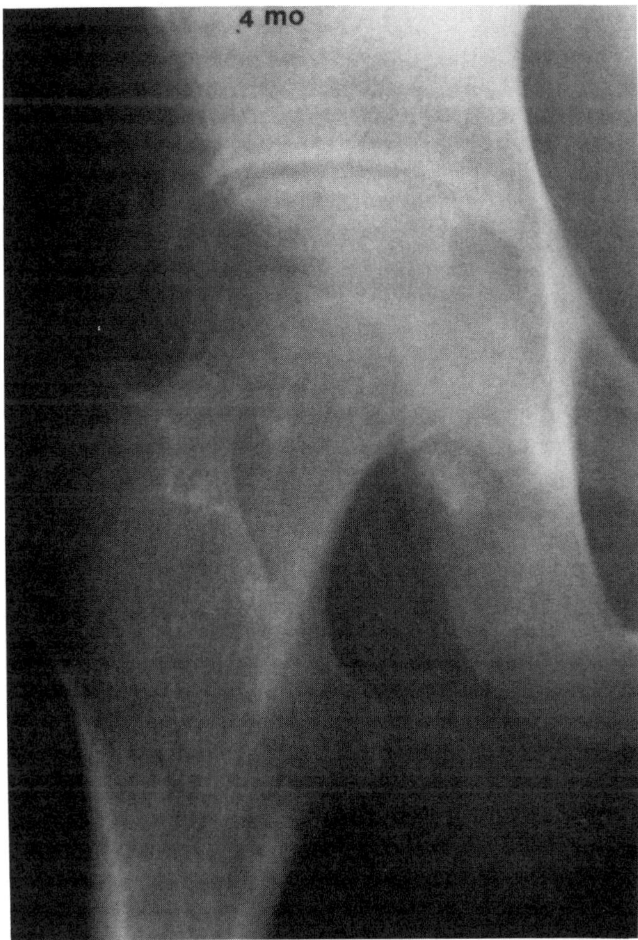

Fig 3–6.—Four months later, anteroposterior view of the right hip joint shows blurring of cortical detail. The femoral head is more flattened than before, and the joint has narrowed further. A slight increase in density is seen at the adjacent bony articular surface between the acetabulum and femoral head, especially at the weight-bearing areas. (Courtesy of Yin Y, Gilula L: *Orthop Rev* 22:943–949, 1993.)

Arthroscopic Management of Septic Arthritis of the Hip

Blitzer CM (Orthopaedic and Trauma Specialists, Somersworth, NH)
Arthroscopy 9:414–416, 1993   129-94-3–21

Objective.—Arthroscopy has been effectively used for septic arthritis of the ankle, knee, and shoulder. The arthroscopic management of septic arthritis of the hip was examined in 5 patients.

Treatment.—Between 1988 and 1991, 5 patients with suspected septic arthritis of the hip were treated with arthroscopic irrigation, débridement, and drainage. The duration of symptoms ranged from about 24 hours to 2 weeks. All patients underwent emergent aspiration of the hip under fluoroscopy, with findings either confirmatory or highly suggestive for pyarthrosis.

Outcome.—During an average follow-up of 20.4 months (range, 6–47), all 3 patients with early diagnosis had excellent results. One child had a final diagnosis of juvenile rheumatoid arthritis. Arthroscopic irrigation and drainage were performed rather than risk the severe sequelae of potentially undertreating a septic hip. Diagnosis was late in 2 patients. One patient had well-controlled infection, but she had progression of arthritis. The other patient had severe damage to the articular cartilage at the time of arthroscopy.

Implication.—Arthroscopy offers an effective alternative to open arthrotomy for septic arthritis of the hip, with much less morbidity. Early diagnosis remains important in the successful management of septic arthritis of the hip.

▶ Arthroscopic irrigation, débridement, and drainage were found to be effective in 4 patients with septic arthritis of the hip. As with open arthrotomy, early intervention and diagnosis is essential.—R. Poss, M.D.

Evaluation of Painful Hip Arthroplasties: Are Technetium Bone Scans Necessary?

Lieberman JR, Huo MH, Schneider R, Salvati EA, Rodi S (Univ of California, Los Angeles; Yale Univ, New Haven, Conn; Hosp for Special Surgery, New York)
J Bone Joint Surg (Br) 75-B:475–478, 1993   129-94-3–22

Objective.—The value of technetium bone scanning in evaluating the painful hip arthroplasty was examined in 54 patients who also had plain radiographs taken, hip aspiration performed, and underwent surgical exploration. The 32 women and 22 men had an average age of 65 years. A 3-phase bone scan was obtained an average of 10 years after primary hip arthroplasty.

Findings.—Forty-three hips were revised for loosening, 10 for infection, and 1 for chronic dislocation. In 30 hips both the acetabular and femoral components were reviewed. Both the bone scan and serial radiography detected loosening with reasonable accuracy. Bone scanning had greater accuracy for femoral than for acetabular loosening. The 2 studies agreed on the femoral side in 93% of patients and on the acetabular side in 90%. Bone scanning did not provide information on loosening that was not available from the plain radiographs. Bone scanning detected 7 of 10 infections, but plain radiographs never led to a diagnosis of infection. Hip aspiration was positive in all 10 patients confirmed as having infection and negative in 39 of 41 uninfected patients. There were 2 dry taps.

Recommendations.—Hip aspiration is indicated if plain radiographs are consistent with loosening. If the x-ray tests are negative, a bone scan can rule out loosening, and an aspirate may be examined if infection is suspected. Any area of focal nuclide uptake requires close follow-up. If symptoms persist during partial weight-bearing, serial radiography and repeat bone scanning are indicated. If the scan shows no increase in uptake, other causes of pain, such as trochanteric bursitis and spinal pathology, should be considered.

▶ Technetium bone scanning did not provide additional information when compared with the accuracy, sensitivity, and specificity of serial radiographs. The authors found that evaluation of a painful hip arthroplasty is adequately conducted with serial plain radiographs and that bone scans are useful only when a diagnosis of loosening or infection cannot be made with routine studies.—R. Poss, M.D.

Osteonecrosis

Avascular Necrosis of the Femoral Head: Natural History and Magnetic Resonance Imaging
Takatori Y, Kokubo T, Ninomiya S, Nakamura S, Morimoto S, Kusaba I (Univ of Tokyo; Shizuoka Children's Hosp, Japan)
J Bone Joint Surg (Br) 75-B:217–221, 1993   129-94-3–23

Background.—Magnetic resonance imaging is more sensitive than radiography in detecting segmental collapse in an osteonecrotic femoral head. Magnetic resonance imaging reveals a hypointense zone of fat that delineates the proximal necrotic lesion, revealing the site and extent of necrosis. The prognostic value of MRI in early-stage avascular necrosis of the femoral head was prospectively evaluated.

Methods.—The study included 25 patients with 32 asymptomatic hips at risk for osteonecrosis. Spin-echo MRI revealed bandlike hypointense zones; plain anteroposterior and lateral radiographs were normal. Two groups of femoral heads were identified based on the MR findings. In group 1, fat intensity was confined to the medial anterosuperior portion of the femoral head, and the bandlike hypointense zone was confined to the zenith of the femoral head on the midsagittal MR scan. Group 2 had greater fat intensity than group 1 and had a bandlike hypointense zone extending beyond the zenith of the femoral head. Patients did not undergo core decompression or biopsy. Disease progression was monitored radiographically. Content and timing of segmental collapse were recorded as survival time from MRI diagnosis.

Results.—Fifteen patients were assigned to group 1; 17 were assigned to group 2. No subsequent segmental collapse occurred in group 1. Fourteen collapses occurred in group 2, with a mean survival of 15 months. The risk of segmental collapse was significantly higher in group 2 femoral heads.

Conclusion.—The risk of segmental collapse is heightened if the necrotic lesion occupies most of the weight-bearing area. Early MRI can predict the probability of subsequent segmental femoral head collapse.

▶ Magnetic resonance imaging was shown to be of predictive value in patients at high risk for osteonecrosis of the hip. In these asymptomatic patients with normal plain radiographs, the degree to which the necrotic lesion occupied the weight-bearing area of the femoral head was directly correlated to the subsequent likelihood of collapse. If these findings are confirmed in future studies, patients at high risk may be candidates for surgical intervention earlier in the natural history of the disease.—R. Poss, M.D.

Bone-Marrow Oedema Syndrome and Transient Osteoporosis of the Hip: An MRI-Controlled Study of Treatment by Core Decompression
Hofmann S, Engel A, Neuhold A, Leder K, Kramer J, Plenk H Jr (Univ of Vienna; Rudolfinerhaus Hosp, Vienna; Orthopaedic Hosp, Vienna)
J Bone Joint Surg (Br) 75-B:210–216, 1993   129-94-3–24

Background.—Bone marrow edema syndrome (BMES) of the hip has a specific MRI pattern related to increased fluid in femoral head marrow cavities. Other characteristics of BMES include severe pain, a nonspecific focal loss of radiologic density, and a positive bone scan. This MRI-controlled study verified the histomorphology of BMES and concomitant bone and marrow changes.

Methods.—Ten cases of BMES were diagnosed in 9 patients with no other signs of avascular necrosis. All 10 patients were treated with core decompression. At initial diagnosis and latest evaluation, the hips were graded using the Harris hip score. At 6- to 12-month intervals, patients underwent standard anteroposterior and frog-leg lateral radiographs as well as MRI.

Results.—Core decompression provided immediate relief in all patients; MRIs returned to normal after 3 months. Bone core specimens confirmed BMES. Specimens contained necrotic cells and remnants, as well as a fibrous matrix and new dilated vessels suggestive of active repair. Trabecular bone contained extended osteoid seams covered by active osteoblasts; osteoclastic resorption was rare. One of 8 hips had Arlet and Durroux type 1 changes; 3 had type 2 changes, and 4 had type 3 changes. Volume density was normal with no sign of osteoporosis, although quantitative microradiography revealed a distinct loss of hydroxyapatite content in all patients.

Conclusion.—Bone marrow edema syndrome may be the initial phase of nontraumatic avascular necrosis. Although these patients would have improved under conservative treatment after 6–12 months, core depression dramatically reduced the average duration of symptoms. Thus, all nontraumatic BMES of the femoral head should be treated by core decompression. The risk of progression to full avascular necrosis with femoral head collapse after conservative treatment outweighs the minimal surgical risk associated with the procedure.

▶ The advent of MRI has made it possible to observe subclinical and sometimes spontaneously reversible pathologic events. Bone marrow edema syndrome gives a characteristic MRI pattern that may represent an initial phase of avascular necrosis, but in most patients it will spontaneously resolve over time *without* intervention.—R. Poss, M.D.

Early Detection of Avascular Necrosis of the Femoral Head by MRI
Fordyce MJF, Solomon L (Kent and Sussex Hosp, Kent, England; Bristol Royal Infirmary, England)
J Bone Joint Surg (Br) 75-B:365–367, 1993   129-94-3–25

Introduction.—By the time radiographic changes appear in patients with avascular necrosis (AVN), they reflect the formation of new bone on the surfaces of dead trabeculae, which may occur weeks to months after bone death. Magnetic resonance imaging has the potential for very early diagnosis of bone ischemia and necrosis, perhaps before symptoms develop; however, this has never been established in a prospective study. Such a study was performed in a group of patients at high risk for AVN—kidney transplant patients receiving high-dose corticosteroid immunosuppressive therapy.

Methods.—Hip MRI scans were obtained in 32 such patients 9–21 months after transplantation. The average corticosteroid dose was 1,680 mg of prednisolone in 30 days. Patients with abnormal scans were followed up by clinical examination, plain radiography, CT, radionuclide bone scanning, and repeat MRI at 2 and 3 years after the initial examination.

Results.—Magnetic resonance image changes indicating ischemia—namely focal areas of decreased signal intensity in the subarticular area of the femoral head on both T1- and T2-weighted images—were seen in 5 hips in 3 patients. All of these patients had normal radiographic, CT, and bone scan findings. One patient became symptomatic 9 months later; the other diagnostic investigations became positive as well. He was found to have increased intraosseous pressure in both hip joints, which showed necrotic bone on a core biopsy specimen. No symptoms or changes in the MRI findings have been seen in the other 3 hips.

Conclusion.—At least during the medium term, the early MRI appearance of femoral head AVN does not indicate inevitable bone collapse. During 3 years of follow-up, patients may remain asymptomatic and the MRI picture may remain unchanged. Such patients are good candidates for the evaluation of nondestructive treatments intended to prevent or alleviate the effects of bone ischemia.

▶ In a series of patients at high risk for osteonecrosis (all of whom were asymptomatic, plain radiographs, CT scans, and bone scans were negative. Magnetic resonance imaging was found to be the most sensitive instrument to establish a diagnosis of osteonecrosis. Not all patients progressed to segmental collapse. A hypothesis as to why some patients might not have progressed to collapse is offered in Abstract 129-94-3–23.—R. Poss, M.D.

Mechanical Consequences of Core Drilling and Bone-Grafting on Osteonecrosis of the Femoral Head
Brown TD, Pedersen DR, Baker KJ, Brand RA (Univ of Iowa, Iowa City; Texas Scottish Rite Hosp for Children, Dallas)
J Bone Joint Surg (Am) 75-A:1358–1366, 1993   129-94-3–26

Introduction.—Patients with symptomatic osteonecrosis of the femoral head most often have eventual collapse, but many of them are relatively young adults for whom total hip replacement is not optimal. The availability of MRI for detecting early marrow changes in involved cancellous bone has made preservation of the natural femoral head a realistic possibility for many patients. Both core drilling and cortical bone grafting have been used to alter the pattern of load transmission in the necrotic femoral head.

A Model.—Changes in stress transmission consequent to both core drilling and bone grafting were examined using a three-dimensional finite-element model of the proximal femur. Areas of osteonecrosis were represented by uniform relative attenuation of the local mechanical properties of normal cancellous bone. Elastic modulus was reduced 75%, and strength was reduced by 50%. A geometric preprocessing algorithm was developed to automatically rezone parts of the finite-element mesh of the natural head to align interelement boundaries with the periphery of the modeled core or graft tract.

Observations.—Cores that penetrated deeply into the body of the lesion placed nearby necrotic bone at a considerably increased risk of structural collapse compared with no treatment (Fig 3–7). This effect was most evident in the bone overlying the tip of the core and that beneath the proximal underside of the tract. Peak stress: strength ratios for the central tract were consistently less than those for the lateral tract, and they were not very dependent on the depth of penetration. Stress patterns were sensitive to the placement of fibular grafts 8 mm in diameter. Grafts directed into the medial one third of the lesion were ineffective, but both centrally and laterally directed grafts enhanced the stress: strength ratio of the untreated lesion (Fig 3–8). Grafts uniting with the subchondral plate achieved substantial unloading at the lesion. A laterally

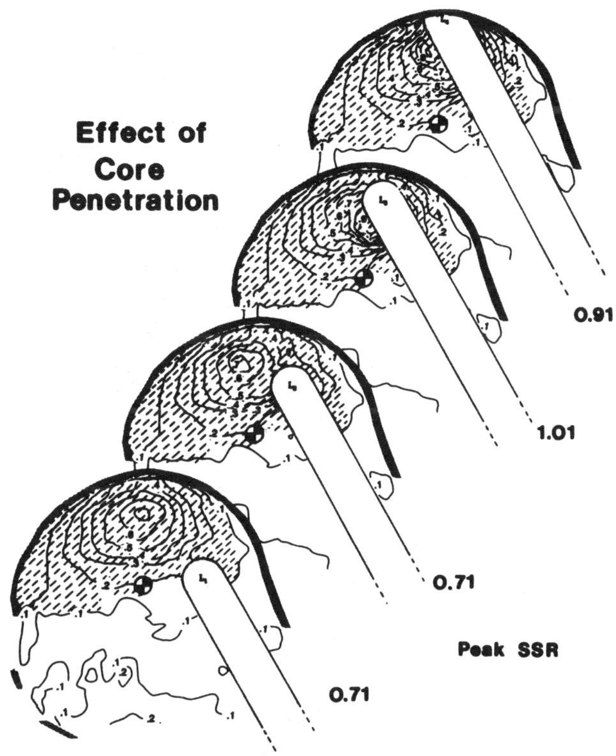

Fig 3–7.—Effect of the depth of penetration of the core for laterally directed cores (L_1 through L_4). Cores that penetrated deeply into the lesion caused substantial elevations in the stress: strength ratio (SSR), whereas cores that penetrated only into the midsubstance of the lesion did not. (Courtesy of Brown TD, Pedersen DR, Baker KJ, et al: *J Bone Joint Surg (Am)* 75-A:1358–1366, 1993.)

directed graft that penetrated only midway through the lesion, however, substantially increased the global peak stress:strength ratio.

Suggestions.—Adequate graft length is as critical as the direction of its placement. Coring is relatively inconsequential structurally as long as the tract stops well below the subchondral plate. It appears best to direct the core tract toward the center of the lesion. A graft should make direct mechanical contact with the subchondral plate. An improperly placed graft may be worse than no graft at all.

▶ This intriguing study suggests the importance of placing cortical bone grafts to provide the greatest structural support for osteonecrotic femoral heads. When a cortical graft abuts the subchondral plate and is placed in the superior central or lateral aspect of the femoral head, the best improvement in structural support is obtained.—R. Poss, M.D.

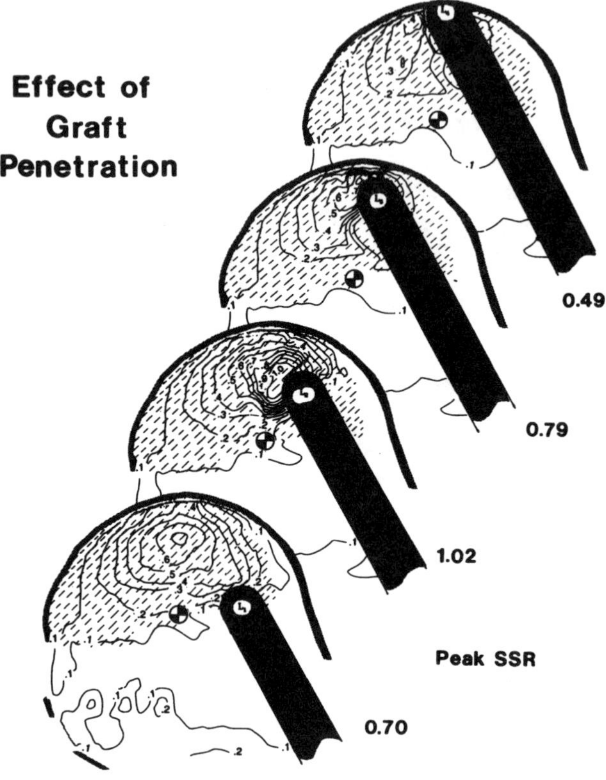

Fig 3–8.—*Abbreviation: SSR*, stress:strength ratio. Effect of penetration of an 8-mm graft for the lateral tract. A substantial structural benefit was realized only with flush engagement of the subchondral plate. (Courtesy of Brown TD, Pedersen DR, Baker KJ, et al: *J Bone Joint Surg (Am)* 75-A:1358–1366, 1993.)

The Effect of Fracture on Femoral Head Blood Flow: Osteonecrosis and Revascularization Studied in Miniature Swine

Swiontkowski MF, Tepic S, Rahn BA, Cordey J, Perren SM (Harborview Med Ctr, Seattle; Lab for Experimental Surgery, Davos, Switzerland)
Acta Orthop Scand 64:196–202, 1993   129-94-3–27

Objective.—The effects of femoral neck fracture on blood flow in the femoral head were investigated in miniature swine, which have a femoral vascular anatomy resembling that of human beings.

Methods.—Blood flow was assessed by laser Doppler flowmetry before and after injury, after internal fixation, and 8 weeks after injury. The fracture was created by scoring the mid–femoral neck with a saw and completing the cut with an osteotome. Fluorescent bone labeling was done 2, 4, and 6 weeks after injury using Xylenol Orange, Calcein Green, and Oxytetracycline.

Observations.—Blood flow in the femoral head consistently decreased after the fracture was created. Flow decreased to 40% of baseline. Disruption of venous drainage was partly responsible. Internal fixation with Kirschner wires did not alter femoral head blood flow. Bone density decreased in the operated femoral head, especially when gross collapse of the femoral head was present. Fluorescence microscopy demonstrated early neovascularization when gross collapse did not occur.

Conclusion.—These findings suggest that a femoral neck fracture disrupts arterioles and distorts venous drainage channels, leading to relative ischemia of the femoral head. Reduction and internal fixation augment blood flow and limit ischemia to some extent.

▶ In this swine model, fracture of the femoral neck resulted in decreased blood flow to the femoral head, leading to relative femoral head ischemia. Internal fixation improved femoral head blood flow. Gradual improvement in femoral head blood flow occurred by vascular dilation and neovascularization. Prolongation of the ischemic period was associated with an increased incidence of collapse of the femoral head.—R. Poss, M.D.

Association of Alcohol Intake, Cigarette Smoking, and Occupational Status With the Risk of Idiopathic Osteonecrosis of the Femoral Head
Hirota Y, Hirohata T, Fukuda K, Mori M, Yanagawa H, Ohno Y, Sugioka Y-i (Kyushu Univ, Fukuoka, Japan; Kurume Univ, Japan; Jichi Med School, Tochigi, Japan; et al)
Am J Epidemiol 137:530–538, 1993   129-94-3–28

Background.—Ischemic necrosis of bone, especially of the femoral head, appears to be an increasing cause of musculoskeletal disability. A number of studies have suggested an association between alcohol intake and idiopathic osteonecrosis. The association between idiopathic osteonecrosis of the femoral head and alcohol consumption, cigarette smoking, occupation, and other factors was investigated in a national multicenter case-control study in Japan.

Methods.—From 1988 to 1990, a total of 118 patients were compared with 236 control subjects matched for sex, age, ethnicity, clinic, and date of initial examination. The patients had no history of systemic corticosteroid use. The risks of femoral head necrosis associated with potential risk factors were estimated by adjusted relative odds obtained by a conditional logistic regression model.

Findings.—The relative odds for occasional and regular drinkers were 3.2 and 13.1, respectively. There was a significant dose-response relationship. For current drinkers, the relative odds were 2.8 for less than

320 g/wk of ethanol consumption, 9.4 for weekly consumption of 320–799 g, and 14.8 for weekly consumption of 800 g or more. Current smokers also had an increased risk of femoral head necrosis developing (relative odds, 4.7), but there was no linear increasing trend in the cumulative effect of smoking at 20 pack-years or more. There was a weak but significant dose-response relationship with daily occupational energy consumption.

Conclusion.—Alcohol intake is strongly associated with the development of femoral head necrosis. Cigarette smoking also appears to be positively associated with it. In addition, heavy physical work may play a role.

▶ Japanese patients with high cigarette consumption or alcohol intake were compared with matched controls. There was a significantly increased risk of osteonecrosis in both the smoking group and the drinking intake group. In the alcohol-intake group, there was a dose-response increased risk. An increased risk was found for current smokers, but the risk did not increase over time. Those who performed heavy physical work were at somewhat less risk of osteonecrosis when compared with the other 2 groups.—R. Poss, M.D.

Osteolysis

Studies of the Mechanism by Which the Mechanical Failure of Polymethylmethacrylate Leads to Bone Resorption
Horowitz SM, Doty SB, Lane JM, Burstein AH (Univ of Pennsylvania, Philadelphia; Hosp for Special Surgery, New York)
J Bone Joint Surg (Am) 75-A:802–813, 1993   129-94-3–29

Objective.—In implant components that are loose without associated infection, tissue changes at the bone-cement interface suggest some relationship between fragmentation of the cement, the associated biological response, and the development of aseptic loosening. The evidence supports the view that the fatigue failure of the cement leads to generation of particles that initiate a biological response, and it eventually leads to bone resorption and aseptic loosening. The association between mechanical failure of polymethylmethacrylate and bone resorption at the bone-cement interface of a total hip prosthesis was explored.

Methods.—Tissues were examined from the bone-cement interface of 18 femoral components from total hip prostheses that had loosened without associated infection. The presence of very small (1–12 μm) particles that were phagocytized by macrophages was noted. An in vitro study of this phenomenon was set up by exposing macrophages in tissue culture to 3 preparations of polymethylmethacrylate cement. A new method of cement preparation that controlled for solid and soluble contaminants was used that accurately determined which mediators were released from the macrophages.

Results.—All 3 types of cement showed phagocytosis of the very small particles, as documented by electron microscopy. All 3 cements were toxic, as indicated by the inhibition of ^{3}H-thymidine incorporation. Although exposure to cement increased release of tumor necrosis factor, it did not prompt release of prostaglandin E_2. Only exposure to particles small enough to be phagocytized, and not to larger particles, led to the inhibition of ^{3}H-thymidine incorporation and the release of tumor necrosis factor. Neither small nor large particles induced the release of prostaglandin E_2.

Conclusion.—Cement failure leading to bone resorption and aseptic loosening appears to result from a 2-phase macrophage-mediated response. Mechanical failure of the cement mantle results from production of 1–12 μm particles, which are small enough to be phagocytized by macrophages. The resulting biological response consists of a repetitive cycle of particle phagocytosis and cell death, with release of bone-resorbing mediators such as tumor necrosis factor. These mediators are the cause of bone resorption at the bone-cement interface. Prostaglandin E_2 at the interface may be produced by osteoblasts stimulated by tumor necrosis factor, rather than by macrophages.

▶ The ingestion of particulate debris by macrophages initiates a cascade of biochemical responses that can result in bone resorption. In this model, the authors demonstrate that particles of polymethylmethacrylate ranging in size from less than 1 μm to 12 μm result in cell toxicity as expressed by an inhibition of ^{3}H-thymidine incorporation and release of tumor necrosis factor. Particles too large to be phagocytized had no adverse effects.—R. Poss, M.D.

The Differences in Toxicity and Release of Bone-Resorbing Mediators Induced by Titanium and Cobalt-Chromium-Alloy Wear Particles
Haynes DR, Rogers SD, Hay S, Pearcy MJ, Howie DW (Univ of Adelaide, South Australia, Australia; Royal Adelaide Hosp, South Australia, Australia)
J Bone Joint Surg (Am) 75-A:825–834, 1993   129-94-3–30

Purpose.—Recent research suggests that a tissue response to prosthetic wear particles is an important cause of loosening in patients with total hip and other arthroplasties. The inflammatory effects of these particles may be more harmful than their toxic effects. The association between the toxic effects of metal wear particles and their ability to stimulate the release of inflammatory mediators that play a role in bone resorption was examined.

Methods and Results.—In vitro studies were performed using rat peritoneal macrophages exposed to particles milled from the metal components of hip prostheses. Particles from either cobalt-chromium-alloy or titanium-aluminum-vanadium particles were tested. The particles were about the size and concentration of those found in the tissues around failed prostheses in human beings. Toxicity was low with the titanium-aluminum-vanadium particles, even at high concentrations, whereas the cobalt-chromium particles demonstrated very high toxicity. However, across a range of concentrations, the titanium-aluminum-vanadium particles induced significantly greater release of prostaglandin E_2. This alloy also increased the release of interleukin-1, tumor necrosis factor, and interleukin-6; and cobalt-chromium particles were associated with decreased release of prostaglandin E_2 and interleukin-6 and had no important effect on release of interleukin-1 and tumor necrosis factor.

Conclusion.—Different types of metal wear particles, even of the same size, elicit different cellular responses. Although cobalt-chromium particles show greater tissue toxicity, titanium-aluminum-vanadium particles are more likely to induce release of inflammatory mediators of osteolysis. These results mandate special attention to the design of titanium-aluminum-vanadium implants to minimize the potential for wear particles, especially in modular implants.

▶ In this in vitro study using rat macrophages, cobalt-chromium particles were found to be toxic when compared with titanium-aluminum-vanadium particles of the same size and concentration as those found in human tissues that are adjacent to failed implants. However, the titanium particles resulted in the release of more prostaglandin E_2 than did the cobalt-chromium particles. This study demonstrates a differing cellular response to particles of similar size and concentration. At least in this model, titanium particles are associated with the release of those inflammatory mediators that can result in osteolysis.—R. Poss, M.D.

Tumor Necrosis Factors α and β Can Stimulate Bone Resorption in Cultured Mouse Calvariae by a Prostaglandin-Independent Mechanism

Lerner UH, Ohlin A (Univ of Umeå, Sweden; Univ of Lund, Malmö, Sweden)
J Bone Miner Res 8:147–155, 1993   129-94-3–31

Introduction.—Tumor necrosis factors (TNF) α and β stimulate bone resorption both in vitro and in vivo. This ability appears to result from a paracrine interaction between osteoblasts and osteoclasts, rather than from a direct effect on osteoclasts. Tumor necrosis factor can induce prostaglandin E_2 (PGE_2)—a potent stimulator of bone resorption—in mouse and rat osteoblasts. Whether the stimulatory action of TNF-α and TNF-β on bone resorption required the TNF-induced formation of PGE_2 was determined.

Observations.—Experiments were performed in cultured calvarial bone tissue from neonatal mice. Addition of human recombinant TNF-α and TNF-β, at concentrations of 1 ng/mL and above, resulted in a time- and dose-dependent release of ^{45}Ca. Tumor necrosis factor also stimulated PGE_2 formation in a dose-dependent fashion and enhanced the biosynthesis of prostaglandin I_2. Stimulation of PGE_2 by TNF was maximal at 12 hours.

Whereas the unrelated nonsteroidal anti-inflammatory drugs indomethacin, flurbiprofen, and meclofenamic acid were able to abolish TNF-induced PGE_2 production, they reduced ^{45}Ca release only slightly. The partial inhibitory effect of indomethacin was seen across a wide range of TNF-α concentrations, with no effect on the concentration producing a half-maximal stimulatory response. Studies in bone prelabeled with [^{3}H]proline suggested stimulation of bone matrix breakdown by TNF; this effect was reduced somewhat by indomethacin. Tumor necrosis factor–induced PGE_2 production was abolished by hydrocortisone and dexamethasone. Unlike the cyclooxygenase inhibitors, corticosteroids did not affect TNF–induced ^{45}Ca release.

Conclusion.—This in vitro study suggests that TNF-α and TNF-β can both induce bone resorption by some prostaglandin-independent mechanism. This mechanism is essentially unknown, but it may be mediated by an initial action on osteoblasts that results in paracrine stimulation of osteoclasts.

▶ Tumor necrosis factors α and β were found to stimulate bone resorption through a process independent of prostaglandin production. Abstracts 129-94-3–29 through 129-94-3–31 suggest the complexity of the mechanism by which biochemical mediators induce bone resorption. It seems clear that the process is initiated by phagocytosis of small particles that, in bulk form, are relatively nontoxic and noninflammatory. The cellular response of these particles to phagocytosis produces both cell toxicity and mediators of inflammation, of which either or both can result in the loss of bone.—R. Poss, M.D.

Total Hip Replacement

Histological and Radiographic Assessment of Well Functioning Porous-Coated Acetabular Components: A Human Postmortem Retrieval Study
Engh CA, Zettl-Schaffer KF, Kukita Y, Sweet D, Jasty M, Bragdon C (Anderson Orthopaedic Research Inst, Arlington, Va; Sapporo Med College, Japan; Armed Forces Inst of Pathology, Washington, DC; et al)
J Bone Joint Surg (Am) 75-A:814–824, 1993   129-94-3–32

Purpose.—In total hip arthroplasty, porous-coated acetabular components become fixed through fibrous tissue and bone growth into the porous surface. Fixation is good, but studies of actual bone ingrowth have given disappointing results. Most of these studies have analyzed components removed at revision operation because of malposition. These studies may not reflect the bone ingrowth characteristics of a prosthesis with good long-term function. A postmortem study of bone ingrowth in well-functioning porous-coated acetabular components was evaluated.

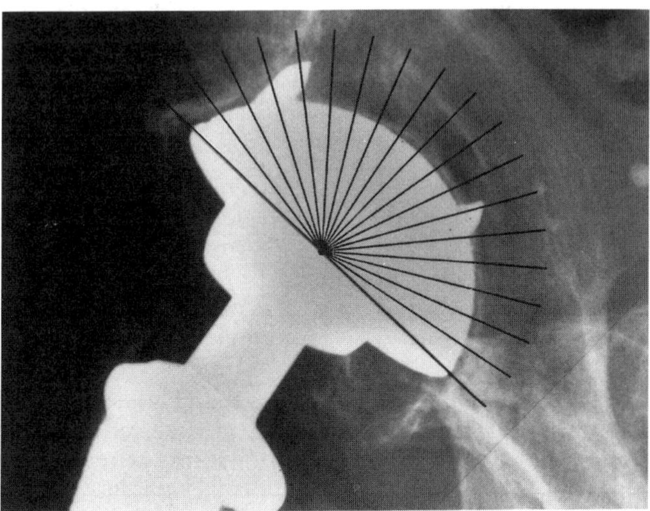

Fig 3–9.—All of the anteroposterior and iliac oblique radiographs were evaluated with use of a 10-degree-increment grid. The final follow-up iliac oblique radiograph of patient is shown. There is a complete radiolucent line around the hemispherical surface of the component. (Courtesy of Engh CA, Zettl-Schaffer KF, Kukita Y, et al: *J Bone Joint Surg (Am)* 75:A:814–824, 1993.)

Methods.—Nine components from patients undergoing total hip arthroplasty at the authors' institution were retrieved after the patients had died. There were no apparent clinical problems with the components, all of which were radiographically stable. The components had been in place for a mean of 50 months. Bone ingrowth into the porous coating of the metal component was measured by standard back-scattered electron microscopy. The histologic appearance of the interface was compared with its clinical radiographic appearance (Fig 3–9), and nonossified areas were studied by light microscopy.

Results.—Bone ingrowth was seen in all components, occupying a mean of 32% of the fields examined. Areas of bone ingrowth had an even higher mean area density (48%). The clinical radiographic data consistently underestimated the presence of gap areas and overestimated the occurrence of bone apposition. The fibrous tissue found in nonossified areas was very dense and well organized. Light microscopic examination found no signs of granulomatous formation in the nonossified regions.

Conclusion.—This postmortem study gives encouraging results regarding the bone-implant interfaces of well-functioning porous-coated acetabular components. Only about one third of the surface of the components is in contact with bone, but the fibrous tissue in the nonossified gaps is consistently dense and well organized. These areas have no signs of granulomas; the depth and orientation of the fibrous tissue appear to impede the flow of particulate debris and protect the areas against early osteolysis.

▶ Plain radiographs consistently underestimate the area of porous ingrowth acetabular cups that are actually bone ingrown. In this postmortem study, a mean of only 32% of the available area was fixed by bone. Fibrous tissue ingrowth was found to be dense and well organized in these cups, which were functioning well at the time of the patients' death.—R. Poss, M.D.

Roentgenographic Densitometry of Bone Adjacent to a Femoral Prosthesis

Engh CA, McGovern TF, Schmidt LM (Anderson Orthopaedic Research Inst, Arlington, Va)

Clin Orthop 292:177–190, 1993
129-94-3–33

Purpose.—The authors previously reported a radiographic study of the stress-related bone mass changes occurring in the proximal femur after total hip arthroplasty (THA). The radiographic technique used was useful in describing early, obvious differences in bone remodeling. However, it left many important questions unanswered (e.g., whether the proximal bone resorption that occurs with large-diameter stems is progressive over the long term and whether bone remodeling patterns can be followed quantitatively over time). Toward answering these questions, the authors have developed a digital imaging method to measure stress-related changes in radiographic bone density after THA.

Findings.—The investigators' technique—histogram-directed equalization—attempted to isolate and quantify image brightness over defined zones adjacent to the implant. The technique was used to compensate for differences in the quality of images resulting from variations in delivered energy. Significant decreases were obtained in quantitative change resulting from variation in delivered energy: 7% for radiographs obtained with a 2-kVp variation and 31% for those obtained with a 4-kVp variation.

The technique also allowed accurate description of changes depicted in annual postoperative radiographs. Fifteen patients with fully porous-coated implants were analyzed, 5 with small-diameter stems and 10 with large-diameter stems. Radiographic bone density in the medial and lateral proximal regions decreased significantly—from 11% to 28%—in both groups. At both 2 and 5 years, the patients with large-diameter stems had larger decreases in radiographic bone density. Bone remodeling was greatest in the first 2 years, slowing down thereafter. The technique was also able to confirm the predicted effect of stem diameter on bone remodeling patterns.

Conclusion.—Histogram-directed equalization as a new method of radiographic measurement of stress-related changes in bone density after THA was studied. Further study will be needed to define the relationship of measured radiographic density to actual changes in bone mineral content.

▶ How clinically important is the proximal stress shielding that occurs in the presence of canal filling, fully porous-coated femoral components? By this densitometric method, all 15 patients who were measured sustained a decrease in bone density ranging from 11% to 28%. The large-diameter stem group had a larger decrease in bone density than did patients who received stems of smaller diameter.—R. Poss, M.D.

Femoral Component Offset: Its Effect on Strain in Bone–Cement
Davey JR, O'Connor DO, Burke DW, Harris WH (Massachusetts Gen Hosp, Boston; Harvard Med School, Boston)
J Arthroplasty 8:23–26, 1993   129-94-3–34

Background.—After total hip arthroplasty, the magnitude of the offset of the femoral prosthesis greatly affects the mechanics of the hip. Increased offset increases the moment arm of the abductor muscles, which reduces the abductor force needed in normal gait. Consequently, the resultant force across the hip joint is decreased. However, increased offset also increases the bending moment on the implant, which may adversely increase the strain in the medial cement mantle.

Methods and Findings.—Cadaveric femora were studied to assess the relative advantages and disadvantages of the conflicting results of increasing the offset of the femoral component. The effects of differing offsets of the femoral component on strain in the cement mantle were measured in vitro. The intact femora were tested, the femoral prostheses were cemented in place, and the abductor force, resultant force, and strain in the cement mantle under loading conditions that simulated single-limb stance at different femoral offset levels were then quantified. The decrease in abductor and resultant force was substantial with increased femoral component offset. However, the strain in the cement of the proximal medial portion of the cement mantle was not increased significantly.

Conclusion.—Under conditions simulating single-legged stance, the strain in the cement mantle is not adversely influenced by an increase in femoral component offset from 33 mm to 53 mm. The present findings confirm that the measured abductor force and calculated joint reactive force are reduced with an increase in femoral component offset and the accompanying increased abductor angle. Therefore, although the lever arm of the bending moment is raised by the increased offset, the bending moment is only marginally increased, and the net change in strain in the medial cement mantle is not compromising.

▶ An increased offset confers biomechanical advantages to the prosthetic hip by increasing the abductor moment and reducing the joint reactor force. Two concerns regarding stem design with increased offset are the possibility of stem breakage and increased strains on cement. The improved alloys of the past 10 years have virtually eliminated the possibility of stem breakage because of increased offset. In this study, increased offset did not significantly increase the strain in the proximal medial cement.—R. Poss, M.D.

Penetration and Shear Strength of Cement–Bone Interfaces In Vivo
Macdonald W, Swarts E, Beaver R (Royal Perth Hosp, Australia)
Clin Orthop 286:283–288, 1993   129-94-3-35

Background.—The continuing problem of loosening has prompted further development of polymethylmethacrylate cement (PMMA) for total joint arthroplasty. The focus has been on improving mechanical interdigitation of the PMMA cement with cancellous bone. However, all previous studies of cement penetration and fixation strength have been done in vitro, and interface bleeding may compromise the cement–bone attachment.

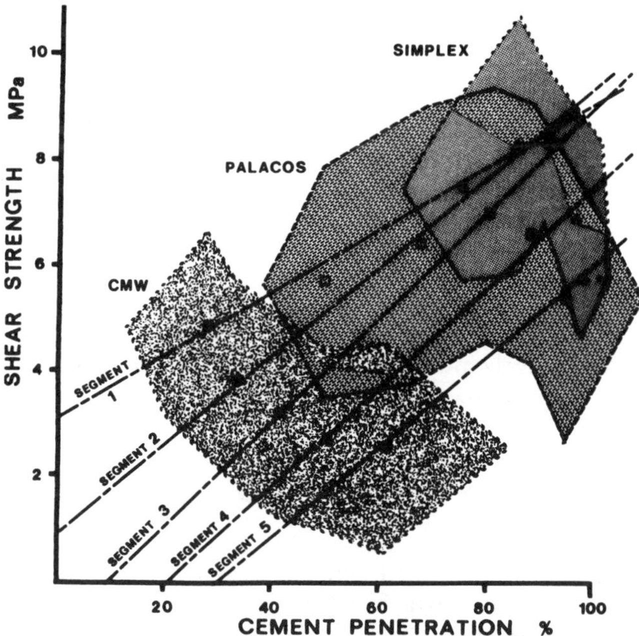

Fig 3–10.—Interfacial shear strength plotted against cement penetration. The *shaded areas* represent mean ± standard deviation for both variables. (Courtesy of MacDonald W, Swarts E, Beaver R: *Clin Orthop* 286:283–288, 1993.)

Methods.—Twenty-one mongrel dogs were used to study the relationship between interfacial shear strength and the degree of cement penetration into bone in the presence of confounding factors such as bleeding. The dogs underwent bilateral implantation of a sham proximal femoral component.

Findings.—Shear strength at the interface between PMMA bone cement and cancellous bone was linearly dependent on the depth of penetration of the cement into the bone. When distal bone plugging, pressure lavage, and pressurized insertion of cement were used, shear strength at the interface was increased by 82% and penetration by 74%. When a cement with lower viscosity was used, penetration and shear strength were increased by a further 18%. No film of blood was found at the cement–bone interface with pressurized insertion of Simplex P and Palacos R cements. The interfacial shear strength plotted against cement penetration for 3 types of cement is shown in Figure 3–10.

Conclusion.—Blood ingress in vivo may not compromise the cement–bone attachment, as had been suggested. Thus, technical and material improvements aimed at increasing cement–bone penetration should result in improved fixation strength.

▶ Increased penetration of cement into cancellous surfaces increases the shear strength at the interface. Modern cementing techniques—including distal bone plug, pressure lavage, and pressurized insertion of cement—enhance penetration and increase shear strength.—R. Poss, M.D.

General

Hip Joint Loading During Walking and Running, Measured in Two Patients

Bergmann G, Graichen F, Rohlmann A (Free Univ Berlin)
J Biomech 26:969–990, 1993   129-94-3–36

Background.—Continued advances in the design of hip prostheses and their clinical use will require precise data on in vivo loading of the prostheses. Inductively powered, telemetering total joint implants are now available for in vivo study of 3-dimensional hip joint forces. Data from 2 patients with implanted telemetering total hip prostheses were analyzed.

Methods.—The first patient was a healthy, active elderly man who required bilateral hip joint replacement for severe arthritis. The other patient was an elderly woman who received a single implant for idiopathic femoral head necrosis; she had cerebellar atrophy and axonal polyneuropathy in her right leg, which caused atactic gait patterns. Hip joint force, its orientation, and moments were measured during walking, running, and stumbling in both patients.

Findings.—In the first patient, walking speeds to $1-5$ km/h^{-1} increased median peak forces from 280% to 480% of the patient's body weight (BW). These forces increased to about 550% BW during jogging and very fast walking, and up to 720% BW during an episode of stumbling. The second patient had median forces of 410% BW while walking at 3 km/h^{-1} and of 870% BW during stumbling. In both patients and during all activities, high magnitudes of force made only slight changes in the direction of the peak force in the frontal plane. Peak force acted mainly from medial to lateral, perpendicular to the long femoral axis, whereas the ventral-to-dorsal component increased at the higher magnitudes of force. The direction of large forces came close to the average anteversion of the natural femur in 1 joint in the first patient and in the second patient. Torsional moments around the implant stem were 40.3 and 24 N/m, respectively.

Conclusion.—These detailed telemetric data on loading of total hip prostheses will find useful applications in prosthetic design, surgical technique, postoperative physical therapy, and counseling patients about which activities to avoid. Only 2 elderly patients, representing extremes in physical activity and condition, have been studied so far. The results to date suggest that torsional moments probably increase with a smaller anteversion angle.

▶ Two patients who underwent hip replacement received instrumented devices that recorded the magnitude of forces on their hips. The forces measured by these authors were higher than previous theoretical and experimental results. Activities such as jogging, fast walking, or a mis-step can cause multiples between 5 and 8 times a patient's body weight. The magnitude of these forces should be understood by surgeons and patients alike when the longevity of a total hip replacement is discussed.—R. Poss, M.D.

Effects of Oral Administration of Type II Collagen on Rheumatoid Arthritis
Trentham DE, Dynesius-Trentham RA, Orav EJ, Combitchi D, Lorenzo C, Sewell KL, Hafler DA, Weiner HL (Harvard Med School, Boston; Harvard School of Public Health, Boston)
Science 261:1727–1730, 1993   129-94-3–37

Background.—No satisfactory treatment has been found for rheumatoid arthritis (RA). Current treatments control established disease only in part, and the side effects limit their use early in the course of illness. Oral administration of native type II collagen has been reported to improve RA in 2 animal models in which arthritis was induced by type II collagen or complete Freund's adjuvant.

Study Design.—Sixty patients with severe, active RA were enrolled in a double-blind phase II trial of chicken type II collagen. Immunosuppressive treatment was stopped. Twenty-eight of the 59 evaluable patients were fed .1 mg of solubilized type II collagen daily for 1 month, followed by .5 mg daily for the next 2 months. The other 31 patients received a placebo.

Results.—The collagen-treated patients had fewer swollen joints and less joint tenderness and pain in the first 3 months of the trial. Disease resolved completely in 14% of actively treated patients but not in any of the placebo recipients. Four placebo patients, however, benefited substantially and achieved a functional class I ranking. No side effects were ascribed to collagen treatment, and there was no evidence of sensitization to collagen.

Conclusion.—The oral use of solubilized heterologous type II collagen in small amounts was shown to be a safe means of lessening the symptoms of active RA. If longer-term efficacy is confirmed, collagen will be preferable to immunosuppressive drug therapy because of its lack of toxicity.

▶ In this clinical investigation, patients with RA were found to have a good response to type II collagen when it was given orally. The concept of oral tolerization, if confirmed in further human trials, presents an exciting new approach to the therapy of RA and other autoimmune diseases.—R. Poss, M.D.

Osteoporosis and Hip Fractures

Hip Fracture Rates in Hong Kong and the United States, 1988 Through 1989
Ho SC, Bacon WE, Harris T, Looker A, Maggi S (Chinese Univ, Hong Kong; Ctrs for Disease Control, Hyattsville, Md; World Health Organization Research Program on Aging, Bethesda, Md)
Am J Public Health 83:694–697, 1993   129-94-3–38

Objective.—Hip fracture reportedly is less frequent in Asian countries than in the United States, but recent data are not available and differences in case definition make the comparison problematic. Accordingly, trends in hip fracture by age and sex were examined by reviewing hospital discharge data in Hong Kong and the United States from 1988 through 1989.

Findings.—There were 3,205 hip fractures in Hong Kong and 2,881 in the United States sample during the 2-year period. Age-adjusted rates of fracture per 100,000 population were significantly higher in the United States than in Hong Kong for both males and females. Typically, rates were 1.5–2.5 times higher in the United States across age and gender groups. In both populations, fracture rates were higher in females and increased with advancing age. For the oldest age groups, males in the United States had a higher rate of hip fracture than females in Hong Kong.

Conclusion.—Hip fracture is becoming more prevalent in Hong Kong, but it still is less frequent than in the United States. Clarifying the reasons for this difference might prove helpful in identifying preventive measures.

Admission Rates for Hip Fracture in Australia in the Last Decade: The New South Wales Scene in a World Perspective

Lau EMC (Royal Newcastle Hosp, New South Wales, Australia)
Med J Aust 158:604–606, 1993   129-94-3–39

Background.—Hip fractures, a major cause of mortality and morbidity among elderly individuals, is associated with substantial health expenditure in developed nations. Admission rates for hip fracture in New South Wales in the past decade were determined and compared with rates in Europe, the United States, and Asia.

Methods.—New South Wales hospital discharge data were obtained for the years 1981, 1986, and 1989–1990. The number of patients discharged with hip fracture as 1 diagnosis was determined, and age-specific rates were calculated using census population information.

Findings.—Men in New South Wales had hip fracture incidence rates of 148 per 100,000 in 1981, 181 per 100,000 in 1986, and 182 per 100,000 in 1989–1990. The corresponding rates among women were 437, 537, and 500 per 100,000, respectively. For both sexes, the age-adjusted rates were high, comparable to the rates in the United States and New Zealand (table).

Age-Adjusted Incidence Rates (per 100,000) of Hip Fracture by Sex in the Population Older Than 50 Years of Age, by Geographical Area

Geographic area and year(s)	Age–adjusted rates			Female:male ratio
	Women	Men	Total	
White population				
Norway 1983–1984	1293	551	968	2.3
Sweden 1972–1981	701	310	530	2.3
Denmark 1973–1979	620	203	437	3.1
New Zealand 1973–1976	620	151	414	4.1
California, US 1983–1984	559	207	402	2.7
Texas, US 1980	530	205	384	2.6
Rochester, US 1965–1974	510	174	364	2.9
NSW, Australia 1981	437	148	289	3.0
NSW, Australia 1986	537	181	409	3.0
NSW, Australia 1989–1990	500	182	360	2.7
Southampton, UK 1985	255	71	174	3.6
Non–white population				
Hong Kong, Chinese 1986	353	181	277	2.0
California, Blacks 1983–1984	219	144	185	1.5
California, Hispanics 1983–1984	197	90	151	2.2
New Zealand, Maoris 1973–1976	107	182	149	0.6

Note: Rates directly standardized to 1985 United States population.
(From Lau EMC: *Med J Aust* 158:604–606, 1993. Courtesy of Maggi S, Kelsey JL, Litvak J, et al: *Osteoporosis Int* 1:232-241, 1991.)

Conclusion.—By world standards, the incidence of hip fracture in New South Wales in the past decade has been very high. As the population ages, preventing hip fracture will be essential.

▶ The incidence of hip fracture varies around the world. The rate of fracture in Hong Kong is lower than that in the United States. In Australia, the incidence is increasing and approaches that of the United States.—R. Poss, M.D.

Risk of Hip Fracture After Osteoporosis Fractures: 451 Women With Fracture of Lumbar Spine, Olecranon, Knee or Ankle

Lauritzen JB, Lund B (Univ of Copenhagen; Rigshospitalet, Copenhagen)
Acta Orthop Scand 64:297–300, 1993   129-94-3-40

Objective.—Fractures of the distal radius and the proximal humerus in postmenopausal women are associated with an increased risk of subsequent hip fracture. Women with fractures related to osteoporosis and their subsequent risk for hip fracture were evaluated.

Patients.—Between 1976 and 1984, 451 female patients, aged 60–99 years, were hospitalized with fracture involving the lumbar spine in 70, olecranon in 52, knee in 129, and ankle in 200. The observed number of hip fractures during an observation time of 241, 180, 469, and 779 person-years after fracture of the lumbar spine, olecranon, knee, and ankle, respectively, was compared with the age-specific incidence of hip fracture in a female background population in the same area during the same period.

Results.—The relative risk of subsequent hip fractures in postmenopausal women was increased by 3.8 after fracture of the lumbar spine, 2.6 after fracture of the olecranon, 2.4 after fracture of the knee, and 1.3 after fracture of the ankle, compared with the background population. The risk was most pronounced in women, aged 60–79 years, and highest within the first years after the primary fractures, with a tendency to level off 3 years after the primary fractures.

Implications.—The relative risk for subsequent hip fracture after osteoporosis fractures may not appear to be dramatically increased in these women, but a twofold increased relative risk for a common disease is obviously important. Because the increased risk may be caused by imbalance and a greater propensity to fall, rather than by osteoporosis, the goals of intervention should address lifestyle, home environment, medications that interfere with balance and postural capability, medication against osteoporosis, and trauma-reducing arrangements.

▶ Women with osteoporosis who had sustained a fracture of either the lumbar spine, the olecranon, or fractures about the knee or ankle were found to be about 1.5–5 times more likely to sustain a hip fracture. The highest likelihood of hip fracture was in patients who had sustained a previous vertebral compression fracture. Of interest, the increased risk of hip fracture diminished 3 years after the fracture at the remote site. Is osteoporosis a cyclic disease during which an increased resorptive phase renders patients more likely to sustain a fracture?—R. Poss, M.D.

Strength Training Increases Regional Bone Mineral Density and Bone Remodeling in Middle-Aged and Older Men
Menkes A, Mazel S, Redmond RA, Koffler K, Libanati CR, Gundberg CM, Zizic TM, Hagberg JM, Pratley RE, Hurley BF (Univ of Maryland, College Park; Johns Hopkins Univ, Baltimore, Md; Univ of Maryland, Baltimore; et al)
J Appl Physiol 74:2478–2484, 1993   129-94-3-41

Introduction.—The bone loss associated with aging is a problem in men as well as in women. Treatment of osteoporosis has centered on factors that affect the balance between bone resorption and bone formation and result in bone mass and bone mineral density (BMD). The effects of strength training (ST) on BMD and bone remodeling were examined in middle-aged and older men.

Methods.—The study participants were 18 healthy, untrained men (mean age, 59 years), all of whom were nonsmokers and free of cardiovascular disorders. Eleven of the men volunteered for the ST program and 7 served as inactive controls. The participants were studied before and after 16 weeks of ST or no exercise. Supervised training sessions were held 3 times per week using Keiser K-300 equipment.

Results.—The training program resulted in a small but significant decrease in percentage of body fat, but there were no significant changes in body weight or fat free mass. Training increased muscular strength by an average of 45% on a 3-repetition maximum test and by 32% on an isokinetic test of the knee extensors performed at 60 degrees/sec. Bone mineral density was increased in the femoral neck by 3.8% and in the lumbar spine by 2.0%. Changes in BMD of the lumbar spine, however, did not differ significantly from those in the control group. Total body BMD showed no significant change. Training significantly increased levels of osteocalcin and skeletal alkaline phosphatase isoenzyme, but not levels of tartrate-resistant acid phosphatase.

Conclusion.—Epidemiologic studies have shown an association between higher BMD and reduced fracture risk. This is the first report to demonstrate a significant increase in regional BMD as a result of ST in older men. The findings suggest that ST may stimulate bone remodeling, with a greater effect on bone formation than on bone resorption.

▶ Bone mineral density was found to increase in a group of 60-year-old men who participated in 16 weeks of ST exercises.—R. Poss, M.D.

Impact Near the Hip Dominates Fracture Risk in Elderly Nursing Home Residents Who Fall

Hayes WC, Myers ER, Morris JN, Gerhart TN, Yett HS, Lipsitz LA (Beth Israel Hosp, Boston; Hebrew Rehabilitation Ctr for Aged, Boston; Boston Orthopaedic Group, Inc, Brookline, Mass)

Calcif Tissue Int 52:192–198, 1993   129-94-3–42

Background.—Each year more than 250,000 hip fractures occur in the United States, and more than 90% occur in the 31 million individuals older than age 70 years. Most hip fractures are believed to be the result of age-related bone loss or osteoporosis. However, because more than 90% of these fractures are caused by falls, a fall surveillance study was done to determine whether factors relative to the mechanics of falling are associated with the increased risk of hip fracture.

Patients and Methods.—A total of 395 elderly patients from a chronic care facility who fell during the study period were included in the study. The mean age of the residents was 87 years. Eighty-two patients sustained a hip fracture after a fall. The remaining 313 patients fell, but they did not experience a fracture. Patients and reliable witnesses (when available) were asked several open-ended questions about the falls. In addition, medical records for each patient were examined, and brief physical examinations were performed to obtain further information. Multivariate logistic regression was used to analyze the information.

Results.—Impact on the hip or side of the leg, as well as potential energy associated with the fall, were correlated with an increased risk of hip fracture. Quetelet, or body mass index, was inversely related to fracture risk. For falls involving impact on the hip region, the adjusted odds ratio for fracture was 21.7. The potential energy associated with these falls was greater than the average energy necessary to fracture elderly, cadaveric, proximal femurs in previous in vitro experiments.

Conclusion.—A fall from standing height should be considered traumatic enough to pose a high risk of hip fracture when impact occurs on the hip and energy-absorbing processes are insufficient. Among the elderly, fall mechanics are an important factor in the etiology of hip fracture.

▶ The potential energy associated with falls is an order of magnitude greater than the energy required to fracture the proximal femurs of elderly individuals. The authors have found that fall mechanics must be considered when approaching the problem of preventing hip fractures.—R. Poss, M.D.

Predicting Results of Rehabilitation After Hip Fracture: A Ten-Year Follow-Up Study

Thorngren K-G, Ceder L, Svensson K (Lund Univ Hosp, Sweden; Helsingborg

Hosp, Sweden)
Clin Orthop 287:76–81, 1993   129-94-3–43

Objective.—Data on the outcome of rehabilitation after hip fracture were acquired from 103 consecutive patients older than 50 years of age. An easy-to-use predictive system based on clearly defined clinical and social parameters was sought to help in planning rehabilitation and to avoid both prolonged hospitalization and unnecessary institutional after-care.

Patients and Treatment.—The 75 women and 28 men in the study had a mean age of 75 years at the time of injury. Sixty-five had cervical fractures and 38 had trochanteric fractures. Typically, early surgery was followed by immediate weight-bearing. Cervical fractures were nailed by the Rydell method. Trochanteric fractures were both nailed and plated. The patients were followed up at 3 weeks, 4 months, and at 1, 5, and 10 years after fracture. Background and functional variables were analyzed by multivariate discriminant statistical techniques.

Findings.—The 3 most important variables for discharge directly to the patient's home were walking ability 2 weeks after surgery, whether the patient lived alone, and general medical condition. The only variables relevant to the outcome at 4 months to 5 years were age, the ability to visit someone before injury, and walking ability within 2 weeks after surgery. The ability to visit someone also was a factor in the 10-year outlook, as were age, sex, and type of fracture. Adjusting for general medical status did not alter the variables that were significant in the long-term outlook.

Implications.—By using "soft" data, it is possible to reliably predict both the short- and long-term outlook after hip fracture. The patient and society will both benefit from early rehabilitation at home.

▶ The authors have identified physical and social factors that were predictors in determining the outcome of rehabilitation after hip fracture.—R. Poss, M.D.

Biochemical Markers of Nutrition in Osteoporosis
Rico H, Relea P, Revilla M, Hernandez ER, Arribas I, Villa LF (Alcaldá de Henares Univ, Madrid)
Calcif Tissue Int 52:331–333, 1993   129-94-3–44

Objective.—Several nutritional deficiencies have been reported in osteoporosis, but no studies have assessed the biological markers of nutrition in patients with osteoporosis. The possible existence of nutritional deficiency in patients with postmenopausal osteoporosis was investigated by studying the markers of nutrition.

Methods.—Prealbumin (PAb), retinol binding-protein (RBP), transferrin (TF), and fibronectin were measured in 36 women (mean age, 71 years) with postmenopausal vertebral osteoporosis. For control, 40 healthy women of similar age were also studied.

Results.—Women with vertebral osteoporosis had significantly decreased levels of PAb, RBP, TF, and fibronectin compared with the healthy women. Serum albumin and total body mineral content were significantly lower in patients than in controls. Multiple regression analysis showed a significant correlation between total body mineral content and the biochemical markers of nutrition in the patients with osteoporosis, but not in the control group.

Conclusion.—Postmenopausal osteoporosis may be associated with a nutritional deficiency. Zinc is essential for the synthesis of collagen, albumin and TF, and RBP. Zinc has also been correlated with bone mass and enhances the effect of estrogens on bone. Zinc levels have been shown to be reduced in patients with osteoporosis, and a deficiency of zinc and TF, PAb, and RBP has been shown in diseases featuring osteopenia. Given these data, the deficiency in RBP, PAb, and TF in women with osteoporosis may be secondary to or associated with zinc deficiency.

▶ The study cohort with vertebral osteoporosis was found to have markers for poor nutrition. Patients with postmenopausal osteoporosis may also have nutritional deficiencies.—R. Poss, M.D.

Costs

The Hospital Cost of Total Hip Arthroplasty: A Comparison Between 1981 and 1990

Barber TC, Healy WL (Lahey Clinic, Burlington, Mass)
J Bone Joint Surg (Am) 75-A:321–325, 1993   129-94-3–45

Objective.—Total hip arthroplasty is one of the operations targeted for cost control because of its high cost and the increasing rate at which it is being performed. The changes in hospital costs for this procedure were examined during a 10-year period at the Lahey Clinic.

Methods.—The hospital bills for 44 hip replacements performed in 1981 were compared with the bills for 104 similar operations done in 1990. Each hospital charge was converted to cost using the government-mandated, hospital-specific cost-to-charge ratios. The 2 patient groups were similar in age and diagnosis.

Findings.—Hospital costs for total hip arthroplasty remained quite constant from 1981 to 1990. The inflation-adjusted cost increased only 1.9%, although the actual cost increased 46.5%. During the same period, the consumer price index increased 43.8%. The most marked reduction was in the cost of a patient room, which was 50% of the total cost in 1981 but only 37% in 1990 (Fig 3–11). The cost of using an operating room and that of a hip prosthesis increased. Expenditures for blood

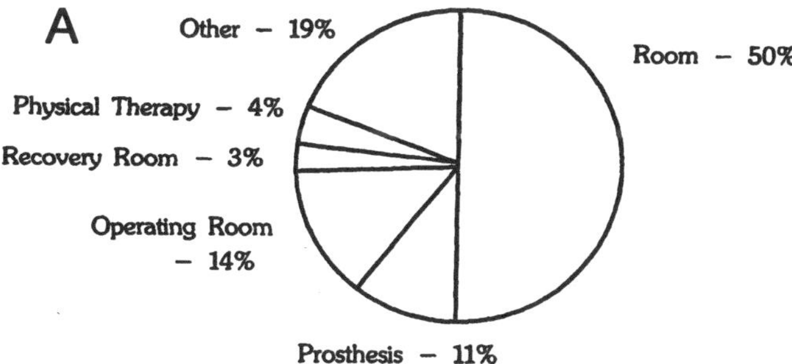

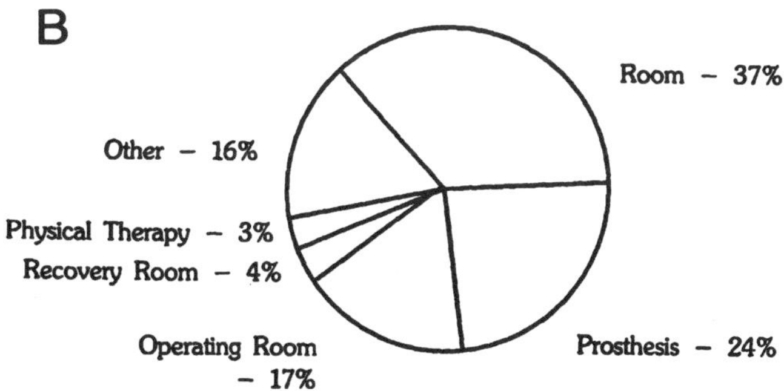

Fig 3–11.—**A,** allocation of costs for total hip arthroplasty in 1981 at the Lahey Clinic. **B,** allocation of costs for total hip arthroplasty in 1990 at the Lahey Clinic. (Courtesy of Barber TC, Healy WL: *J Bone Joint Surg (Am)* 75-A:321–325, 1993.)

products decreased 59% during the interval, and those for radiology services decreased by 36%.

Conclusion.—Hospital costs for total hip arthroplasty were kept under control in the 1980s through a reduced use of hospital resources. To continue this trend in the current decade, it will be necessary to lower the costs of hip prostheses and operative supplies without compromising patient care.

▶ During the past decade, hospital savings associated with total hip arthroplasty have been offset by the unit cost of supplies and the cost of hip prostheses. One seemingly attractive solution to this problem is to use lower-cost, so-called "generic" hips for elderly or less active patients. Before such a strategy can be used, it must be shown to be cost-effective. Currently, our best total hip replacements have an average longevity of 20 years or less, whereas the life span of patients who are currently in their 60s may be more than 20 years. If the cost of hip replacement is looked at globally, the most expensive event is that associated with revision surgery. We must be certain that the prostheses that are used (even in elderly patients) are built to stand the test of time.—R. Poss, M.D.

4 Spinal Disorders

Introduction

For the past five years, I have had the distinct privilege of serving as a reviewer for the YEAR BOOK OF ORTHOPEDICS. Now, I have assumed the duties of Editor-in-Chief for the newly formed *Journal of the American Academy of Orthopaedic Surgeons,* which demands my full attention.

As I look over the progress in the diagnosis and treatment of spinal disorders during the past five years, a number of trends have become evident. The newer imaging techniques, particularly MRI, continue to unveil less common etiologic factors, as well as give information about the often minimal anatomical changes that follow therapeutic interventions such as disk excision. For example, 2 abstracts this year show that many patients with successful results after lumbar disk excision have major residual lesions.

The focus of the literature continues to dwell far more on operative than on nonoperative treatment. In fact, it is a real challenge to find well-designed studies that rigorously evaluate nonoperative treatment, although this is what most of our patients require.

Two techniques continue to receive particular attention—percutaneous diskectomy and internal fixation for spinal fusion, particularly pedicle fixation. Only now are we getting information based on prospective, randomized clinical trials. One article presented here by Revel and co-authors (Abstract 129-94-4–14) shows that percutaneous suction diskectomy has far less efficacy than chymopapain. Although the study has been criticized for its design, it now seems incumbent for others to undertake similar studies. Another article shows fairly clear evidence for enhanced fusion with pedicle fixation. At the same time, the compilation of risks attendant to fixation devices and the less than glowing reports of the clinical outcomes for spinal fusion continue to grow.

In the past, I have noted that in many ways the care of patients with spinal disorders will be shaped less by our technology and more by the events surrounding health care reform. Large databases are being evaluated that give a clearer picture of how often surgery is performed and its attendant risks and complications. Another of these nationally based studies appears in this edition (Abstract 129-94-4–29). This information already is being used in national policy decision-making. This should not be surprising, as spinal disorders have huge costs to society. Although spinal surgeons should hold themselves accountable for the results of their interventions, the biggest factor for these costs—disability—is driven by far more complex societal and legal forces, which the medical profession can influence only at the periphery.

John W. Frymoyer, M.D.

Cervical Spine

TRAUMA

Diagnosis and Etiology

Acute Injuries to Cervical Joints: An Autopsy Study of Neck Sprain
Taylor JR, Twomey LT (Univ of Western Australia, Nedlands; Curtin Univ of Technology, Bentley, Western Australia)
Spine 18:1115–1122, 1993   129-94-4–1

Background.—Pathologic changes in soft tissue associated with neck sprain are difficult to characterize. Standard radiography does not reveal soft tissue injuries, and many neck sprains are symptomatic for more than 2 years despite little or no evidence of organic disease. A comparative autopsy study characterized soft tissue lesions in cervical spines without fractures or dislocations to distinguish typical soft tissue lesions.

Methods.—Sixteen cervical spines from victims of recent trauma were compared with those of 16 subjects who had died of natural causes. Only spines without radiologically visible cervical fractures or dislocations were included; all spines were removed by an experienced postmortem technician.

Results.—Antemortem traumatic lesions were found in 15 spines from victims of major trauma. These spines showed linear clefts within the cartilage plate in an average of 3 affected disks. The linear clefts varied from 3 mm to 2 cm in length, running close and parallel to the vertebral end-plate. The lesions most often affected the disk periphery, near the vertebral rim where the cartilage plate lamellae are continuous with the lamellae of the anulus fibrosus, and resembled lumbar disk "rim lesions." In addition to these lesions, 6 traumatic disk ruptures with posterior herniation, 10 bruises within the outer anulus, and 21 soft tissue synovial joint injuries were found. Most of the synovial joint injuries were hemarthroses from small capsular or synovial tears. Two control spines had a single, apparently long-standing rim lesion in a single disk.

Conclusion.—In this study, rim lesions were strongly associated with trauma, but not with degeneration. These lesions are painful at the time of injury and progress to early disk degeneration, with cleft extension and vascularization. These degenerative changes contribute to chronic pain and dysfunction of the cervical spine.

▶ The quest to establish the pathologic basis for cervical sprains continues. This study provides fairly convincing evidence for a significant soft tissue injury affecting the disks, and the investigators create a plausible set of hypotheses about how the rim lesion could produce acute and continuing symptoms. Of course, there is no way to reconstruct whether or not the autopsied victims had trauma consistent with the more usual vehicular causes of cervical sprain.—J.W. Frymoyer, M.D.

The Etiology of Missed Cervical Spine Injuries

Davis JW, Phreaner DL, Hoyt DB, Mackersie RC (Univ of California, Fresno; Univ of California, San Diego; Trauma Research and Education Found, San Diego, Calif)
J Trauma 34:342–346, 1993   129-94-4-2

Introduction.—Missed or delayed diagnoses of cervical spine (C-spine) injuries may result in paralysis or death. Previous studies of the incidence of missed C-spine injuries have failed to determine the cause of the errors or the extent to which these errors are avoidable. The frequency of delayed or missed diagnoses of C-spine injuries, the frequency of adverse sequelae from these delays, and the factors involved in the diagnostic errors in an organized trauma system were investigated.

Methods.—From August 1985 through February 1991 a total of 32,117 trauma patients were admitted to the 6 centers of the San Diego County Trauma System. The patient data collected included age, gender, mechanism of injury, Trauma Score, Injury Severity Score, level of injury, stability of injury, and neurologic sequelae. All patients who died of their injuries were autopsied. Errors were classified as inadequate standard

TABLE 1.—Distribution of Error Types

Error Type	Number of Errors
Inadequate standard C-spine series	15
Lateral view only	12
Nonvisualization of T-1	2
No cervical roentgenograms in unconscious patient	1
Misread roentgenograms	16
With adequate standard series	8
With inadequate standard series	8
Lateral view only	7
Nonvisualization of C-7–T-1	1
Technically adequate/negative roentgenographic findings	1
Indeterminable	2
Total	34

(Courtesy of Davis JW, Phreaner DL, Hoyt DB, et al: *J Trauma* 34:342–346, 1993.)

TABLE 2.—Complications of Missed Cervical Spine Injuries

Error	Attributed Complication				Total
	Death	Quad/Hemiplegia	Deficit	None	
Inadequate C-spine series	1	1	1	13	17
Misread roentgenograms	1	2	2	10	14
Error in judgment	0	1	0	0	1
Indeterminable	0	0	1	1	2
Totals	2	4	4	24	34

(Courtesy of Davis JW, Phreaner DL, Hoyt DB, et al: *J Trauma* 34:342–346, 1993.)

C-spine series, misread studies, or errors in patients with properly interpreted (negative) radiographs with technically adequate cervical radiographs.

Results.—Injuries to the C-spine were identified in 740 (2.3%) patients. In 34 (4.6%) of these patients the diagnosis was delayed or missed (Table 1). The delays ranged from less than 1 day to 30 days. All patients were significantly injured, most (25) in motor vehicle crashes. The C-spine injuries consisted of 29 fractures and 10 subluxations or dislocations. Most missed injuries were in the lower C-spine and at C2. The dominant error in 15 patients was failure to obtain an adequate standard C-spine series. There were 16 misread roentgenograms, 8 with an adequate standard series and 8 with an inadequate standard series. Two cases of error were classified as indeterminable because the initial roentgenograms could not be located. Missed C-spine injuries resulted in 2 deaths, 4 patients with quadriplegia or hemiplegia, and 4 patients with permanent extremity paresis (Table 2).

Conclusion.—Up to 10% of patients with C-spine injuries arrive intact at the hospital, but deficits occur during the course of their care. All patients at risk for such injuries should have a technically adequate 3-view C-spine series interpreted by skilled reviewers. Had this protocol been followed, delayed diagnosis could have been avoided in at least 31 of these 34 patients.

▶ Diagnostic failures often are not the result of some esoteric problem, but a failure to adhere to fundamental principles. This article clearly shows that failure to detect serious cervical spine injuries occurred when standard radiographs were not obtained in trauma patients. The results were catastrophic for many of these patients.—J.W. Frymoyer, M.D.

Transverse Process Fractures of the Cervical Vertebrae: Are They Insignificant?
Woodring JH, Lee C, Duncan V (Univ of Kentucky, Lexington)
J Trauma 34:797–802, 1993   129-94-4-3

Background.—Transverse process fractures of the cervical vertebrae are considered rare and of little clinical significance. However, recent reports suggest an increasing frequency of significant vascular and neurologic injuries associated with these fractures.

Study Design.—In a retrospective study, the frequency and clinical significance of transverse process fractures of the cervical vertebrae were evaluated among 216 patients seen with 453 proven cervical fractures.

Findings.—Transverse process fractures were seen in 24% of the patients with cervical fractures and accounted for 13.2% of all cervical fractures. All but 1 of the transverse process fractures were identified on CT, but only 7 were detected on plain x-ray films. The fractures occurred most often at C7 and C2 (table) and were associated with other cervical fractures in 82%. Cervical radiculopathy and brachial plexus palsy occurred in 10% of the patients. In 78% of the patients, CT scanning showed that the transverse process fractures extended into the transverse foramen (Fig 4-1). Vertebral angiography showed dissection or occlusion of the vertebral artery in 7 of 8 patients (88%) who had 1 or more fractures of the transverse processes extending into the transverse foramen, including 2 (29%) with clinical evidence of vertebral-basilar artery stroke. There was no apparent difference in the outcome for patients with vertebral artery injury who received anticoagulation and those who did not.

Conclusion.—Transverse process fractures of the cervical vertebra are much more common than previously believed. These fractures appear to be associated with a significant potential for nerve root injury as well as vertebral artery injury among those with fractures that extend into the transverse foramen. However, vertebral angiography should be limited

Anatomical Level of Transverse Process Fractures

Level	Number	Percentage
C1	1	1.6
C2	13	21.6
C3	4	6.6
C4	5	8.3
C5	6	10
C6	10	16.6
C7	21	35
Totals	**60**	**100**

(Courtesy of Woodring JH, Lee C, Duncan V: *J Trauma* 34:797–802, 1993.)

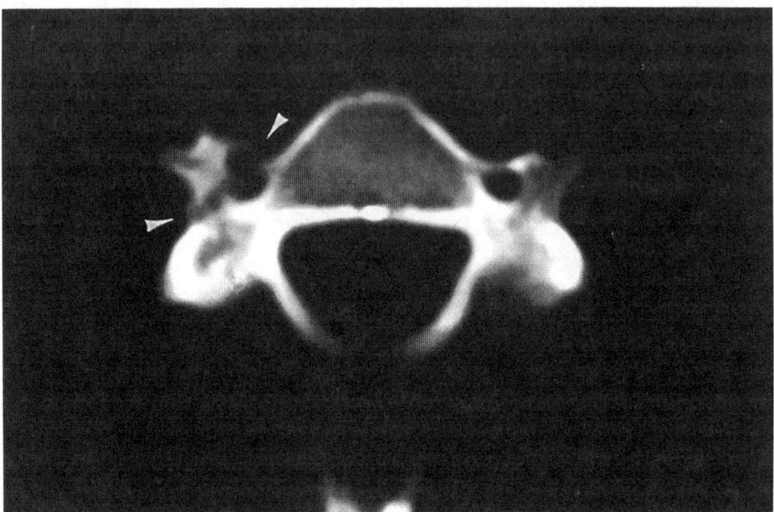

Fig 4–1.—A CT scan of a boy, aged 16 years, with neck pain and tenderness after an automobile crash shows fractures of the anterior and posterior roots (*arrowheads*) of the right C3 transverse process extending into the transverse foramen. Note the sharp edge of the fractured posterior root projecting into the transverse foramen. Vertebral angiography demonstrated occlusion of the right vertebral artery at this level. (Courtesy of Woodring JH, Lee C, Duncan V: *J Trauma* 34:797–802, 1993.)

to patients with fractures extending into the transverse foramen who have signs and symptoms of vertebral-basilar artery stroke.

▶ Based on the question posed by this article's title, the answer is "no." This article shows that transverse process fractures accompanying cervical trauma are common and may be the source of significant symptoms. The most impressive injuries relate to the vertebral artery. The authors speculate but cannot prove that these "incidental" fractures may also be a source of neurologic injury. An important point is that transverse process fractures usually are overlooked on the plain radiographs, but they are evident on well-performed CT scans.—J.W. Frymoyer, M.D.

Treatment and Risks

Magnetic Resonance Imaging Documentation of Coexistent Traumatic Locked Facets of the Cervical Spine and Disc Herniation
Doran SE, Papadopoulos SM, Ducker TB, Lillehei KO (Univ of Michigan, Ann Arbor; Johns Hopkins Univ, Baltimore, Md; Univ of Colorado, Denver)
J Neurosurg 79:341–345, 1993   129-94-4-4

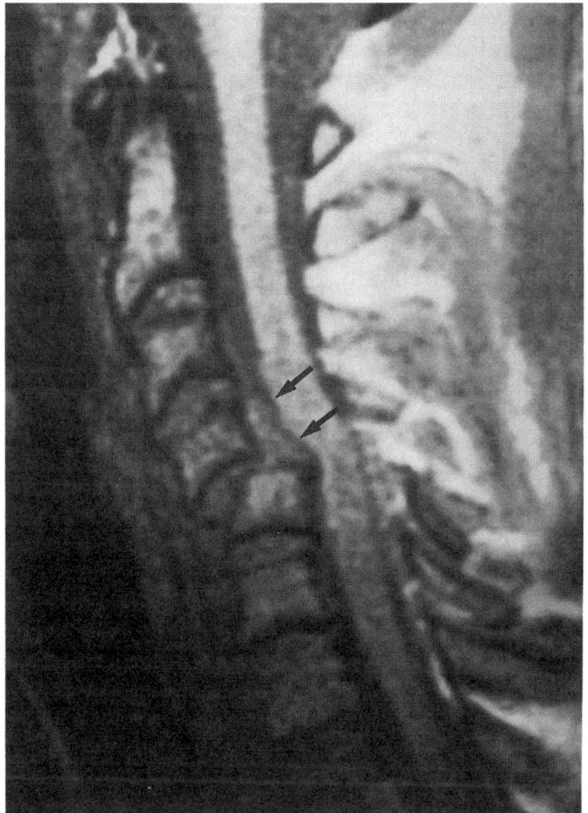

Fig 4–2.—A T1-weighted MR image in a man, aged 19 years, showing a C4–5 unilateral locked facet and concurrent C6–7 disk herniation (*arrows*) before reduction of the locked facets. (Courtesy of Doran SE, Papadopoulos SM, Ducker TB, et al: *J Neurosurg* 79:341-345, 1993.)

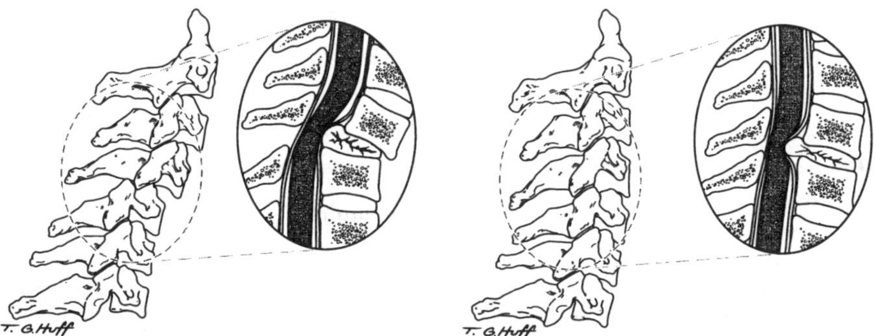

Fig 4–3.—Illustrations showing bilateral locked facets with concurrent disk herniation (**left**) resulting in increased canal compromise after closed reduction (**right**). (Courtesy of Doran SE, Papadopoulos SM, Ducker TB, et al: *J Neurosurg* 79:341-345, 1993.)

Introduction.—Although traumatic locked facets of the cervical spine may coexist with a herniated disk, there have been few reports of this situation. Disk disease in patients with trauma of the cervical spine may be safely and reliably assessed by MRI. Data were reviewed on 13 patients with locked facets of the cervical spine in whom MRI demonstrated a high incidence of associated disk herniation.

Patients.—The 12 male and 1 female patient had a mean age of 31 years. Nine had bilateral and 4 had unilateral locked facets of the cervical spine. The first 9 patients were managed with immediate closed reduction by traction or manipulation, or both. The attempt was successful in only 3 patients. In another 3, it had to be abandoned because of deterioration in neurologic condition. In the last 4 patients, MRI was done before closed reduction was attempted. All patients had MRI at some point, which demonstrated frank disk herniation in 10 patients and pathologic bulging in the other 3. Figure 4–2 shows a prereduction cervical spine x-ray film and the corresponding MRI illustrating frank disk herniation in association with a C4–C5 unilateral locked facet. All patients with frank herniation were managed with anterior cervical diskectomy, followed by reduction of the persistent facet dislocation and anterior fusion or by posterior reduction and arthrodesis. The 3 patients with bulging disks had no significant cord compression.

Conclusion.—For patients with traumatic locked facets of the cervical spine, MRI must be performed during the initial evaluation to look for a herniated disk. For those with an associated disk rupture, closed reduction may increase spinal cord compression and neurologic deficit (Fig 4–3). Patients with a herniated disk should undergo anterior diskectomy and fusion rather than attempted closed reduction or operative posterior reduction.

▶ This article makes a compelling case for MRI before an attempted closed reduction of unilateral or bilateral locked facets, particularly in patients with an incomplete spinal cord lesion. If MRI is not available, it is essential that serial neurologic examinations be performed while closed reductions are being attempted. Any worsening in neurologic status is sufficient reason to abandon the attempted reduction.—J.W. Frymoyer, M.D.

Neurological Complications of the Reduction of Cervical Spine Dislocations

Mahale YJ, Silver JR, Henderson NJ (Stoke Mandeville Hosp, Aylesbury, Buckinghamshire, England)
J Bone Joint Surg (Br) 75-B:403–409, 1993   129-94-4–5

Background.—Traumatic facet dislocation of the cervical spine, regardless of fracture, causes severe neurologic damage. Nevertheless, some patients sustain little or no spinal cord or nerve root damage. Neurologic damage secondary to treatment may cause considerable morbid-

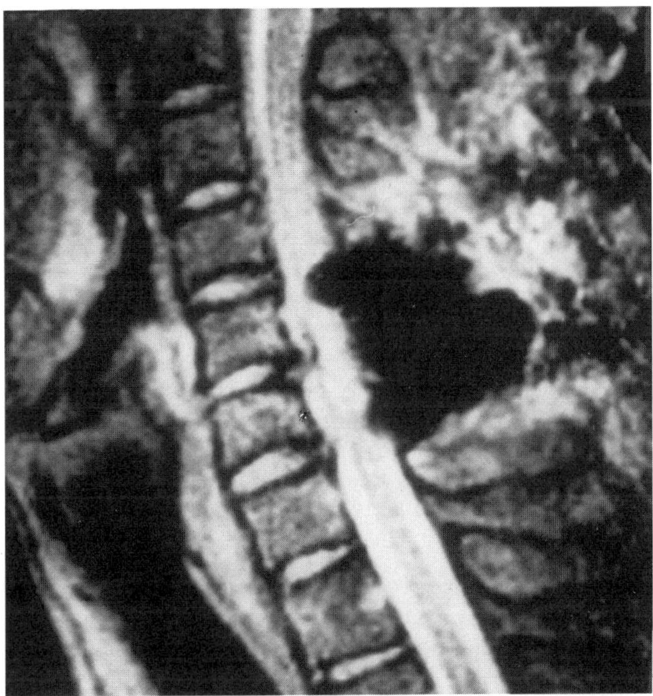

Fig 4–4.—Magnetic resonance image of a 41-year-old man who sustained unilateral facet dislocation at C5–C6 with no neurologic involvement. Operative reduction using Halifax clamps resulted in severe cord involvement. Magnetic resonance imaging at the National Spinal Injury Center revealed a disk prolapse. Treatment was conservative, and there has been slow but incomplete neurologic recovery. (Courtesy of Mahale YJ, Silver JR, Henderson NJ: *J Bone Joint Surg (Br)* 75-B:403–409, 1993.)

ity. The causes of neurologic damage secondary to cervical spinal injury were investigated.

Methods.—The medical records of 16 patients who had cervical spine dislocation with minimal spinal cord involvement and sustained postreduction cord damage were reviewed.

Results.—Before reduction, 8 patients had minimal cord damage; 1 had nerve root palsy; and 2 had transient paralysis. Complete paralysis occurred in 6 patients after reduction and in 1 after manipulation. Additional treatment-related complications included 1 cerebellar infarction and 5 complete sensation-sparing motor paralyses. Radiography revealed 8 bilateral facet dislocations, 5 unilateral dislocations (Fig 4–4), one C1–C2 dislocation secondary to nonunion of a previous odontoid process, and 2 fractures secondary to C2–C3 dislocations. Postreduction radiographs revealed 8 complete reductions, 2 partial reductions, and 2 failures, as well as 2 repeat dislocations and 2 progressions from unilateral to bilateral dislocation or the reverse. Definitive reduction was attempted between 4 and 72 hours after injury in 11 patients, and up to 8 weeks after injury in 5. All patients became paralyzed within 48 hours of the final reduction attempt, although only 5 had immediate neurologic deterioration. After comprehensive rehabilitation, complete recovery was achieved in 5 of 7 patients with complete paralysis and in 3 patients with partial paralysis; recovery was substantial in all 6 with motor paralysis and in 3 of the 4 patients whose dislocations could not be completely reduced.

Conclusion.—Patients with cervical injury should be admitted immediately to specialized centers for appropriate diagnosis and treatment.

▶ This article demonstrates that catastrophic neurologic worsening can follow dislocation of the cervical spine. In this retrospective study, many patients were included whose injury antedated sophisticated imaging. In addition to disk herniation, the investigators speculate that other factors are contributory, including congenitally narrow spinal canal, hematoma, misapplication of skeletal traction, and ischemic damage.—J.W. Frymoyer, M.D.

Internal Fixation

Anterior Cervical Fusion With the Caspar Instrumentation System
Naito M, Kurose S, Oyama M, Sugioka Y (Saiseikai Yahata Hosp, Fukuoka, Japan; Fukuoka Municipal Hosp, Japan; Kyushu Univ, Fukuoka, Japan)
Int Orthop 17:73–76, 1993 129-94-4-6

Background.—Internal fixation of vertebral bodies using plates and screws may prevent complications associated with anterior cervical diskectomy. Excellent stabilization with low morbidity and mortality has been achieved with Caspar's instrumentation system for anterior cervical fixation. The outcomes of 106 patients who underwent anterior cervical fusion with Caspar's instrumentation system were evaluated.

Methods.—All patients had signs of spinal cord compression: 73 had cervical spondylosis; 12 had a traumatic lesion; 9 had ossification of the posterior longitudinal ligament; 6 had cervical disk herniation; and 6 had tumors or other lesions of the cervical spine. Seventy patients were treated using the Smith-Robinson technique. Twenty patients with posterior instability received an additional posterior procedure; 16 underwent adjunctive corpectomy followed by a graft. Postoperatively, each patient was fitted with a soft collar or Somi brace. Follow-up averaged 4.5 years. The Japanese Orthopedic Association "17-point" scoring system, which records neurologic deficits in the arms and legs as well as urinary disturbance, was used for preoperative and postoperative assessments.

Results.—Among the 106 patients, 103 had radiologic evidence of fusion by 5 months (Fig 4–5). The average postoperative point score was 14.1, an improvement of 5 points from the average preoperative score. Ten patients had postoperative complications that required implant removal. In 6 patients, loosening necessitated screw removal. Three of 83

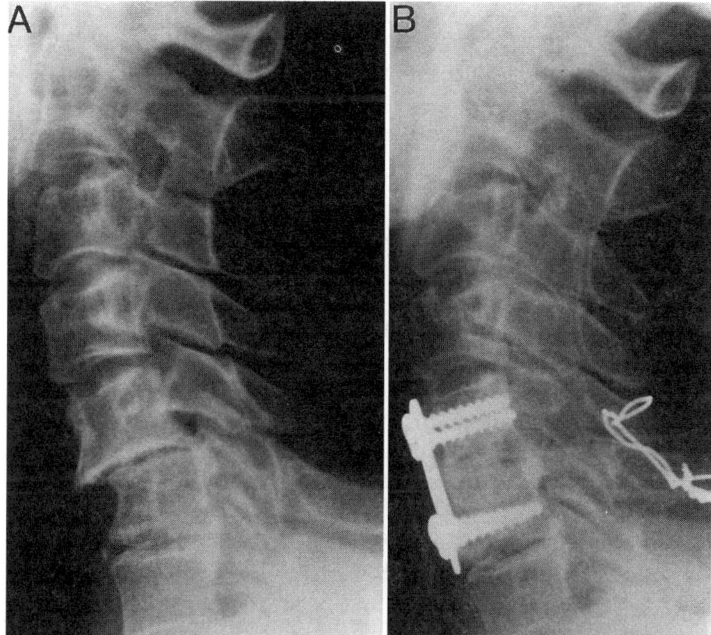

Fig 4–5.—A, C5–C6 subluxation with unilateral locked facets, anterior spinal cord injury, and left C6 radiculopathy in a 44-year-old man. Lateral view of the spine, under skull traction (20 kg), shows C5–C6 subluxation with unilateral locked facets. **B,** radiograph 7 months after anterior cervical fusion with Caspar's plating system in combination with posterior wiring shows solid bony fusion and good alignment. (Courtesy of Naito M, Kurose S, Oyama M, et al: *Int Orthop* 17:73–76, 1993.)

patients with multilevel fusions underwent an additional anterior procedure because of nonunion.

Discussion.—Screw loosening may be a devastating complication of anterior cervical fusion. In this series, 6 of 8 screw loosenings resulted from failure to engage the posterior cortex. To provide maximal stability at the fusion site, screws must engage both the anterior and posterior vertebral body cortices. When care is taken to affix the screws properly, anterior cervical fusion using Caspar's plating system is a good operation for symptomatic cervical instability.

Anterior Cervical Plate Fixation With the Titanium Hollow Screw Plate System

Kostuik JP, Connolly PJ, Esses SI, Suh P (Johns Hopkins Hosp, Baltimore, Md; Toronto Hosp)
Spine 18:1273–1278, 1993   129-94-4–7

Background.—The titanium hollow screw plate (THSP) system was designed for use in mandible reconstruction and has been modified for use in cervical spine surgery. The system uses a conical expansion bolt that locks a cross-split screw into the plate, preventing screw loosening and migration and obviating posterior cortex purchase. The clinical usefulness of THSP in cervical spine stabilization was evaluated.

Patients.—The THSP system was used in 42 patients with disabling cervical spondylosis, cervical myelopathy, recurrent meningioma, ossification of the posterior longitudinal ligament, postlaminectomy cervical kyphosis, post-traumatic instability or cervical kyphosis, acute fracture dislocation, cervical fracture, or C2 nonunion.

Technique.—An anterior Southwick-Robinson approach to the cervical spine is used. A plate is chosen that will allow arthrodesis screw placement in the upper region of the vertebral body. Once the plate is positioned, screw holes are drilled using a guide with a 16-mm stop. The holes are tapped and hollow screws are placed. The screws are locked into place with a conical expansion bolt. Postsurgical immobilization is achieved with either a soft neck roll, Philadelphia collar, or 4-poster cervical orthosis.

Results.—Operative time ranged from 70 to 360 minutes. The average follow-up was 18 months. Fusion was achieved in all patients within a mean of 13 weeks; 1–4 levels were fused. No deaths or neurologic complications occurred, although 3 patients had early, self-limiting persistent dysphagia. Seven hardware-related problems occurred, including broken screws, plate migration, and plate and screw loosening. Three patients had lucency around 1 of the screws at the most recent follow-up, but all achieved solid fusion.

Conclusion.—The THSP system facilitates reliable fusion with minimal complication. Immediate, stable fixation is achieved without risk of posterior cortex penetration. Screw and plate migration occur only with improper screw placement.

Esophageal Penetration by an Anterior Cervical Fixation Device: A Case Report
Yee GKH, Terry AF (John Peter Smith Hosp, Fort Worth, Tex)
Spine 18:522–527, 1993   129-94-4–8

Background.—Supplemental internal fixation with anterior or combined posterior stabilization may prevent graft dislodgement and late angulation after cervical fracture-dislocation repair. Few complications have been reported for anterior cervical plating. A unique complication—migration of a loose screw into the esophagus and through the gastrointestinal tract—was reported.

Case Report.—Man, 24, sustained a flexion compression injury at C5 resulting in complete C6 quadriplegia. The patient underwent a C5 corpectomy and spinal cord decompression with anterior stabilization, autogenous iliac grafting

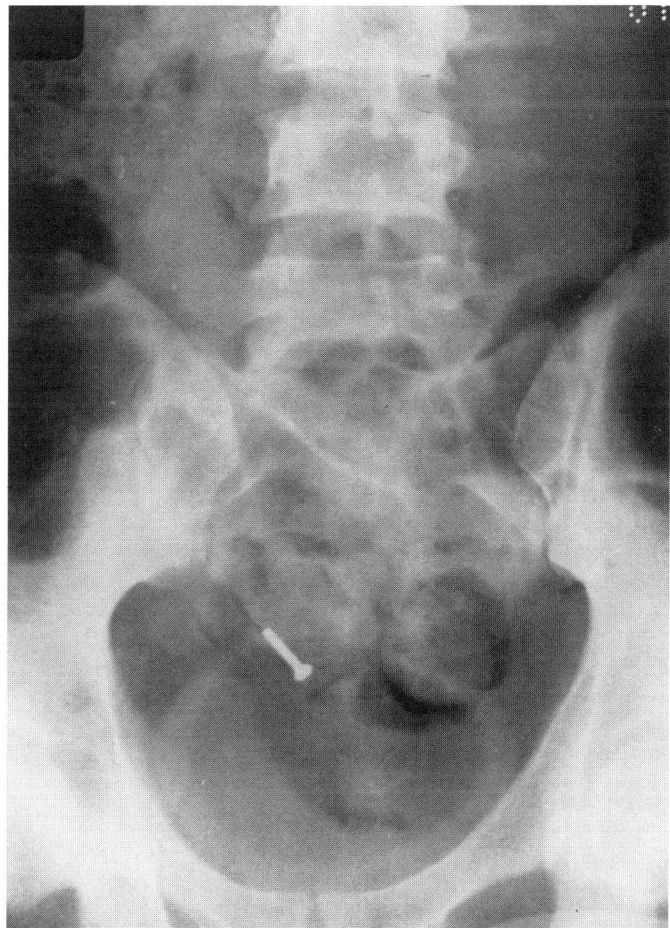

Fig 4–6.—Missing screw in the lower gastrointestinal tract. (Courtesy of Yee GKH, Terry AF: *Spine* 18:522–527, 1993.)

from C4 to C6, and application of an anterior cervical plate from C4 to C7. Three months after injury, the patient had not recovered motor or sensory function. Cervical spine radiographs and tomograms indicated fusion from C4 to C6. However, on subsequent films, 1 screw was missing from the cervical plate. The patient recalled no symptoms; however, a subsequent routine radiograph revealed the screw in the lower gastrointestinal tract (Fig 4-6). The screw subsequently passed without complication.

Discussion.—The principal problem with anterior cervical plate fixation is screw loosening as a result of technical difficulties. In this patient, the loose screw failed to enter the posterior cortex. Apparently, it entered the intervertebral disk instead, an error that could have been prevented with high-quality intraoperative radiography. Esophageal perforation is one of several surgical complications of anterior cervical procedures. The resulting cellulitis may resolve; more commonly, it evolves into a serious infection with 20% to 50% mortality.

Conclusion.—Screw loosening is a complication of anterior cervical plate fixation that may be averted by paying strict attention to the technique of screw placement, depth of screw insertion, and proper postoperative immobilization, if indicated.

▶ There is growing popularity for anterior internal fixation as a method to achieve early stabilization in a variety of degenerative, neoplastic, and traumatic conditions. Enhanced rates of fusion are the suspected outcome, but this benefit has not been proven scientifically. Abstracts 129-94-4–6 and 129-94-4–7 detail the experience with different systems. The Caspar system requires fixation to the posterior cortex. As the authors note, failure to obtain that fixation was the major determining factor in later implant failure. The THSP system overcomes this need and its attendant risks for spinal cord injury by an ingenious screw design. Failures in this patient series related largely to malplacement of screws. Both articles emphasize the risks, particularly esophageal perforation. That such events can occur is demonstrated by Abstract 129-94-4–8, although the outcome was benign. What remains unclear to me is when these devices are clearly indicated and when the risks attendant to their use outweigh the benefits.—J.W. Frymoyer, M.D.

Thoracic Spine

TRAUMA

Conservative Care

Acute Injuries of the Upper Dorsal Spine
Grootboom MJ, Govender S (Univ of Natal, Durban, Republic of South Africa; King Edward VII Hosp, Durban, Republic of South Africa)
Injury 24:389–392, 1993   129-94-4-9

Introduction.—There are few reports in the English literature on the management of injuries of the upper dorsal spine. The records of 50 patients with acute injuries of the upper dorsal spine seen between January 1983 and July 1988 were reviewed.

Clinical Features.—Most of the injuries were caused by road traffic accidents, followed by falls from heights and train accidents. The level of injury varied from T3 to T9. Twenty-nine patients had associated injuries, including 4 that were missed because of coexistent head injury or multiple trauma. Twenty-three patients had neurologic deficits, most of whom had burst fractures and fracture-dislocations.

Treatment/Outcome.—Four patients with partial neurologic deficit underwent anterior spinal decompression and strut grafting. Two patients with significant instability had posterior stabilization and fusion.

The remaining patients were treated conservatively. At follow-up 1–3 years later, only 1 patient, a child with multiple compression fractures initially, had significant deformity. All patients with partial neurologic deficit improved, but none of those with complete neurologic lesions improved. Five patients had significant back pain that required analgesics.

Conclusion.—Most acute injuries of the upper dorsal spine are stable and can be treated without operation. Surgery is indicated in patients with partial neurologic deficit and significant spinal canal compromise or those with significant instability. Children with compression fractures should be followed up until maturity to look for late spinal deformity.

▶ This article is self-explanatory and complimentary to the following article (Abstract 129-94-4–10), which also advocates conservative therapy for the majority of patients with thoracic and thoracolumbar fractures.—J.W. Frymoyer, M.D.

Thoracolumbar Burst Fractures: The Clinical Efficacy and Outcome of Nonoperative Management

Mumford J, Weinstein JN, Spratt KF, Goel VK (Univ of Iowa, Iowa City)
Spine 18:955–970, 1993   129-94-4–10

Background.—Many authors advocate surgical management of a failure of the middle osteoligamentous complex, particularly with retropulsion of fragments into the spinal canal (the burst fracture), but others advocate conservative management by postural reduction and prolonged bed rest. The clinical outcome and efficacy of nonoperative treatment for middle column failure were reviewed on the hypothesis that conservative management yields an acceptable clinical outcome. The remodeling, if any, that occurred in the bony canal was measured by serial CT.

Method.—Forty-one patients with a burst fracture of the thoracolumbar spine at a single level without neurologic deficit were reviewed clinically and radiographically after nonoperative management. The patients were treated with a mean of 4 weeks of strict bed rest, followed by ambulation in a custom-molded, acrylic thoracolumbosacral orthosis (TLSO). Follow-up included neurologic evaluation and a questionnaire on work status, pain location, intensity and interference, disability, and activity. Plain roentgenograms and CT scans were obtained at the time of injury and during follow-up.

Findings.—During an average follow-up of 2 years, 49% of the patients had excellent outcomes relative to pain and function; 17% had good, 22% had fair, and 12% had poor outcomes. Approximately 90% had a satisfactory work status. Progression in body collapse averaged 8% from injury to follow-up, but serial CT showed significant improvement for canal compromise and midsagittal diameter. No patient had canal deterioration over time and only 1 patient had neurologic deterioration requiring surgery. Nearly two thirds of the fragment occluding the canal resorbed, with most remodeling complete within 1 year. Most patients experienced some pain, predominantly back pain, but most were able to perform a majority of basic activities.

Conclusion.—Patients with burst fractures who were neurologically intact were managed with strict bed rest and a custom-molded acrylic TLSO. Results were acceptable for neurologic function, complications, work status, disability, and pain. The incidence of subsequent neurologic deficits was very low. Bony deformity progressed marginally relative to the canal area remodeling. Nearly two thirds of the fragment occluding the canal resorbed, with most remodeling complete within 1 year. There was no correlation between initial severity of injury or residual deformity on radiography and symptoms at follow-up.

▶ The abstract does not capture the complex statistical analyses and the detailed outcome measures used in this study. Further, the article also contains a very complete analysis of radiologic variables at injury and follow-up. The key points to emphasize are that patients entering this study did not have neurologic injuries. This is intriguing given the high prevalence of associated laminar fractures. The subsequent collapse of vertebral body height as measured radiographically averaged 8%.

The authors also performed CT scans, confirming that over time the canal remodels, with resorption of the retropulsed fragments. All of this was accomplished with a reasonable period of hospitalization, and the clinical outcomes were fairly impressive. Obviously, what we now need is a randomized, prospective study comparing nonoperative and operative treatment.—J.W. Frymoyer, M.D.

Operative Complications

CT Analysis of Pedicles and Screw Tracts After Implant Removal in Thoracolumbar Fractures

Sjöström L, Jacobsson O, Karlström G, Pech P, Rauschning W (Univ Hosp, Uppsala, Sweden; Elisabeth Hosp, Uppsala, Sweden)
J Spinal Disord 6:225–231, 1993   129-94-4-11

Background.—Pedicle screw fixation is increasingly popular as a method for spinal fixation. Pedicle screws are not supposed to encroach on the spinal canal, as this presents risks for the dura, spinal cord, and cauda equina. The risk of screw encroachment was examined by studying the pedicles and screw tracts for positioning, lesions, and postoperative changes after the removal of the implant.

Patients.—This patient series was composed of 21 of 22 consecutive patients who underwent surgery for burst fractures of the thoracolumbar junction and had their internal fixation devices removed within 2 years

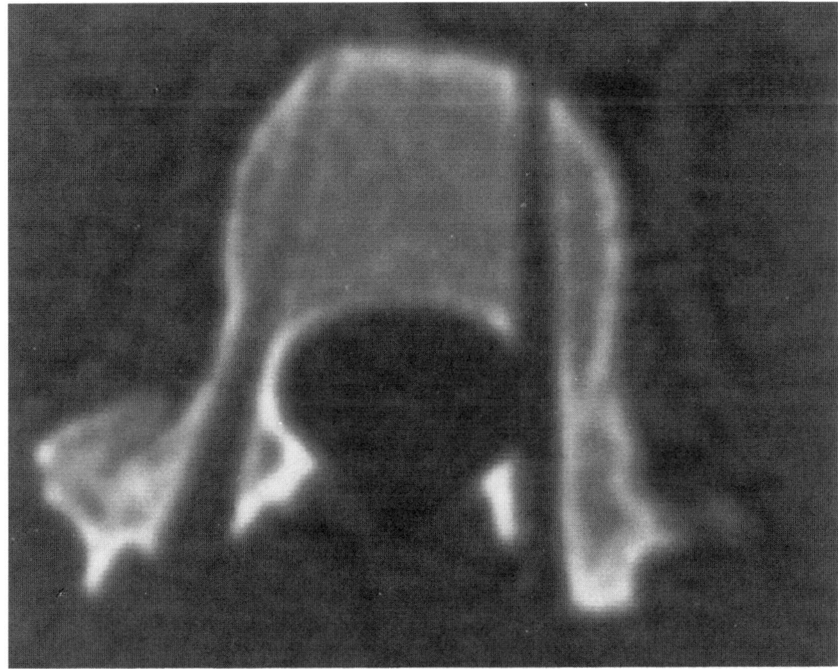

Fig 4–7.—A CT scan of T12 after screw removal in a 19-year-old woman. The left screw caused a medial cortical defect in the pedicle; the screw had encroached 1.5 mm into the spinal canal. The patient had no neurologic symptoms before or after the operation. (Courtesy of Sjöström L, Jacobsson O, Karlström G, et al: *J Spinal Disord* 6:225–231, 1993.)

(Fig 4–7). There were 11 men and 10 women with an age range of 20 to 63 years.

Methods.—A posterior segmental fixator was used for reduction and stabilization of the fracture. Pedicle screws either 5 or 6 mm in diameter were inserted into the pedicles. Axial CT scans were obtained on the second postoperative day of 82 screw tracts in 41 vertebrae.

Findings.—Of the 82 screw tracts examined, 66 were safely within the cortical boundaries of the pedicle. Five screws had caused a pedicle defect without intruding into the spinal canal, and 5 screws had penetrated medially to a maximum of 3.5 mm. Three screws had partly cut off the pedicles laterally and traversed the costotransverse joints. No inferior or superior screw penetrations were detected. Of the 82 screws, 48 had purchase in the vertebral anterior wall, 24 penetrated the cortex, 10 did not reach the wall, 1 had perforated the vertebra laterally, and 23 had perforated anteriorly.

Conclusion.—The use of pedicle screws at the thoracolumbar junction, even by an experienced surgeon, is associated with a risk of misplacement and damage. A mismatch between pedicle dimension and screw size results in pedicle expansion and lateral wall fracture. Preoperative CT examination should be used to choose screws of the appropriate diameter before surgery.

▶ Not all pedicle screws are placed where they belong! Although there are obvious neurologic and potential vascular risks, this high rate of misplacement did not result in any obvious problems for the patients treated.—J.W. Frymoyer, M.D.

Lumbar Spine

EPIDEMIOLOGY/ETIOLOGY

Back Pain in Primary Care: Outcomes at 1 Year
Von Korff M, Deyo RA, Cherkin D, Barlow W (Group Health Cooperative of Puget Sound, Wash; Univ of Washington, Seattle)
Spine 18:855–862, 1993   129-94-4–12

Background.—In primary care, back pain is frequently viewed as either acute or chronic, resolving after a time-limited episode or continuing indefinitely. To date, favorable prognostic estimates have been associated with the typical patient with back pain seen in primary care. However, back pain is often a recurrent problem that is neither acute nor chronic. When viewed as a recurrent illness, back pain prognosis appears less favorable. This study was undertaken to improve understanding of back pain outcomes in primary care patients.

Patients and Methods.—A sample of patients with back pain seen by a primary care physician during a 1-year period (including prevalent and recent-onset patients) was identified. From 3 to 6 weeks after the index visit, eligible individuals were asked to participate in a 30-minute interview. One year after the initial interview, 1,128 patients were reinterviewed by telephone. One-year outcomes were described in terms of characteristic severity of pain and the total days of pain during a 6-month interval. The prognostic value of participant characteristics (age, sex, race, education, and compensation status) and pain characteristics (intensity, disability, days in pain, and onset recency) was evaluated. Pain status improvements were related to changes in depressive symptoms.

Results.—One year after initial care was sought, most recent- and nonrecent-onset patients reported experiencing back pain during the previous month (69% vs. 82%) (Table 1). A significant minority of the recent- and nonrecent-onset patients had either a poor functional outcome (14% vs. 21%) or continued to experience high-intensity pain without substantial disability (10% vs. 16%). Pain-related disability, days in pain, lower educational levels, and female gender were identified as predictors of poor outcome. Fifty percent of the initially dysfunctional patients with persistent pain were improved at the 1-year follow-up, and one third had a good outcome. Table 2 shows the percentage of patients who reported no back pain in the previous 6 months, the median num-

TABLE 1.—Baseline Status and 12-Month Outcome of Primary Care Back Pain: Recent vs. Prevalent Cases

	Recent Onset Cases (N = 177)		Prevalent Cases (N = 889)	
	Baseline	1 Year Follow-up	Baseline	1 Year Follow-up
Pain grade				
0: Pain-free	—	20.9	—	12.2
I: Low disability–low intensity	36.2	54.8	34.7	51.7
II: Low disability–high intensity	22.6	10.2	28.3	15.6
III: High disability–moderately limiting	21.5	6.2	20.5	11.3
IV: High disability–severely limiting	19.8	7.9	16.6	9.2
Days in pain (past 6 mo)				
0	—	21.0	—	12.0
1–30	48.8	43.2	39.8	42.1
31–89	27.3	11.9	18.2	10.1
90+	23.8	23.9	42.0	35.8
Most recent back pain (cumulative %)				
Within 24 hr	—	32.8	—	51.4
Within 1 wk	—	49.8	—	65.5
Within 1 mo	—	69.0	—	82.2

Note: Data were missing for 62 patients. Values are percentages.
(Courtesy of Von Korff M, Deyo RA, Cherkin D, et al: *Spine* 18:855–862, 1993.)

TABLE 2.—Back Pain Outcomes at 1 Year Follow-Up by Baseline Pain Grade and Days in Pain (no. = 1,059)

Baseline Pain Grade	Baseline Pain Days	Pain-Free (%)	Median Pain (days) *	Good Outcome (%)	Poor Outcome (%)	(N)
I	1–30	30.3	8	89.7	2.6	(234)
II	1–30	25.5	7	77.6	6.4	(94)
III + IV	1–30	17.0	21	67.0	17.8	(118)
I	31–89	3.7	25	94.4	1.9	(54)
II	31–89	10.4	14	70.8	10.4	(48)
III + IV	31–89	3.9	30	57.8	34.3	(102)
I	90–180	7.7	100	78.0	13.2	(91)
II	90–180	7.4	150	46.6	20.3	(148)
III + IV	90–180	4.7	125	33.5	49.4	(170)

Note: Data were missing for 69 cases. N values are in parentheses.
* Excluding individuals who were completely pain-free for 6 months.
(Courtesy of Von Korff M, Deyo RA, Cherkin D, et al: *Spine* 18:855–862, 1993.)

ber of back pain days in the previous 6 months, the percentage of patients with a good outcome, and the percentage with a poor outcome. Elevated depressive symptoms returned to normal levels at follow-up among the initially dysfunctional patients who experienced a good outcome.

Conclusion.—In this study, back pain outcomes were predicted by pain-related disability and days in pain rather than by recency of onset. Therefore, it may be more useful to differentiate characteristic levels of pain intensity, pain-related disability, and pain persistence, than to classify patients as either acute or chronic.

▶ The epidemiologic data suggest most patients with low back pain have a satisfactory outcome. In actual practice, I have found significant and continuing back pain to be a major problem, but I always assumed this was because of the selective nature of my practice. This article suggests that the epidemiologic data may be overly optimistic. Most of the predictors of continuing or recurrent difficulty fall into the psychosocial domain. The article reports nothing on diagnosis; however, it is unlikely the majority of these patients had some major structural disorder. A reassuring point is that "Reductions in pain-related disability were accompanied by reductions in psychological distress."—J.W. Frymoyer, M.D.

Epidural Hematoma of the Lumbar Spine: 18 Surgically Confirmed Cases

Gundry CR, Heithoff KB (Ctr for Diagnostic Imaging, St Louis Park, Minn)
Radiology 187:427–431, 1993
129-94-4-13

Background.—Relatively few cases of spontaneous epidural hematoma involving the lumbar spine have been reported. The largest series of surgically proven cases to date was analyzed.

Patients and Findings.—The cases of 18 patients were reviewed. Sixty-seven percent were male. The average patient age was 42 years, with a range of 22–65 years. The mean time from initial presentation to surgery was 230 days. Forty-four percent of the patients had large encapsulated hematomas at the time of surgery (Fig 4–8). Overall, the clinical findings were identical to those of acute disk herniation. Underlying disk abnormalities were common. Seventy-eight percent of the hematomas were related to small concomitant disk herniations or underlying annular tears. Magnetic resonance imaging and CT results were similar to those of extruded/free-fragment disk herniation images.

Conclusion.—Spontaneous epidural hematoma should be considered in patients with acute radiculopathy and imaging studies showing a ventral extradural soft tissue mass, especially if the mass is largest at the mid-vertebral body level. The apparent association between epidural hematoma and underlying disk disruption suggests that spontaneous epidural

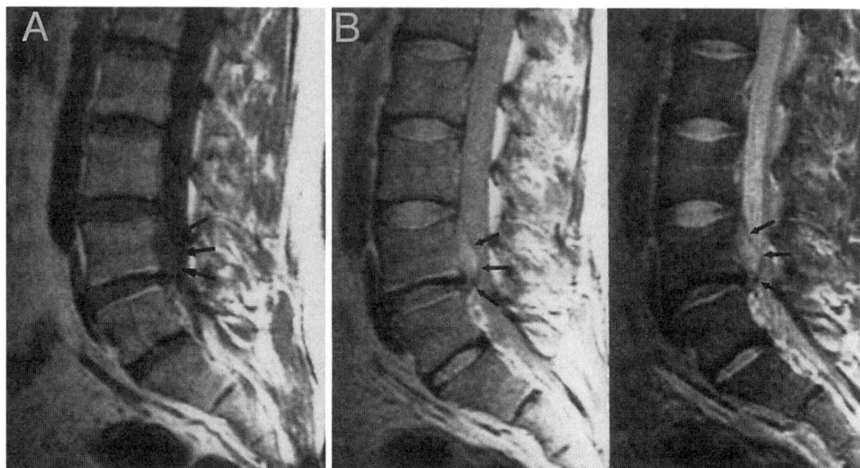

Fig 4–8.—Magnetic resonance images of large cranially dissecting epidural hematoma at the L4 vertebral body level. **A,** sagittal T1-weighted spin-echo image shows a ventral extradural soft tissue mass of relatively low signal intensity that is largest at the midvertebral body level (*arrows*). **B,** sagittal proton-density (*left*) and T2-weighted (*right*) images reveal a cranially dissecting epidural hematoma that compresses the ventral margin of the thecal sac and extends from L4–5 to reach the superior margin of the L4 vertebral body (*arrows*). At surgery, this was noted to represent a large encapsulated epidural hematoma. (Courtesy of Gundry CR, Heithoff KB: *Radiology* 187:427–431, 1993.)

hematomas result from tearing of fragile epidural veins adjacent to the displaced anulus or nucleus.

▶ There is no doubt that the most common cause for lumbar radiculopathy is disk herniation. However, numerous other conditions may mimic this condition, of which spontaneous epidural hematoma is one. In reviewing the authors' cases, there is little in the history or physical examination that differentiates this condition from a typical disk. Therefore, the diagnosis is dependent on careful evaluation of the imaging studies.—J.W. Frymoyer, M.D.

LUMBAR DISK HERNIATION

Surgical Management

▶↓ So you think less is better? Read the following 3 abstracts (Abstracts 129-94-4–14 through 129-94-4–16) and your thinking might change.—J.W. Frymoyer, M.D.

Automated Percutaneous Lumbar Discectomy Versus Chemonucleolysis in the Treatment of Sciatica: A Randomized Multicenter Trial
Revel M, Payan C, Vallee C, Laredo JD, Lassale B, Roux C, Carter H, Salomon C, Delmas E, Roucoules J, Beauvais C, Savy JM, Chicheportiche V, Bourgeois P, Smadja M, Hercot O, Wybier M, Cagan G, Blum-Boisgard C, Fermanian J (Hôpital Cochin, Paris; Hôpital Blaujon, Paris; Hôpital Saint Antoine,

Paris; et al)
Spine 18:1–7, 1993 129-94-4-14

Background.—More than 200,000 patients have been treated via chemonucleolysis since 1964, with a success rate approaching 60% to 70%. However, substantial complications have been reported. In 1975, percutaneous posterolateral intradiskal decompression by partial removal of the nucleus pulposus—percutaneous nucleotomy—was introduced, followed by automated percutaneous diskectomy (APD) in 1985. The latter procedure currently is used worldwide by spinal surgeons and radiologists, and more than 50,000 procedures have been performed to date. However, percutaneous diskectomy has been supported by uncontrolled experiences only, with reported success rates between 29% and 85%. The results of APD were compared with those obtained via chemonucleolysis to assess the relative risks and benefits of each procedure.

Patients and Methods.—A total of 141 patients with sciatica caused by a disk herniation were included in this study. Inclusion criteria comprised a minimum age of 16 years and disk herniation at only 1 vertebral level, verified via CT, MRI, or myelography. In addition, disk herniation had to compress the clinically involved nerve root. Sixty-nine patients were randomly assigned to treatment with APD, whereas the remaining 72 underwent chemonucleolysis. Follow-up was conducted on the day of discharge and at 1, 3, and 6 months after the initial visit. Patients used two 100-mm visual analogue scales to rate the intensity of sciatica and low back pain. Functional impairment was rated using the scales of Waddell and Main. Principle outcome comprised the overall assessment of the patient 6 months after treatment. In addition, patients returned at least 1 year after treatment for examination and lateral roentgenogram.

Results.—Of the 72 patients treated via chemonucleolysis, 61% reported successful results, compared with 44% in the APD group. Subsequent open surgery was performed in 7% of the chemonucleolysis patients and 33% of the APD patients within 6 months of initial treatment. Overall success rates were 66% in the chemonucleolysis patients and 37% in the APD group at 1-year follow-up. The complication rates for each group were low. However, 42% of the chemonucleolysis patients did experience a high rate of low back pain.

Conclusion.—There are no methodological implications that can account for the notably disappointing results obtained with APD. Thus, before APD can be considered a useful intervention, further controlled studies should be conducted. With respect to chemonucleolysis, the results obtained in this study verify those reported in previous investigations.

▶ Percutaneous diskectomy has gained significant popularity for all of the usual reasons (e.g., it may be an outpatient rather than an inpatient procedure, more rapid return to function, fewer complications, etc.). After many years, a randomized, prospective study has been performed comparing automated percutaneous diskectomy with chymopapain, a drug with established therapeutic efficacy. At 1 year, the outcomes for chymopapain were similar to those reported in other prospective, randomized, placebo-controlled trials. In comparison, results using APD were poor. This article is already being criticized for methodological flaws, most notably by those who think the procedure is good. I would submit that the critics need to perform a similar prospective, randomized study. Until they do, they have no leg to stand on, and the current study's conclusion that "the results of our trial suggest that further controlled studies should be carried out before APD can be considered a useful intervention" will stand.—J.W. Frymoyer, M.D.

Does Microscopic Removal of Lumbar Disc Herniation Lead to Better Results Than the Standard Procedure? Results of a One-Year Randomized Study

Tullberg T, Isacson J, Weidenhielm L (St Göran's Hosp, Stockholm; Karolinska Hosp, Stockholm)
Spine 18:24–27, 1993   129-94-4–15

Background.—Standard surgical treatment for intervertebral disk herniation comprises partial hemilaminectomy and partial disk removal, first described in 1934. However, during the past 14 years, a relatively new microsurgical technique has also been used, with good treatment results reported. The clinical results of each surgical approach were compared to determine any differences in either short- or long-term patient outcomes.

Patients and Methods.—A total of 60 patients with CT-verified single-level lumbar disk herniation were included in the study. The patients were randomly assigned to 1 of 2 equal treatment groups. Group 1 underwent surgery via the microscopic technique, and group 2 underwent standard surgical treatment. All operations were performed by the same surgeon, regardless of method. Similar dissection and disk herniation removal methods were used in each group. The smallest possible laminectomy was made, and careful hemostasis was maintained via bipolar diathermy. The average skin incision lengths were 3.5 cm and 7.5 cm in the microsurgical and standard surgical groups, respectively. Patients were followed by an impartial observer at 3 weeks, and at 2, 6, and 12 months. Average patient pain was recorded via a visual analogue scale at each visit, and at 12 months, patient opinion on the surgical result was solicited.

Results.—No between-group differences were noted with respect to perioperative bleeding, complications, inpatient stay, or time off work. In addition, at 12 months, no significant differences in terms of end operative results were noted in either group. Good or satisfactory results were reported by 85% of the patients, which concurred with those of other studies using the standard procedure.

Conclusion.—The decision to use the microsurgical technique should be a matter of personal preference, as no differences in short-term or end-result effects were noted between this method and the standard technique.

Radiographic Changes After Lumbar Discectomy: Sequential Enhanced Computed Tomography in Relation to Clinical Observations
Tullberg T, Rydberg J, Isacsson J (St Görans Hosp, Stockholm; Karolinska Hosp, Stockholm)
Spine 18:843–850, 1993   129-94-4–16

Purpose.—It may be difficult to interpret the radiologic evaluation of a patient with persistent or recurrent symptoms after lumbar diskectomy; it is particularly difficult to differentiate scar tissue from recurrent disk herniation as the cause of radicular leg pain. Data on the radiographic events resulting from disk surgery would be helpful in interpreting the postoperative changes observed and their clinical significance. Serial CT scans were performed to document the course of postoperative disk changes, including the development of scar tissue, and to relate the CT changes to clinical symptoms.

Methods.—The prospective evaluation included 50 patients with single-level disk herniations, all verified by CT. The patients were randomized to undergo either microsurgery or standard surgery. Both groups were followed up postoperatively by contrast-enhanced CT, which was performed during the first postoperative week, after 1–2 months, and after 1 year. Analysis of these images included the measurement of any protrusions and classification of any dural deformation. The patients also were followed clinically by an orthopedic surgeon other than the one who performed the operations.

Results.—None of the patients had any significant leg pain, although 11 had some persistent pain. The CT findings were not significantly related to pain symptoms at any examination. Disk protrusion decreased gradually during follow-up, although 16 patients still had an uneven posterior disk margin at 1 year of follow-up. Dural sac deformation also decreased gradually; at 1 year, no patient had severe deformation but 18 had moderate deformation. Similarly, there were no cases of severe scar tissue, but there were 22 cases of moderate scar tissue at 1 year. Thirteen patients had nerve root displacement at 1 year. The 2 surgical groups were no different in terms of early dural sac formation or in scarring or residual disk herniation at 1 year.

Conclusion.—Sequential CT after lumbar diskectomy reveals that disk protrusion, scar formation, and persistent nerve root displacement are common. However, none of these changes are correlated with the patients' symptoms of leg or back pain. Although some correlations may be detected in a larger group of patients, these findings warrant very careful interpretation of CT findings during the first year after lumbar diskectomy.

▶ Microscopic diskectomy is very popular among some surgeons. The rationale for using it is based on shortened hospital stay, more rapid return to work, and less risk of later scarring. Although the methodology of these studies (Abstracts 129-94-4-15 and 129-94-4-16) could be criticized, they demonstrate little apparent benefit for microscopic diskectomy versus the more traditional approach.

Abstract 129-94-4-16 debunks the notion that less scar formation occurs. The early follow-up CT scans predictably showed little change, but at that interval artifacts are common. At 1 year, scar tissue was present in many patients, but it had no statistical relevance to the clinical outcome. The authors' final admonition that "it is clear that the significance of the postoperative CT findings within 1 year must be regarded with great caution" is important. The same probably can be said for MRI.—J.W. Frymoyer, M.D.

Lumbar Spine Following Successful Surgical Discectomy: Magnetic Resonance Imaging Features and Implications
Deutsch AL, Howard M, Dawson EG, Goldstein TB, Mink JH, Zeegen EH, Delamarter RB (St John's Hosp and Health Ctr, Santa Monica, Calif; Univ of California, Los Angeles)
Spine 18:1054–1060, 1993   129-94-4–17

Introduction.—Few studies have sought to establish the various long-term imaging findings that might be seen in patients after successful lumbar disk surgery. Such information would be useful in patients with persistent or recurrent symptoms. The preoperative and long-term (greater than 1 year) postoperative studies were compared in a group of patients whose surgery was unequivocally successful.

Patients and Methods.—Twenty-three patients, 15 men and 8 women (mean age, 39 years) took part in the study. All had preoperative MRI and were willing to return for a follow-up MRI examination. The patients had undergone surgery at least 1 year before study entry, had experienced pain relief and returned to their presymptomatic functional status, and required no medication for back or leg pain since the time of surgery. Preoperative and postoperative MRI examinations were reviewed by musculoskeletal radiologists who were experienced in spinal imaging. Items of interest were size of disk herniation; thecal sac effacement; nerve root enlargement or displacement; and disk signal intensity. Patients were graded according to the changes in the size of focal convexities in the outer disk contour observed at follow-up.

Results.—The postoperative images of 8 patients (9 disk levels) demonstrated a 75% to 100% diminution in size of the soft focal tissue mass in direct continuity with the disk; the decrease ranged from 25% to 75% in 11 patients (13 disk levels) and was less than 25% in 3 patients. Thus, some patients with a successful outcome had a total resolution of disk herniations, some had moderate but persistent posterior contour defects, and a few showed virtually no change in the apparent contour of the posterior disk margin. Gadolinium contrast examinations demonstrated enhancement of the persistent contour abnormalities in 18 of 19 disk levels, indicating the common presence of fibrosis after successful diskectomy.

Conclusion.—Long-term follow-up imaging studies of patients who have had successful diskectomy are likely to show localized disk contour abnormalities suggestive of recurrent disk herniations. The nature of the material producing the soft tissue masses has yet to be determined, but these findings underscore the importance of factors other than mechanical compression in the production of back pain.

▶ Persistent residual lesions were identified in a significant proportion of patients, all of whom had excellent results after operation. Like the previous abstract (Abstract 129-94-4-16), their observations beg the question, "What are the physiologic and anatomical reasons that disk excision is successful?" —J.W. Frymoyer, M.D.

SPINAL STENOSIS

Conservative Care

Lumbar Spinal Stenosis: Clinical/Radiologic Therapeutic Evaluation in 145 Patients: Conservative Treatment or Surgical Intervention?
Onel D, Sari H, Dönmez Ç (Univ of Istanbul, Turkey)
Spine 18:291–298, 1993   129-94-4-18

Background.—The term lumbar spinal stenosis (LSS) is used to define any condition involving any type of narrowing of the spinal canal, nerve root canals, or tunnels of intervening foramina. It can be classified into 2 categories—congenital or developmental, and acquired. The most prominent clinical sign in LSS is neurogenic claudication, which is defined by pain, aching, and cramping associated with paresthesias in the lower limbs on walking or exercise in the erect position. Impotence, incontinence, or cauda equina may be present. Conservative therapy usually is tried, unless progressive neurologic muscle weakness or symptoms of neurogenic bladder and bowel are evident. Surgery may be performed for relief of pain and the preservation or restoration of neurologic function. In a prospective study, the results of conservative treatment of LSS were evaluated with clinical, radiologic, and CT findings.

Method.—A total of 145 patients with LSS were evaluated by detailed locomotor and neurologic examinations, routine laboratory tests, lumbosacral roentgenograms, and CT scans. Clinical parameters of pain on motion, lumbar range of motion, straight leg raising test, deep tendon reflexes, dermatomal sensations, motor functions, and neurogenic claudication distances were measured at baseline and after completion of conservative therapy. Patients were hospitalized for 1 month and treated with 100 IU of synthetic salmon calcitonin (s-CT) every day for 5 days and every other day for the following 3 weeks; calcium salts were administered daily. They also underwent daily infrared heating, ultrasonic diathermy, and flexion and extension exercises.

Results.—At admission, all the patients had pain on motion and neurogenic claudication, 77% had restriction of extension, 23% had limited straight leg raising, 47% had dermatomal sensory impairment, 29% had motor deficit, and 40% had reflex deficit. With the exception of reflex deficits, all clinical parameters were significantly improved after conservative therapy.

Conclusion.—In 145 patients evaluated for lumbar spinal stenosis, conservative therapy significantly improved all clinical parameters except reflex deficits. In patients with LSS, surgery is indicated for intolerable pain or for the preservation or restoration of neurologic function. In other cases, conservative therapy combining medical and physical therapy should be tested before surgical intervention is undertaken.

▶ Anyone who wants to achieve some balance between conservative and operative interventions for spinal stenosis has to scramble to find any meaningful literature on nonoperative management. This article gives a very short outcome (1 month) for a hodgepodge of conservative techniques, many of which are of dubious value (e.g., ultrasound, diathermy, calcium salts, exercises, etc.). As a result of (or in spite of) therapy, most of the patients improved, as assessed by some fairly objective criteria. Obviously, a longer study is necessary to determine whether patients maintain the improvement. However, the article is one of few addressing the nonoperative issues in a growing segment of patients seeking spinal care.—J.W. Frymoyer, M.D.

Complications of Operative Care

Spondylolysis After Posterior Decompression of the Lumbar Spine: 35 Patients Followed for 3–9 Years
Suzuki K, Ishida Y, Ohmori K (Nagoya Daini Red Cross Hosp, Japan)
Acta Orthop Scand 64:17–21, 1993   129-94-4–19

Background.—Acquired spondylolysis has been reported as a postoperative complication after spinal fusion, but it has not been reported after posterior decompression without spinal fusion. The incidence of spondylolysis after posterior decompression without spinal fusion and possible causative factors were investigated.

Method.—Radiographs were examined from 35 patients who underwent posterior decompression without lumbar spinal fusion. None of the patients had spondylolysis in the segments before surgery. The segmental range of motion, the width of decompression, and the degree of vertebral slippage of each vertebra corresponding to the lamina operated upon were measured.

Findings.—Spondylolysis was found in 10 of the 35 patients who had posterior decompression without fusion of the lumbar spine. Four of the patients had undergone conventional laminectomy and 6 had been treated with suspension laminotomy. The patients with postoperative spondylolysis had greater vertebral slippage than those without. The mean number of laminae operated upon was 3.3 in patients with spondylolysis and 2.4 in patients without. The percentage of decompressed width in laminae was 85% with spondylolysis and 56% without spondylolysis.

Conclusion.—These findings suggest a causal relationship between acquired spondylolysis and the extent of decompression, perhaps because of weakened pars interarticularis. Excessive bony decompression may cause postoperative spondylolysis after posterior decompression without spinal fusion.

▶ Instability after extensive lumbar decompression can be a source of failure. Of the various risk factors, the extent of decompression is most important and may be associated with later acquired spondylolisthesis and fractured facets. The authors describe a much higher prevalence of acquired spondylolysis, with or without later slip, than previously described. The most predictive factor was the extent of the laminectomy. Why the authors found such a high prevalence is uncertain. They suggest it is overlooked because oblique films are not obtained. Like many radiologic abnormalities identified after surgical interventions, the presence of spondylolysis was not usually associated with symptoms. This leads me to conclude that oblique films need not be part of the follow-up films, unless the patient is experiencing symptoms.—J.W. Frymoyer, M.D.

Long-Term Results

Long-Term Results of Surgical Treatment of Lumbar Spinal Stenosis
Herno A, Airaksinen O, Saari T (Kuopio Univ Hosp, Finland)
Spine 18:1471–1474, 1993   129-94-4–20

Background.—To date, little information regarding the long-term outcome of laminectomy for lumbar canal stenosis exists. In this longitudinal study, the Oswestry questionnaire was used to determine alterations in subjective disability in patients who had undergone surgery for lumbar spine stenosis during mean follow-ups of 7 and 13 years.

Patients and Methods.—A total of 108 patients, 50 women and 58 men, were included in this study. All patients underwent initial surgery during 1974–1981. Clinical diagnoses of stenosis were verified primarily by myelography. The mean patient age at surgery was 50.7 years. Most patients underwent surgery for disabling leg pain, progressively limited walking distances, or standing endurance. The surgical procedure was a bilateral laminectomy extended laterally to decompress the nerve roots. In most instances, lateral decompression was accomplished via partial facetectomy, although when necessary, the entire facet was removed. No fusions were performed. The Oswestry questionnaire was completed in both 1985 and 1991 by all 108 patients, at a mean follow-up of 6.8 and 12.8 years, respectively. Evaluations of surgical results were based on subjective disability and were graded as excellent, good, poor, or very poor.

Results.—In 1985, the mean subjective disability was 34.5. In 1991, the mean score was 30.2. Men demonstrated greater improvement than women. In the good-to-excellent disability category, the mean value for men was significantly improved, whereas no improvement was noted for women. In 1985, the mean proportion of good-to-excellent results was 66.7% for all patients. In 1991, those same outcomes were 69.4%. No differences in outcomes were noted with respect to whether patients were older or younger than 50 years at the time of surgery. Both groups showed significant improvement during follow-up. From 1985 to 1991, the subjective disability remained unchanged in 56.5%, improved in 26.9%, and worsened in 16.7% of the patients. During the study, 10 patients underwent repeat decompression because of symptom recurrence and concordant findings at caudography. Repeat surgery was done an average of 7.5 years after the initial operation. In 35 patients with coexisting illness before initial surgery, significant improvement was not noted.

Conclusion.—Overall, patient outcomes improved during the course of the longitudinal follow-up of 7 and 13 years. The incidence of reoperation after initial surgery for lumbar spinal stenosis is low.

▶ The long-term results of decompressive laminectomy for spinal stenosis continue to be debated. This article presents a fairly extensive, long-term surveillance of a sizable cohort, none of whom had spinal fusion. Unlike an earlier article by Katz et al. (1), the results did not deteriorate with time as measured by a variety of functional criteria, nor was advanced age an adverse selection criterion. Like Katz, these authors found that co-morbidities were associated with poorer results.—J.W. Frymoyer, M.D.

Reference

1. Katz IN, et al: *J Bone Joint Surg (Am)* 73-A:809, 1991.

Spinal Fusion

Patient Selection

▶↓ The following 3 articles (Abstracts 129-94-4–21 through 129-94-4–23) attempt to answer the question, "Can we improve on the selection criteria to determine which patients will have a successful outcome from spinal fusion?" None of them are "high science," and the validity of their conclusions are debatable.—J.W. Frymoyer, M.D.

The Value of Facet Joint Blocks in Patient Selection for Lumbar Fusion
Esses SI, Moro JK (Univ of Toronto)
Spine 18:185–190, 1993   129-94-4–21

Purpose.—The association between patient response after the injection of local anesthetic into selected lumbar facet joints and patient outcome after surgical arthrodesis of selected lumbar spine levels was determined.

Patients and Methods.—During a 9-year period, 296 patients with mechanical, activity-related low back pain underwent facet block procedures. Spinal deformities, neoplasia, or significant trauma were not noted in any patient. A 20- or 22-gauge needle was inserted into specific facet joints under fluoroscopic guidance, and a total of 1.5 cc of local anesthetic was injected into each joint. Aseptic technique was used during each procedure. Pain response was evaluated between .5 and 3 hours after injection.

Results.—Of the original 296 patients, 126 were available for full interviews, comprising 50 men and 76 women. The mean time between facet joint block and follow-up was 4.7 years, and mean follow-up time from treatment was 4.6 years. One-, 2-, and 3-level facet joint blocks were performed in 27, 85, and 10 patients, respectively. Records of facet joint blocks were unavailable in the remaining 4 patients. Full pain relief, defined as complete absence of pain for at least 15 minutes postinjection, was achieved in 19 patients. Fifty-two patients experienced partial pain relief, defined as incomplete but significant relief of pain. The remaining 55 patients did not experience any pain relief. Eighty-two patients underwent subsequent single- or multiple-level lumbar fusion operations, which comprised the first low back operation for 52 patients. Laminectomy, diskectomy, or fusion at other levels had been performed previously in 30 patients. Nonsurgical treatment was undertaken in 35 patients, and 9 patients chose not to have any therapeutic intervention. At follow-up, treatment outcome was good in 37, poor in 25, and unimproved in 20 of the 82 surgical patients. Of the 44 patients with nonoperative intervention, outcome was good in 14, poor in 17, and unimproved in 13. After statistical analysis, no significant correlation between the facet block results and surgical and nonsurgical treatment outcomes was noted.

Conclusion.—Because they cannot predict either surgical or nonsurgical success, it is concluded that lumbar facet joint injections should not be used to determine appropriate patient treatment.

▶ Again, facet blocks seem to have little value (in particular, no prognostic value) in determining the outcomes of spinal fusion. The results also call into question the overall efficacy of fusion, particularly when return to work is an outcome measure. Of the 82 surgical patients, 71 were employed before surgery, 27 of whom remained employed.—J.W. Frymoyer, M.D.

Use of the Pantaloon Cast for the Selection of Fusion Candidates in the Treatment of Chronic Low Back Pain
Rask B, Dall BE (Michigan State Univ, Kalamazoo)
Clin Orthop 288:148–157, 1993   129-94-4–22

Background.—It is well established that lateral spinal fusion can be effective in relieving pain-producing instability. However, of the 2.6 million individuals with chronic low back pain, it is difficult to determine whom it may best serve. Temporary lumbosacral stabilization with a cast was used to determine individuals whose symptoms might be caused by lumbar segmental instability. Lateral fusions were subsequently performed on selected patients.

Patients and Methods.—A total of 45 patients with low back pain of at least 6 months' duration were included in this study. Neurologic motor deficits were not noted in any patient, and all were refractory to conservative treatment. Each patient was fitted with a fiberglass pantaloon cast, covering the nipples to the waist and extending over 1 leg to the knee, and all patients were advised to return for cast removal in 2–4 weeks. Lateral, intertransverse process fusion with iliac bone grafts was subsequently performed in patients who had passed the cast trial, in whom pain returned after cast removal, and in whom the levels for fusion were determined via a facet block or a normal saline acceptance test.

Results.—Thirty-one patients experienced significant pain relief while in the pantaloon cast. Of these, 23 were treated via spinal arthrodesis. After an average follow-up of 14 months, 17 of the surgically treated patients reported significant pain relief. The remaining 8 patients did not receive subsequent fusion for various reasons. Of these, 2 patients reported continued pain relief, and 2 others reported improvement in function at an average of 9.4 months after the cast trial.

Conclusion.—In patients with chronic low back pain, the pantaloon cast may be effective in identifying those who could benefit from spinal stabilization procedures.

▶ The experimental design of this study is not great. However, given the choice between pedicle fixation and pantaloon spica, most of our patients would be wise to choose the spica.—J.W. Frymoyer, M.D.

External Transpedicular Fixation Test of the Lumbar Spine Correlates With the Outcome of Subsequent Lumbar Fusion
Soini J, Slätis P, Kannisto M, Sandelin J (Orthopaedic Hosp of the Invalid Found, Helsinki; Kapyla Rehabilitation Ctr, Helsinki)
Clin Orthop 293:89–96, 1993   129-94-4-23

Background.—Both external and internal transpedicular spine fixation are widely used to treat unstable conditions of the spine. A series of patients with chronic back pain underwent a transpedicular lumbar fixation test. Patients were subsequently treated with anterior interbody fixation and were evaluated for no less than 2 years after surgery. The results of treatment were reported.

Patients and Methods.—During a 3-year period, 42 patients underwent testing via temporary external fixation of the lower lumbar spine, caused by chronic low back pain and obvious or strongly suggested radiographic evidence of lower lumbar segment instability. Testing aims included realignment of the involved segments, restoration of disk height, and (when applicable) consideration of subsequent anterior interbody spondylodesis of the affected segments. All tests were performed with a Magerl external fixator and took place during a period of 1–3 weeks. Pain was recorded using a visual analogue scale, and performance was evaluated via the Oswestry disability score. Of those tested, 13 did not experience noticeable pain reduction. The remaining 29 patients (including 12 women and 10 men with a mean age of 43 years) had marked pain relief, improved performance, and good radiographic spinal realignment. These individuals underwent subsequent anterior interbody fusion of the lumbar spine shortly after test completion. Lumbar spine instability was caused by failed disk surgery in 17, spondylolisthesis in 3, and degenerative disk disease in 2 patients who had not undergone previous surgery. Surgery had been performed once in 2, twice in 11, 3 times in 4, and 4 times in 3 patients.

Results.—Twenty-two of the 29 patients completed follow-up examinations for at least 2 years. Nine patients were completely pain-free after 1 year, and 12 patients experienced improvement. The remaining patient was worse after surgery. After 2 years, the same 9 patients remained pain-free, and one third of the patients had returned to work. Pain perception was less incapacitating, and performance levels remained significantly better than before transpedicular fixation testing. The testing results appeared to predict the outcome of lumbar fusion.

Conclusion.—In patients who are being considered for spondylodesis, the temporary external fixation test may be a useful procedure for outcome predictions.

▶ The debate goes back and forth. I would not recommend that this technique be used for anything other than experiments. Like the pantaloon cast study (Abstract 129-94-4-22), this study suggests that a favorable response to immobilization may influence the later outcome of a surgical intervention.—J.W. Frymoyer, M.D.

Benefits of Internal Fixation

A Prospective, Randomized Study of Lumbar Fusion: Preliminary Results

Zdeblick TA (Univ of Wisconsin, Madison)
Spine 18:983–991, 1993   129-94-4-24

Background.—The increased complication rates of pedicle screw fixation systems necessitate that the advantages in using such systems outweigh the risks. The fusion rate and clinical outcome differences in patients with degenerative lumbar spine disorders treated with posterolateral fusion without instrumentation, with semirigid instrumentation, and with a rigid instrumentation system were determined.

Patients and Methods.—A total of 124 patients undergoing lumbar or lumbosacral fusion for various degenerative problems were included in this prospective study. Patients were randomly placed in 1 of 3 treatment groups, including posterolateral fusion using autogenous bone graft (group 1); autogenous posterolateral fusions supplemented with a semirigid pedicle screw/plate fixation system (group 2); or posterolateral autogenous fusion with a rigid pedicle screw/rod fixation system (group 3). The same surgeon operated on all patients, and an identical bone grafting technique was used in each instance. All patients underwent identical postoperative treatment. Anteroposterior, oblique, and flexion-extension radiographs were taken at 1 year to determine fusion status. The average follow-up was 16 months.

Results.—One patient was lost to follow-up, leaving 51 patients in group 1, 35 in group 2, and 37 in group 3. Overall fusion rates comprised 65%, 77%, and 95% for groups 1, 2, and 3, respectively. When compared with that of groups 1 and 2, the increased fusion rate in group 3 was significant. Excellent clinical results, defined as pain-free patients who had returned to work, were noted in 49%, 60%, and 70% of groups 1, 2, and 3, respectively. Good clinical results, defined as patients with mild backaches requiring non-narcotic analgesics who had returned to work, were found in 22%, 29%, and 24% of groups 1, 2, and 3, respectively. Fair results, defined as patients with continuing back pain preventing a return to work, were noted in 29%, 11%, and 5% of groups 1, 2, and 3, respectively. Finally, poor results, defined as patients with worse postoperative pain or patients needing revision surgery, were noted in 8% of group 1, and in 2 of group 2 and none 3 patients. In all 3 groups, fusion rates were lower for smokers than nonsmokers, at rates of 53%, 73%, and 87% for smokers, compared with 69%, 80%, and 100% for nonsmokers in groups 1, 2, and 3, respectively. No infections or neurologic deficits occurred.

Conclusion.—Rigid pedicle screw/rod fixation resulted in a significantly higher rate of fusion in degenerative lumbar disease compared with fusion without instrumentation. However, follow-up is currently short-term. Long-term results will be necessary to fully quantify the effects of rigid instrumentation, particularly with respect to the rate of degeneration at adjacent segments, the incidence of hardware failure, and the necessity for revision surgery.

▶ This is the first study I have seen that prospectively and randomly looks at the effect of fixation on lumbar spinal fusion in human beings. It confirms the earlier experimental data of enhanced fusion with rigid fixation but, as the author points out, does not answer the longer-term issues. Perhaps a more subtle but important message was that the rate of fusion was even more significantly influenced by the smoking status of the patient than by the use of fixation. This is an area that is not influenced by the Food and Drug Administration.—J.W. Frymoyer, M.D.

Reflex Sympathetic Dystrophy After Operative Procedures on the Lumbar Spine
Sachs BL, Zindrick MR, Beasley RD (New England Med Ctr, Boston; Hinsdale, Ill; Concord Hosp, NH)
J Bone Joint Surg (Am) 75-A:721–725, 1993   129-94-4–25

Background.—Reflex sympathetic dystrophy is an unusual complication after surgery on the lumbar spine. The constellation of symptoms includes a painful lesion; an abnormal autonomic reflex rather than a normal sympathetic reflex; and a diathesis, or unusual susceptibility. Carlson et al. hypothesized that motion between the fourth and fifth lumbar segments is associated with an inciting painful stimulus. This report described the occurrence of reflex sympathetic dystrophy in 11 patients after an operation on the lumbar spine and presented the results of treatment.

Patients.—The patients ranged in age from 28 to 60 years, with an average age of 44 years. They underwent a posterior operation on the lumbar spine for lumbar spondylolisthesis or lumbar instability associated with degenerative disk disease or with osteoarthritis of a facet joint. Surgery included at least the level between the fourth and fifth lumbar vertebrae. Ten patients had posterior stabilization with bilateral arthrodesis and interpedicular fixation, with use of plates or screws. One patient had a posterior hemilaminotomy of the fourth and fifth lumbar vertebrae, partial diskectomy, and foraminal decompression of the fifth lumbar nerve root. The symptoms of burning pain, vasomotor dysfunction, and dystrophic changes in the lower limb and foot began 4 days to 20 weeks after surgery. Four patients had bilateral symptoms.

Treatment.—All of the patients had aggressive physical therapy with active and passive range-of-motion exercises of all joints of the lower extremities. Six patients had at least 1 sympathetic nerve block that completely resolved the symptoms in 4 patients. One patient had improvement initially, but slight, persistent pain developed in the lower limb after 10 months. Another patient had no improvement.

Conclusion.—Reflex sympathetic dystrophy is an unusual and rare physiologic response of the autonomic nervous system to a persistent, painful lesion. In 11 patients, reflex sympathetic dystrophy occurred after a posterior operation of the lumbar spine, with symptoms beginning 4 days to 20 weeks after the operation. The constellation of symptoms included burning pain, vasomotor dysfunction, and dystrophic changes in the leg and foot. The most successful treatment was a nerve block of the sympathetic lumbar trunk in addition to physiotherapy.

The Treatment of Chronic Extremity Pain in Failed Lumbar Surgery: The Role of Lumbar Sympathectomy

Wetzel FT, LaRocca SH, Adinolfi M (Pennsylvania State Univ, Hershey)
Spine 17:1462–1468, 1992   129-94-4–26

Background.—Persistent lower extremity pain after failed lumbar surgery may disable patients. Attempts to treat this condition, a chronic radiculopathy, have largely failed. Rhizotomy has produced inconsistent results, and ganglionectomy has not been reliably effective. Chemical deafferentation has proved effective in some instances. The possibility of isolating a reversible component of chronic extremity pain seems attractive.

Objective and Methods.—The frequency of vasomotor symptoms in these patients prompted a study of autonomic function in 17 who had continued to have chronic extremity pain after lumbar surgery. These patients underwent lumbar sympathectomy after an average of 5 previous operations, and they were followed up for at least 2 years afterward. In addition to electromyography and nerve conduction studies, thermography was carried out.

Findings.—Eight of the patients had thermographic findings consistent with autonomic dysfunction. Eight others had mixed findings of autonomic dysfunction and root irritation, and 1 had root irritation only. Sympathetic blockade provided at least partial relief in all patients. Six patients had a satisfactory clinical result at 6 weeks, but in 11 others the outcome was unsatisfactory. The results were comparable after 1 year, but only 2 patients were considered to be clinical successes at 2 years. At

1 year, patients with thermographic findings of autonomic dysfunction were more likely to have a good outcome than those with an element of root irritation, but subsequently no such difference was apparent.

Conclusion.—Surgical sympathectomy has only a limited role in patients who have persistent chronic extremity pain after lumbar surgery.

▶ We have all encountered patients with chronic, burning dysesthetic pain and vasomotor and dystrophic changes after lumbar spine surgery, most often after multiple operations. The first article (Abstract 129-94-4-25) suggests that L4–5 is most often the offending level, but it does not offer any predictable therapy. The authors of Abstract 129-94-4-26 "took the bull by the horns" and performed lumbar sympathectomy after a comprehensive evaluation. Their conclusion is a lesson in stark reality. As one looks over the sagas contained in these detailed case histories, it is natural to ask, "Would these patients have been better off had they never seen a surgeon?"—J.W. Frymoyer, M.D.

Complications/Prevention

A Multicentric Retrospective Study of the Prevention of Thromboembolic Complications After Lumbar Discectomy

Desbordes JM, Mesz M, Maissin F, Bataille B, Guenot M (CHRU Jean Bernard, Poitiers, France)
Neurochirurgie 39:178–181, 1993   129-94-4-27

Purpose.—Spinal surgery to treat herniated disks used to be a complex operation, for which routine prophylactic treatment to prevent deep vein thrombosis (DVT) in the lower extremities and pulmonary embolism (PE) appeared justified. Because there have been many innovations in anesthetic and surgical techniques in recent years, the rate of thromboembolic complications after lumbar disk surgery was studied, and whether the routine use of prophylactic therapy in this setting is still warranted was determined.

Methods.—In 1990, a 9-item questionnaire was sent to 73 public and private neurosurgery services in France requesting data on thromboembolic complications after lumbar disk surgery for the previous year. Fifty neurosurgical units provided data on a total of 16,656 lumbar diskectomies.

Findings.—The average number of operations per center was 333; the average duration of surgery was 55 minutes; and the average hospital stay was 6 days. Of 16,656 patients operated on during 1989 at 50 centers, 10,351 (62.2%) at 27 centers (54%) were not pretreated; 1,001 (6%) at 3 centers (6%) were treated with calciparin; 4,304 (25.8%) at 8 centers (36%) were treated with low-molecular-weight heparin; and 1,000 (6%) at 2 centers (4%) were treated with antiplatelet agents or pentosane polysulfate. The knee-chest position was used for 59.4% of operations, the supine position for 31.8%, and the lateral position for 8.8%.

Outcome.—There were a total of 105 (.63%) thromboembolic complications, including 94 cases of lower extremity DVT and 11 cases of PE. The thromboembolic complications occurred in 68 (0.66%) of the nonpretreated patients and in 37 (0.59%) of the pretreated patients. The difference was statistically not significant.

Conclusion.—The prophylactic use of antithrombotic drugs does not lower the rate of thromboembolic complications after lumbar spine surgery. A prospective, randomized trial is needed to confirm or refute these findings.

▶ When prolonged immobilization was the norm for postoperative care of spinal operations, thromboembolism was a major concern. In recent years, the literature has been relatively silent on this issue, and many of us have assumed this was an unusual complication. In the past year, I have seen a variety of articles, all of which suggest that thromboembolism is, in fact, an issue. This large, multicenter French study demonstrates that thromboembolism occurred in about .60% of patients. In this noncontrolled analysis, anticoagulants were not preventive.—J.W. Frymoyer, M.D.

Vascular Injury in Anterior Lumbar Surgery
Baker JK, Reardon PR, Reardon MJ, Heggeness MH (Baylor College of Medicine, Houston)
Spine 18:2227–2230, 1993   129-94-4–28

Introduction.—Anterior lumbar surgery has gained in popularity for a number of conditions requiring decompressive and reconstructive procedures. There is a potential, however, for vascular complications with this approach to the lumbar spine. A total of 102 consecutive anterior lumbar spinal procedures were reviewed to compare the incidence of vascular injuries in the hypogastric and anterolateral approaches.

Methods.—The operations were performed from July 1990 to August 1991 by 2 vascular surgeons experienced with anterior approaches. Review of the medical records included patient age, diagnosis, approach, number of disk levels exposed, implants used, procedures performed, complications, concurrent medical problems, and history of previous spinal or abdominal procedures. The hypogastric paramedian retroperitoneal approach was used in 76 procedures and the anterolateral approach was used in 26.

Results.—The patient group included 60 men and 43 women; their average age at operation was 44 years. Disk disruption syndrome/degenerative disk disease and pseudarthrosis were the most common admitting diagnoses. One level was exposed in 46 patients, 2 levels in 36, and 3 levels in 17. The average number of levels exposed was 2.3 during the anterolateral approach and 1.6 during the hypogastric approach. Whereas the overall incidence of vascular complications was 15.6%, the incidence was significantly less with the anterolateral than with the hypogastric approach (7.7% vs. 18.4%). In all patients with vascular complications, the orthopedic procedure was anterior interbody arthrodesis. Twelve of the 16 vascular injuries occurred during the exposure. There were no episodes of pulmonary embolism.

Conclusion.—The anterolateral approach is based on a flank incision, with the dissection proceeding through the external and internal oblique muscles as well as the transversus abdominis. These findings suggest that the "small incision" exposure of the hypogastric paramedian approach significantly increases the incidence of vascular injury in anterior lumbar surgery.

▶ There is a growing popularity for anterior lumbar fusion, particularly in combination with posterior fusion. The authors candidly report an overall vascular complication rate of 15.6%. The single most important factor was the incision chosen for their approach. Fortunately, most of the complications had no short- or long-term sequelae, although one suspects the actual events were not particularly favorable to the operating surgeon's coronary arteries.—J.W. Frymoyer, M.D.

Lumbar Spinal Fusion: A Cohort Study of Complications, Reoperations, and Resource Use in the Medicare Population
Deyo RA, Ciol MA, Cherkin DC, Loeser JD, Bigos SJ (Univ of Washington, Seattle)
Spine 18:1463–1470, 1993   129-94-4–29

Background.—Data from the National Hospital Discharge Survey indicates that the frequency of all forms of lumbar spinal surgery increased from 1979 to 1987. Despite controversy regarding surgical indications, the rate of spinal fusion saw a 200% increase during this time. The wide geographic and specialty variety in the use of lumbar spinal fusions suggests a poor consensus on surgical indications. The outcomes of surgery performed with and without fusion were compared in a national cohort of Medicare patients.

Method.—Data were provided by the Health Care Financing Administration for all Medicare patients who underwent lumbar spinal surgery in 1985, with a 4-year follow-up. Patients with primary diagnoses or procedures in the cervical or thoracic spine were excluded, along with those showing a malignancy, spinal infection, inflammatory spondylitis, fracture, or vehicle trauma, or who had undergone another major surgical process. The diagnosis of herniated disk was based on displacement of a lumbar disk, with or without myelopathy. Spinal stenosis included the rubrics lumbar stenosis and spondylogenic compression of lumbar spinal cord. Degenerative disease included degeneration of lumbar disk, lumbosacral spondylosis, and unspecified disk disorders.

Short-Term Outcomes and Resource Use for Patients Undergoing Lumbar Spine Surgery With and Without Spinal Fusion

	Any Lumbar Surgery		Discectomy		Laminectomy		
	With Fusion (n = 1,524)	Without Fusion (n = 25,587)	With Fusion (n = 380)	Without Fusion (n = 12,042)	With Fusion (n = 730)	Without Fusion (n = 10,490)	Fusion Alone (n = 317)
6-Week postoperative mortality, %	1.2[†]	0.7	1.1	0.6	1.1	0.9	1.6
In-hospital complications, %	14.7*	7.7	12.1*	5.8	15.8*	9.8	16.4
Blood transfusion, %	46.7*	12.5	49.0*	8.9	45.3*	16.6	45.7
Discharged to nursing home, %[§]	4.2*	2.4	8.2*	1.7	3.0	3.1	1.6
Mean length-of-stay, days	15.7*	13.2	15.8*	12.9	15.5*	13.4	15.9
Mean inpatient hospital charges, 1985 dollars[‡]	10,091*	6,754	9,631*	6,336	10,162*	7,152	10,198

* Significantly different from surgery without fusion ($P < .0005$).
† Significantly different from surgery without fusion ($P = .04$).
‡ Does not include professional fees.
§ Includes only patients not admitted from a nursing home.
(Courtesy of Deyo RA, Ciol MA, Cherkin DC, et al: *Spine* 18:1463–1470, 1993.)

Results.—Within a study population of 27,111, 5.6% underwent lumbar fusion. The mean patient age was 72 years, and the most common diagnosis was spinal stenosis, followed by possible instability (primary spondylolisthesis). Six weeks after surgery, mortality was twice as high in the patients who had undergone fusions as in those who had surgery without fusions (table). In addition, the complication rate was nearly twice as high in the fusion group, and the blood transfusion rate was 3.7 times greater than the nonfusion group. The mean length of hospital stay for the fusion patients was almost 20% longer, and their hospital charges were almost 50% greater. Finally, the likelihood of morbidity, mortality, or nursing home placement was twice as high in patients who had undergone fusion compared with those who had not, and the risk of needing blood transfusion was 6 times higher. One year after surgery, reoperation rates were slightly higher in the nonfusion group than in patients with fusions. However, after 4 years, 11.9% of patients who had undergone fusion had undergone reoperations, compared with 10.2% of patients who had not undergone fusion.

Conclusion.—In older patients, lumbar spinal fusion brings greater morbidity, mortality, and in-hospital resources than spinal surgery without lumbar fusion. The data indicate an urgent need to standardize the definition of spinal instability and the indications for lumbar spinal fusion. Because of the hazard of non-randomized comparisons, it is suggested that lumbar fusion be tested in randomized trials comparing long-term risks and benefits with other procedures for well-defined patient samples.

▶ The Seattle PORT study group continues to collect a national database regarding the incidence, costs, complications, and outcomes of the treatment of lumbar spine disorders. This study focuses on the older age group and presents the national picture on what is happening. The results are not all bad, but reoperation rates are consequential, and complications are significant. The overwhelming conclusion I have reached is that it is not the operation that is the problem: rather, it is the decision-making process we use in determining which patients are candidates for the operation. This article tells us this question is of even greater importance in the elderly and very elderly.—J.W. Frymoyer, M.D.

Call Mosby Document Express at **1 (800) 55-MOSBY** to obtain copies of the original source documents of articles featured or referenced in the YEAR BOOK series.

5 Foot and Ankle

Introduction

The community of foot and ankle surgeons lost a great leader this past year. Kenneth A. Johnson was an inspired teacher and passionate researcher. He will be missed in many ways, not the least of which is in the splendid job he has done editing this section of the YEAR BOOK OF ORTHOPEDICS for the previous 5 years.

When Dr. Sledge asked me to step in as the new editor of the Foot and Ankle section, I was very pleased and readily accepted. The YEAR BOOK OF ORTHOPEDICS is a worthwhile endeavor that does what it is meant to do very well. Besides, the editorship offers one more enjoyable means for me to routinely review the pertinent literature. The articles that Dr. Johnson and I chose for the Foot and Ankle section this year cover a wide array of topics. Forefoot anatomy is revisited with discussions of the vascular anatomy of the first metatarsal head (Abstract 129-94-5-1), the soft tissue support of the second metatarsophalangeal joint (Abstract 129-94-5-2), and the soft tissue stabilizers of the longitudinal arch (Abstract 129-94-5-3). These articles affect the treatment of forefoot problems commonly encountered in the office as well as potential complications of plantar fasciotomy.

The next 4 articles (Abstracts 129-94-5-4 through 129-94-5-7) cover elective reconstruction of the subtalar complex. The work on calcaneal lengthening and correction of planovalgus deformity holds significance not only for the treatment of early stage posterior tibial problems, but also possibly for the prevention of this very common ailment. The currently popular "double arthrodesis," as well as triple arthrodesis—the gold standard for end-stage posterior tibial involvement and arthritis of the hindfoot—are discussed in following articles. Finally, a classic review of triple arthrodesis in the rheumatoid population is provided. Two more articles, one an extensive review of the Brostrom ankle ligament repair (Abstract 129-94-5-8) and a basic science discussion of Achilles tendon injuries (Abstract 129-94-5-9), cover more sports-related topics.

Several articles concern themselves with salvage of the distal limb, either after tibial nerve interruption (Abstract 129-94-5-11) or when diabetes causes dysvascularity, infection, or a neuropathic arthropathy (Abstracts 129-94-5-12 through 129-94-5-14).

Traumatic injuries to the foot and ankle can be particularly challenging for the orthopedist. Two particularly challenging, and perhaps heretofore unsolved, injuries are those of the tibial plafond and the calcaneus.

A wealth of literature dealt with these topics this past year and we have highlighted them for our readers (Abstracts 129-94-5-17 through 129-94-5-22). Included is the current classic on classification and surgical treatment of acute calcaneal fractures.

The area of foot and ankle research continues to expand, covering a wide range of topics using excellent scientific methods and being represented in a wide range of journals. As academic foot and ankle research centers become more prevalent across the country, the intensity of the research effort will continue to increase. Soon, perhaps, some of the answers to common problems discussed within this issue of the YEAR BOOK may become evident. This continues to be an exciting era in foot and ankle research.

Michael G. Wilson, M.D.

Avascular Necrosis of the First Metatarsal Head: Incidence in Distal Osteotomy Combined With Lateral Soft Tissue Release

Peterson DA, Zilberfarb JL, Greene MA, Colgrove RC (Naval Med Ctr, San Diego, Calif; Kaiser Permanente Hosp, San Diego, Calif)
Foot Ankle 15:59–63, 1994   129-94-5-1

Background.—The incidence of avascular necrosis (AVN) of the metatarsal head has been found to be very low after distal osteotomy of the first metatarsal for hallux valgus treatment. However, the incidence of AVN of the metatarsal head after this procedure combined with adductor tendon release has not been documented in a large series.

Methods and Findings.—Eighty-two consecutive procedures were performed in 64 patients between 1986 and 1988. Forty-two patients, undergoing 58 procedures, were available for clinical and radiologic follow-up. Follow-up ranged from 1 to 4.2 years (mean, 2.5 years). Thirty-five L-shaped and 23 Chevron osteotomies were combined with a lateral soft tissue release, including adductor tenotomy. The mean preoperative hallux valgus angle was 25 degrees and intermetatarsal angle was 12 degrees. At follow-up assessment, the correction averaged 13 degrees and 5 degrees, respectively. Results were satisfactory to 84% of the patients. One case of AVN occurred in a patient who was asymptomatic at 4.2 years of follow-up. Of the remaining patients, 2 had infections and 1 had hallux varus. There were no nonunions.

Conclusion.—Distal first metatarsal osteotomy combined with a lateral soft tissue release is effective in the correction of hallux valgus deformity. The incidence of AVN of the metatarsal head associated with this combined procedure was only 2% in this series.

▶ The authors describe a large series of Chevron osteotomies performed by one surgeon who was not one of the authors. Only one of their patients (2%

of their cases) displayed radiographic evidence of AVN. It should be noted that one third of their patients were lost to follow-up, and the true frequency of AVN in their series may be larger.

In their discussion of the relevant vascular anatomy, the authors explain how lateral soft tissue release can be performed without disrupting the capital blood supply. With meticulous technique, a disruption of blood supply certainly should be a rare occurrence. Unfortunately for those of us who perform bunion surgery frequently, the goal ultimately becomes eliminating complications rather than simply minimizing them. In the field of purely elective forefoot surgery, even 2 or 3 cases of AVN per 100 surgeries may be an unacceptable rate.

Furthermore, the main proponent of Chevron osteotomy during the past decade—our late editor, Kenneth A. Johnson—agreed that lateral soft tissue release is theoretically possible without endangering the blood supply, but that such soft tissue release is rarely necessary given the proper preoperative indications for the Chevron osteotomy. In cases of joint incongruence, perhaps other procedures, such as distal soft tissue realignment combined with proximal osteotomy, would be more appropriate.—M.G. Wilson, M.D.

Second Metatarsophalangeal Joint Instability in the Athlete

Coughlin MJ (St Alphonsus Regional Med Ctr, Boise, Idaho)
Foot Ankle 14:309–319, 1993   129-94-5-2

Objective.—Nine athletic patients in whom second metatarsophalangeal (MTP) joint instability was diagnosed were studied. Areas of interest were the demographics associated with second MTP instability, the results of conservative and surgical treatment, and the value of a positive drawer sign as a predictive factor in the preoperative examination.

Patients and Methods.—Second MTP joint instability was bilateral in 2 patients. Seven toes underwent surgical reconstruction and 4 were treated nonsurgically. The initial evaluation consisted of a physical examination, weight-bearing anteroposterior and lateral radiographs, and a drawer test. Patients were questioned regarding characteristics of the onset of pain, length of symptoms, and type and level of athletic activity. Surgery was recommended for patients with deformity or unrelenting pain. Conservative treatment consisted of a period of taping. Surgical patients were followed for an average of 20.4 months and nonsurgical patients for an average of 15 months.

Results.—The average duration of symptoms was 11 months. All patients reported an insidious onset of pain, at first isolated to the plantar aspect of the second MTP joint. Two patients had previously undergone a total of 5 forefoot surgeries. All had taken part in athletic activities at a high level and were prevented from participation by intractable metatarsalgia. Ten of 10 toes tested had a positive drawer sign. Radiographic examination revealed all second metatarsals to be excessively long in comparison to adjacent metatarsals. Three of the 4 toes treated nonsurgically had a good result. In the fourth case, the second MTP joint eventually dislocated and the patient experienced a severe fixed hammertoe deformity. Two of the surgical patients rated their results as excellent, 3 as good, 1 as fair, and 1 as poor. Those with good results had mild pain with sports activity. The patient with a poor result had undergone several other forefoot operations and eventually had to have the second toe amputated.

Conclusion.—The drawer test was the most useful clinical finding in the initial evaluation of patients with suspected second MTP joint instability. Another common finding was excess length of the second metatarsal compared with the first and third metatarsals. Early diagnosis and intervention may prevent eventual progression of deformity and dislocation, but many patients may have to decrease their level of athletic activity.

▶ The accurate diagnosis of the underlying cause of lesser metatarsophalangeal pain is critical to achieving a good outcome. As the author points out, pain in the area of the second MTP joint is caused by a limited number of pathologic processes, one of which—instability of the joint—can be difficult to determine early in the process when radiographic evaluation is normal. The positive drawer sign appears to be the best early indicator of instability of the second MTP joint.

Soft tissue realignment and adjustment in this high-activity, high-demand population can be seen as a potentially reconstructive procedure, in contrast to traditional salvage procedures that remove part of the metatarsal head. Six of 7 athletes who underwent soft tissue reconstruction returned to moderate-to-vigorous sports activity without further surgery. Although the authors speculate on the relative length of the second metatarsal as an etiologic factor in instability, they acknowledge that a larger series with controls is required. It appears that continued taping and modification of activity level are required for patients who are treated conservatively.—M.G. Wilson, M.D.

Biomechanical Evaluation of Longitudinal Arch Stability
Huang C-K, Kitaoka HB, An K-N, Chao EYS (Mayo Clinic and Found, Rochester, Minn)
Foot Ankle 14:353–357, 1993   129-94-5–3

Background.—Pes planus, or flatfoot, is the most common foot condition in patients of any age. Despite its common occurrence, and the many operations described to relieve its associated symptoms, little information is available on the various structures' relative contribution to the stabilization of the arch.

Methods and Findings.—In this biomechanical assessment of longitudinal arch stability, 12 fresh-frozen cadaveric feet were studied. The feet were loaded along the tibial axis with compressive loads of 230, 460, and 690 newtons intact and after sequential sectioning of plantar fascia, plantar ligaments, and spring ligament. The structures were sectioned in 6 different sequences. Changes in the vertical and horizontal dimensions of the medial arch were measured. The plantar fascia provided the greatest relative contribution to arch stability, followed by the plantar ligaments and spring ligament. The plantar fascia was a primary factor in maintaining the medial longitudinal arch. Arch stiffness in these cadaveric feet was reduced by 25% after plantar fascia division.

Conclusion.—These observations may be very relevant clinically. Plantar fasciotomy apparently will not result in immediate collapse of the arch, with associated dysfunction, in many patients. However, this procedure should be used only in carefully selected patients. Plantar fasciotomy may significantly affect arch stability in patients at risk for pes planus, such as those with posterior tibial tendinitis, systemic ligamentous laxity, and rheumatoid arthritis. In patients with pes planus deformity undergoing soft tissue reconstruction, other static stabilizers might also be reconstructed.

▶ The authors investigated a very common condition, flattening of the longitudinal arch of the foot, from a biomechanical standpoint. To investigate the cause of pes planus, the authors examined the effect of sectioning each of 3 static supportive structures in the plantar foot. Of the 3 structures sectioned (the plantar ligaments, spring ligament, and plantar fascia), the plantar fascia played the greatest role in the maintenance of arch height. However, even when all 3 were sectioned, two thirds of the arch height was maintained.

Clearly, a good deal of arch stability depends on the bony architecture and intact capsular tissues. This may explain why plantar fasciotomy may lead to flattening of the arch when capsular insufficiency is potentiated by other disease processes such as rheumatoid arthritis or general ligamentous laxity. Also, the effect of the relative length of the lateral bony column of the foot impacts on the degree of valgus in the hindfoot, which impacts on the apparent height of the longitudinal arch. Correction of the symptomatic flatfoot requires evaluation of both the bony and ligamentous factors. Iatrogenic pes planus appears to be one additional potential complication of heel pain surgery; this reinforces the principle that patients should undergo plantar fasciotomy only after extensive conservative treatment has failed.—M.G. Wilson, M.D.

Effect of Calcaneal Lengthening on Relationships Among the Hindfoot, Midfoot, and Forefoot
Sangeorzan BJ, Mosca V, Hansen ST Jr (Univ of Washington, Seattle)
Foot Ankle 14:136–141, 1993   129-94-5-4

Background.—In flatfoot, or pes planus, the longitudinal arch is depressed and there may, in addition, be hindfoot valgus and/or an abducted forefoot. The Evans operation is based on the invariably excessive length of the lateral column in intractable cases of clubfoot and the finding that the lateral column is short in some cases of pes planus. The procedure involves sectioning the calcaneus 1.5 cm proximal to the calcaneocuboid joint, elongating the calcaneus, and filling the osteotomy with grafted bone.

Objective and Methods.—The correction achieved by the Evans operation was quantified by examining radiographs of 7 postoperative feet. Each foot had had an osteotomy made 1.5 cm proximal to the calcaneocuboid joint, and the gap was filled with a 1-cm iliac crest corticocancellous bone graft. The lateral talocalcaneal and talometatarsal angles and calcaneal length were measured on a lateral view of the foot, and the relationship between the talus and navicular was assessed on a dorsoplantar view.

Findings.—The average measured increase in calcaneal length was 4 mm, despite the fact that all patients received a 1-cm graft. The lateral talocalcaneal angle increased by 6.4 degrees on average when the long calcaneal axis was measured, or by 6.8 degrees when using the inferior calcaneal surface. The lateral talometatarsal angle improved from 19.7 to 8.4 degrees postoperatively. The dorsoplantar talometatarsal angle, a measure of forefoot adduction/abduction, decreased by an average of 15.8 degrees. The calcaneal pitch angle increased from 3.2 to 14 degrees. The position of the talonavicular joint, reflecting talonavicular coverage, improved by 26 degrees on average.

Conclusion.—The Evans operation for pes planus can be expected to succeed when the navicular is lateral and plantar to the talus, the pitch angle is flat, and the forefoot is abducted.

▶ Symptomatic pes planus is frequently encountered and may be caused by developmental abnormalities, posterior tibial insufficiency, rheumatoid arthritis, neuroarthropathy, or various neuromuscular diseases. This paper supports other current evidence that most of the deformity is occurring through the talonavicular joint rather than at the subtalar joint axis. In this series with lateral column lengthening, the greatest radiographic correction was seen in terms of improved coverage at the talonavicular joint. Relatively minor alterations were noted in the lateral talocalcaneal axis, which reflects subtalar joint adjustment.

Whereas planovalgus deformities traditionally were corrected by triple arthrodesis, more and more investigators are striving to correct deformity while maintaining a supple, pliant hindfoot. Lateral column lengthening, either through calcaneal lengthening or lengthening at the time of calcaneocuboid fusion, holds great promise for achieving these goals. Because the planovalgus foot predisposes to posterior tibial deterioration, lateral column lengthening should be considered in combination with medial soft tissue repair for those patients with supple planovalgus deformities. This article examines a very different set of radiographic parameters compared with the previous article (Abstract 129-94-5–3), which examined longitudinal arch height. I would assume that an improved lateral talometatarsal angle would be associated with increased arch height, but direct measurements would be helpful.—M.G. Wilson, M.D.

Simultaneous Calcaneocuboid and Talonavicular Fusion: Long-Term Follow-Up Study
Clain MR, Baxter DE (Univ of Texas, Houston)
J Bone Joint Surg (Br) 76-B:133–136, 1994   129-94-5–5

Background.—The current trend in the treatment of painful and deformed hindfoot is to perform limited hindfoot arthrodeses in certain patients. The use of simultaneous calcaneocuboid and talonavicular fusion, developed by DuVries, has not been widely reported. Although this approach is not recommended for symptomatic flexible flatfoot, it has other indications.

Methods.—From 1980 to 1988, 19 patients underwent 20 simultaneous calcaneocuboid and talonavicular fusions for a variety of painful hindfoot disorders. Sixteen patients with 16 treated feet were available for review. The mean follow-up was 83 months.

Findings.—Objective results were excellent in 4 feet, good in 8, and fair in 4. None of the patients had poor outcomes. One asymptomatic nonunion of the talonavicular joint occurred. Progressive degenerative arthritis of the ankle was observed in 6 patients and of the naviculocuneiform joint in 7.

Conclusion.—Simultaneous calcaneocuboid and talonavicular arthrodesis is a simple, effective alternative to triple arthrodesis. Biomechanically, this combined approach is better than an isolated talonavicular fusion.

▶ Pain relief is reliably achieved with the authors' described technique of double arthrodesis through the talonavicular and calcaneocuboid joints. Bone grafting was not performed in the lateral joint at the time of fusion, so the described technique is only appropriate for patients with a mild degree of peritalar subluxation. This double arthrodesis technique restricts hindfoot motion to the same degree as a triple arthrodesis; none of the patients displayed any hindfoot inversion/eversion at the time of follow-up. Six of the patients displayed some radiographic progression of ankle arthritis.

The advantage of this technique over a triple arthrodesis is solely technical: the decreased morbidity for the patient results from decreased operative time and less extensive dissection. An alternative procedure, subtalar fusion, preserves a useful degree of inversion/eversion; however, as the data from Abstract 129-94-5–4 suggest, correction of subtalar joint deformity alone may have a limited impact on the planovalgus deformity. The goal of correcting a planovalgus foot while maintaining flexibility remains elusive.—M.G. Wilson, M.D.

Triple Arthrodesis in Older Adults: Results After Long-Term Follow-Up

Graves SC, Mann RA, Graves KO (Campbell Clinic, Memphis, Tenn; San Leandro, Calif)

J Bone Joint Surg (Am) 75-A:355–362, 1993

129-94-5–6

Introduction.—It has been suggested that triple arthrodesis should be considered only as a salvage procedure in older patients with severe, rigid, painful deformities. To investigate further, the results and complications of triple arthrodesis were reviewed in 18 feet of 17 patients who had the procedure at an average age of 66 years (range, 52–88 years).

Indications.—Triple arthrodesis was performed to correct deformities of the hindfoot and midfoot caused by an untreated rupture of the posterior tibial tendon in 10 patients, rheumatoid arthritis in 3, and neuropathic arthropathy (associated with diabetes mellitus), trauma, old poliomyelitis, and a stroke in 1 patient each. The average duration of follow-up was 42 months.

Outcome.—Overall, 14 patients were satisfied with the result; the other 3 were dissatisfied with the position of the foot. All 17 patients had less pain postoperatively, achieving maximum relief of pain at an average of 10 months. Eleven patients still reported some discomfort.

At the most recent follow-up examination, 3 patients had a nonunion involving the talonavicular joint in 1 and the calcaneocuboid joint in 2. Six patients had progressive degenerative joint disease involving the ankle and 7 had progressive degenerative changes in the mobile joints of the feet. Two patients had a wound infection that healed. One patient had postoperative collapse of the foot because of premature, unauthorized weight-bearing. One patient had painful impingement of a staple across the talocalcaneal joint on the tip of the fibula; removal of the staple relieved the pain.

Conclusion.—Many patients with painful deformities of the foot in midlife or later can be helped by triple arthrodesis. However, these patients generally continue to have some pain in the foot. Because it is a technically difficult procedure with a relatively high rate of postoperative complications, triple arthrodesis should be used only as a salvage procedure for a painful, unstable foot or a foot that has a fixed disabling deformity.

▶ I included this article because it serves as a clinical benchmark for a commonly performed procedure, triple arthrodesis. This long-term experience of one surgeon accurately depicts triple arthrodesis as a salvage option with definite limitations for short- and long-term outcome. Clearly, even if the surgeon meticulously prepares and stabilizes the fusion and proper alignment is restored with successful bone union, patients experience a prolonged recovery period of up to 1 year. Some mild discomfort is noted by a majority of patients with certain activities, and there is evidence of radiographic progression of degenerative change at the tibiotalar joint in a significant percentage as well.

I believe that, because of these limitations, this surgery is most appropriate in the older adult population. This article is especially relevant in this regard. To avoid associated degenerative change in the remaining major joints of the foot and ankle, other options such as osteotomy and extensive soft tissue releases should be considered in the younger patient with significant deformity. I suspect that triple arthrodesis in the pediatric and adolescent population hastens the inevitable onset of degenerative arthritis by 1 or 2 decades.—M.G. Wilson, M.D.

Triple Arthrodesis in Rheumatoid Arthritis
Figgie MP, O'Malley MJ, Ranawat C, Inglis AE, Sculco TP (Hosp for Special Surgery, New York; Tufts Univ, Boston)
Clin Orthop 292:250–254, 1993   129-94-5-7

Introduction.—For patients with rheumatoid arthritis, pain and deformity of the foot not only limit ambulation but alter the mechanical alignment of the limb. Despite the common involvement of the subtalar joints in patients with rheumatoid arthritis, there have been few reports of surgical treatment of the hindfoot.

Patients.—The results of triple arthrodesis in 55 patients with rheumatoid arthritis were reviewed. A total of 65 operations were performed during a 10-year period. However, 12 patients died and 3 were lost to follow-up, leaving 49 procedures in 40 patients available for evaluation. The patients were 32 women and 8 men (average age at surgery, 50 years) who were followed for an average of 5 years. Operations followed a standardized technique, with medial and lateral incisions with staple fixation and local bone grafting and correction of deformity with closing wedge osteotomies. Indications were moderate-to-severe pain and difficulty walking.

Outcomes.—Eighty-three percent of patients had complete and 94% had significant pain relief. Eighty percent achieved significant improvements in ambulatory status—over half were limited to household ambulation preoperatively, whereas 90% were at least community ambulators at follow-up. There were 4 cases of superficial wound infection, but all responded to local measures. Secondary surgery for pseudarthrosis was required in 1 patient and pantalar arthrodesis was needed for progressive disease in 3 patients. None of the patients had progressive forefoot or knee symptoms, and patients whose hindfeet were corrected to 0–10 degrees of valgus showed no progression of ankle symptoms.

Conclusion.—Good success was reported with triple arthrodesis for patients with rheumatoid arthritis. The union rate is high, with improvement in pain and ambulation. Progressive ankle disease occurs only in feet with a final hindfoot alignment of greater than 10 degrees of valgus.

▶ This report represents the largest series to date evaluating triple arthrodesis in the rheumatoid population. Overall, the authors achieved the expected goals: relief of pain and increased ambulation potential. Their technique is notable for the exclusive use of staple fixation and local bone chips for graft material. A very high rate of union was achieved, with only 2 nonunions of the talonavicular joint reported. It should be noted, however, that 10 feet were undercorrected in terms of the preoperative varus/valgus deformity. Internal fixation with modern cannulated screws may afford better intraoperative control of the hindfoot alignment than staples. Also, a block of iliac crest bone can be useful for correcting the hindfoot with a severe preoperative valgus deformity. Eight of the authors' patients were left in excessive valgus, each of whom sustained further ankle deterioration. Achieving a neutral 5 degrees of hindfoot valgus is especially critical in rheumatoid patients who may have ankylosis of the remaining midfoot joints.—M.G. Wilson, M.D.

The Modified Brostrom Procedure for Lateral Ankle Instability

Hamilton WG, Thompson FM, Snow SW (St Luke's-Roosevelt Hosp, New York)

Foot Ankle 14:1–7, 1993   129-94-5–8

Background.—Since 1980, 1 of the authors has been using the Gould modification of the Brostrom repair for symptomatic lateral ankle instability in professional ballet dancers. The operation, which tightens stretched-out lateral ligaments without the use of a peroneal tendon for reconstruction, is well suited for ballet dancers in that it maintains full plantar flexion and dorsiflexion and preserves the peroneal function needed for dancing en pointe. Based on the results, the use of this operation was extended to other patients.

Technique.—The procedure is done on an outpatient basis and with general or spinal anesthesia. A curvilinear incision is made along the anterior border of the lateral malleolus, preserving the peroneal tendons. After mobilization of the lateral portion of the extensor retinaculum, a capsular incision is made along the anterior fibular border, with a small cuff left on the fibula for reattachment. The anterior talofibular (ATF) ligament appears as a thickening in the anterior capsule and the calcaneofibular (CF) ligament deep to the peroneal tendons in the distal portion of the wound.

With the ankle in valgus and the foot in eversion-abduction, the CF and ATF ligaments are trimmed and repaired with permanent sutures. The ankle is tested for anterior drawer sign, talar tilt, stability, plantar flexion, and dorsiflexion. The extensor retinaculum is pulled over the distal fibula and sutured in place, and the ankle is checked again. After the swelling goes down, the leg is casted for 4 weeks and splinted for another 2–4 weeks. More vigorous rehabilitation starts at

6 weeks, and the patient returns to activity at 8–12 weeks. Complete peroneal rehabilitation is a must.

Experience.—This modified Brostrom procedure has been used in 28 ankles in 27 patients (average age, 28 years). Fifty-four percent were professional ballet dancers, 35% were recreational athletes, and 11% were nonathletes. At an average follow-up of 64 months, there were 26 excellent, 1 good, and 1 fair result. In no case did the operation fail, and no patient experienced a stretch-out or needed reoperation. There were no complications.

Conclusion.—The Gould modification of the Brostrom procedure is recommended for patients with lateral ankle instability. It preserves full plantar flexion and dorsiflexion without sacrificing peroneal function; the success rate is high and the complication rate is low. It is the procedure of choice for professional dancers and is equally effective for other athletes and nonathletes.

▶ The authors describe the Gould modification of the Brostrom repair, which incorporates the extensor retinaculum. Because the extensor retinaculum originates along the calcaneus laterally, the repair provides stability of the subtalar joint as well, thus addressing subtle cases of combined subtalar and tibiotalar instability. The procedure maintains nearly normal hindfoot motion, and morbidity is minimal given the small incision and preservation of normal anatomy of the peroneal tendons. The modified Brostrom is an excellent choice for reconstruction of most cases of mechanical as well as functional lateral ankle instability.—M.G. Wilson, M.D.

Achilles Tendon Injuries: A Comparison of Surgical Repair Versus No Repair in a Rat Model
Murrell GAC, Lilly EG III, Collins A, Seaber AV, Goldner RD, Best TM (Hosp for Special Surgery, New York; Duke Univ, Durham, NC)
Foot Ankle 14:400–406, 1993   129-94-5-9

Background.—Authorities disagree on the best way to treat ruptures of the Achilles tendon. Surgical repair of the Achilles tendon was compared with no repair in rats.

Methods.—Thirty-two male Sprague-Dawley rats were used. The Achilles tendon and plantaris tendon were divided completely, and the animals received internal splint, Achilles repair with a modified Kessler-type suture, or no repair. A fourth group was subjected to sham operation, involving skin incision only. On the fifteenth day, the rats were killed, and biomechanical and histologic assessments were done on the injured and uninjured tendons.

Findings.—All rats subjected to Achilles tendon division were significantly functionally impaired initially, then gradually improved so that, by day 15, no functional or failure load impairments were noted in any group. Injured tendons in all 3 groups subjected to tendon division had a 13-fold increase in the cross-sectional region. Compared with uninjured and sham-operated tendons, the injured tendons were less stiff and more deformable on the fifteenth day. The magnitude of the biomechanical and morphological changes on day 15 and the initial impairment and functional recovery rate were comparable for the groups receiving no repair, internal splint, and Achilles repair.

Conclusion.—In the rat, surgical repair of the Achilles tendon does not provide any advantages over nonsurgical treatment. These findings concur with previous clinical findings suggesting that Achilles tendon ruptures should be treated nonoperatively.

▶ This elegant animal experiment demonstrates the rather surprising fact that surgically divided Achilles tendons in rats are identical in terms of failure strength and morphological appearance, whether they are surgically repaired or not. The authors conclude that the experimental results support clinical studies advocating nonoperative treatment of these injuries.

Limitations of their design include the fact that a surgical division of the Achilles tendon may not fully simulate a clinical rupture, and that mechanical testing was performed at one point in time (day 15 postinjury). The 13-fold increase in cross-sectional area and disorganized morphology of the specimen suggest that sacrifice took place relatively early in the healing process. Perhaps differences in the experimental groups might have been demonstrated later in the healing process.

Some patients clinically seem to lose push-off strength after nonoperative repair of their Achilles rupture. Surgically divided tendons in this experimental construct were twice as deformable and half as stiff as the uninjured tendons. This suggests that the degree to which the normal resting length of the tendon is restored may determine the functional outcome. Surgical repair may achieve this more reliably, but clearly further work both in terms of animal experiments such as these and randomized prospective studies are needed to clarify the role of surgical repair.—M.G. Wilson, M.D.

The Plantar Incision for Procedures Involving the Forefoot: An Evaluation of One Hundred and Fifty Incisions in One Hundred and Fifteen Patients
Richardson EG, Brotzman SB, Graves SC (Univ of Tennessee, Memphis)
J Bone Joint Surg (Am) 75-A:726–731, 1993   129-94-5-10

Purpose.—Despite the traditional teaching against plantar incisions, several studies have shown good results with plantar incisions for various procedures. However, there have been no extensive investigations specifically addressing the results of such incisions. A large retrospective study was conducted to examine the results of plantar incisions for the treatment of various forefoot disorders.

Methods.—In a 6-year period, 172 plantar incisions were performed in 137 patients. Eighty-five percent of the incisions were longitudinal. Surgical indications included excision of interdigital neuroma, release of the adductor hallucis, and resection of the metatarsal heads. A personal interview and examination were conducted for 89 of the patients: the average follow-up was 25 months. Of the remainder, 26 were interviewed by telephone and 22 were lost to follow-up.

Findings.—Subjective assessments indicated that 96% of the patients examined were pleased with the results of their incision. None of them reported having to alter their activities, and only 3 had made changes in footwear. Three fourths of longitudinal scars were nearly invisible. Of the patients interviewed by telephone, the same percentage (96%) reported satisfaction with their result.

Conclusion.—Excellent results were reported in most patients operated on with plantar incisions. If a procedure can be adequately performed through some other area of the foot, avoiding the plantar incision is recommended. However, a plantar incision may be used for a variety of indications, including resection of interdigital neuroma, drainage of an abscess, removal of a foreign body, sesamoidectomy, lateral release of the first metatarsophalangeal joint, or excision of an invaginated keratotic plug, metatarsal head, or intermetatarsal bursa.

► The authors evaluated 137 patients who underwent a variety of procedures through plantar incisions. The outcome was based solely on the condition of the scar in terms of quality of healing and local tenderness. Although the results of the study are encouraging, 7 patients had poor results, 3 of whom required operative excision of a keratosis within the scar. Seven additional patients who had fair results either had difficulty with shoe wear or delayed wound healing. Six more patients with good results had keratosis that caused occasional tenderness.

Clearly, patients who undergo plantar incisions should be aware that there is a significant risk of thickening of the scar and that in a small percentage of cases painful thickening might result. Planning of these incisions is critical, as satisfactory scar revision is difficult to achieve in the face of underlying bony prominence. Of note, no patient in the series had a Tinel sign relating to the incision; thus, a common complication of dorsal incisions in the foot is not usually encountered with the plantar approach. Keratotic scar healing can occur with dorsal approaches as well, particularly over bony prominences such as the medial eminence. The foot and ankle surgeon should not be afraid to make a plantar approach when the anatomy and deep dissection are facilitated by this exposure.—M.G. Wilson, M.D.

Tibial Nerve Grafting for Restoration of Plantar Sensation

Nunley JA, Gabel GT (Duke Univ, Durham, NC; Baylor College of Medicine, Houston)
Foot Ankle 14:489–492, 1993   129-94-5–11

Background.—Injuries to the tibial nerve can result in plantar anesthesia, which can lead to significant trophic and ulcerative changes on the weight-bearing areas of the foot. The uncommon tibial nerve injury resulting in segmental loss has been treated with interfascicular nerve grafting, with marginal results.

Methods.—Interfascicular nerve grafting was performed to restore plantar sensation in 5 patients with traumatic segmental defects of the tibial nerve. All underwent delayed sural nerve grafting an average of 8 months after their injury. The average graft length was 8 cm, and all were placed in tension-free interfascicular fashion using the operating microscope. Three patients required free tissue transfer. Patients were followed for at least 2 years and assessed for restoration of superficial sensation, healing of plantar ulcers, and absence of neurogenic pain.

Results.—All wounds healed without problems. At an average of 5 years, 4 patients had good results and 1 had fair results. This outcome compared with 1 good and 4 poor results at 2 years. Two patients had had plantar ulcers, which healed at 12–18 months. No patients showed clinical restoration of intrinsic muscle function. All patients but 1 were satisfied with their results; the exception was a patient who gained relief from severe neuropathic pain but was dissatisfied with his sensory recovery.

Conclusion.—Tibial nerve grafting can restore plantar sensation in most patients with disabling segmental tibial nerve injuries. Ensuring an adequate soft tissue environment, including free-tissue transfer if necessary, is a key consideration. The recovery period is prolonged, with full plantar sensation taking at least 2 and up to 4 years to return.

▶ This article sheds new light on the outcome of severe traumatic injuries to the posterior tibial nerve. The described technique is demanding: in each patient, interfascicular grafting using multiple segments of the sural grafts is required. The authors stress the avoidance of tension on the graft at the time of repair and adequate soft tissue coverage, sometimes requiring free tissue transfer in the lower portion of the limb.

Although regeneration took a minimum of 2 years to achieve, all 5 patients regained protective sensation to the plantar aspect of the foot, and no cases of chronic ulceration were noted. In the evaluation of the mangled extremity, posterior tibial nerve disruption still remains one of the most ominous prognostic factors. Nothing in this article changes that fact. Rather, it appears that nerve reconstruction, with or without grafting, is a reasonable option in patients with reconstructible soft tissue defects and less significant bony injury.

The authors make no estimate of the psychological impact of this prolonged rehabilitation period, nor is the functional or vocational impact of the injury assessed. Generally, the patient's best interests are served by one major coordinated attempt at limb salvage. In case of failure, an appropriately timed, early below-knee amputation is far better than repeated unsuccessful attempts to reconstruct the mangled limb.—M.G. Wilson, M.D.

Transcutaneous Oxygen Tension in the Dysvascular Foot With Infection

Pinzur MS, Stuck R, Sage R, Osterman H (Loyola Univ, Maywood, Ill; VA Hosp, Hines, Ill)

Foot Ankle 14:254–256, 1993
129-94-5-12

Introduction.—For patients with peripheral vascular insufficiency, a number of techniques have been recommended to evaluate blood supply to the affected limb and thus predict wound healing. Ultrasound Doppler ankle/brachial index has been the most widely used method, but this method often gives falsely elevated measures of flow in patients with calcified, noncompressible vessels. Measurement of transcutaneous oxygen tension shows promise as a useful technique of measuring the oxygen-delivering capacity of the arterial system in these patients.

Methods.—The transcutaneous oxygen tension at the foot and ankle was evaluated before surgery in 8 adult, insulin-requiring diabetics with peripheral vascular disease. All had foot infection with signs of systemic sepsis that did not respond to initial treatment and so were managed by surgical decompression.

Results.—None of the preoperative measures were judged sufficient to support wound healing. Open ray resection was performed in 4 patients and open midfoot amputation was done in the other 4. After the local infection had resolved, 7 of 8 patients showed significant increases in their transcutaneous oxygen tension values. All of these increased values were considered sufficient to support wound healing.

Conclusion.—Transcutaneous oxygen tension measurements appear to be a reliable means of determining amputation wound-healing capacity in patients with diabetes. Its predictive value in the initial evaluation of patients with deep foot infection appears to be limited. Rather, it may be most useful in the prevention of unnecessary proximal amputation in patients with active, local infection who appear to lack the capacity for healing of a more functional distal amputation.

▶ This report on the recovery of transcutaneous oxygen tension values after initial treatment for infection fills in an important piece of the treatment algorithm for patients with foot infections and decreased vascularity. Evidently, reliable oxygen tension values can only be determined after initial drainage of the soft tissue abscess. Amputation at a more proximal level should be performed during the initial phase of treatment only in cases of extreme morbidity or obvious soft tissue dysvascularity. In more favorable clinical settings, the level for amputation should be determined as a second stage in the treatment algorithm. The findings of this article may ultimately contribute to achieving a higher level of function after definitive treatment for foot infections.—M.G. Wilson, M.D.

Distal Blood Pressure as a Predictor for the Level of Amputation in Diabetic Patients With Foot Ulcer
Larsson J, Apelqvist J, Castenfors J, Agardh C-D, Stenström A (Univ Hosp, Lund, Sweden)
Foot Ankle 14:247–253, 1993   129-94-5–13

Purpose.—For patients with diabetic foot disease, the decision whether to amputate is still clinical. There is a need for some objective, reliable method of assessing the chances that the limb will survive. The predictive value of distal blood pressure measurements was analyzed.

Methods.—The study sample included 161 consecutive patients with diabetes mellitus and foot ulcers who required amputation. All patients had systolic ankle and toe blood pressure levels taken by strain gauge and Doppler techniques at their first visit and every 6 months thereafter until healing. The decision to perform amputation was made on clinical grounds only, with the indications being progressive gangrene, intolerable pain, and refractory septic and/or toxic conditions. Patients were treated on an outpatient basis, except during surgery and periods of complications, by the same multidisciplinary foot care team.

Findings.—Ankle or toe blood pressure measurements were available for 86% of patients. In about one fourth of patients, pressures could not be taken at 1 site or the other because of incompressible arteries, ulcer or gangrene at the site, previous amputation, poor general condition, or an emergency situation. Below an absolute lower ankle pressure of 50 mm Hg, minor amputation was never sufficient to obtain healing. The same was usually true below a pressure of 75 mm Hg; at or above that level, no prediction could be made. Minor amputation usually was not sufficient when toe pressure was below 15 mm Hg. No further predictive information could be gained from pressure indices at either site.

Conclusion.—Ankle and toe pressure thresholds were identified below which minor amputation is unlikely to achieve healing in patients with diabetic foot disease. No upper limit, above which major amputation is not required, can be identified from this study. A number of clinical factors may limit the use of ankle and toe blood pressure measurements.

▶ The levels and timing of amputation in this series were based on clinical grounds. The surgeons were aware of the absolute systolic pressures measured at the ankle and toe, but they attempted not to be swayed by these data in selecting their level of amputation. We do not know whether true blinding of the blood pressure data would have affected the outcome. Nevertheless, the authors successfully defined the threshold systolic pressure below which no minor amputation healed. This work takes us one step closer to the creation of reliable guidelines for level of amputation in dysvascular patients with diabetes.—M.G. Wilson, M.D.

Deformity Following Fracture in Diabetic Neuropathic Osteoarthropathy: Operative Management of Adults Who Have Type-I Diabetes
Thompson RC Jr, Clohisy DR (Univ of Minnesota, Minneapolis)
J Bone Joint Surg (Am) 75-A:1765–1773, 1993   129-94-5-14

Purpose.—Deformities of the extremities may follow fractures in patients with various types of neuropathies, including diabetic neuropathy. Despite a rational approach to therapy, progressive skeletal deformities may develop as the result of fracture nonunion or malunion, particularly when treatment includes weight-bearing. In 1 series of patients with type I diabetes, reconstructive surgery was performed in an attempt to salvage lower extremities with fracture-associated deformities.

Patients.—Fifteen lower extremities in 14 adults with type I diabetes and neuropathic osteoarthropathy were treated. All fractures were in the region of the ankle or tarsal bones. In 13 patients, the deformity occurred after treatment by means other than non–weight-bearing and immobilization. In the other 2 patients, the deformity was diagnosed late. All of the deformities, which were severe and were the result of fracture nonunion or malunion, were managed by surgical reconstruction.

In 11 patients, the deformity was difficult to manage even with a custom orthosis; the other 4 cases were associated with persistent ulcers. Criteria for the success of reconstruction included healing of ulcerations, a plantigrade foot, and the ability to bear weight on the extremity with a patellar tendon-bearing orthosis.

Results.—A plantigrade, ulcer-free foot was achieved after reconstruction in 10 patients. The foot was plantigrade but with a persistent draining ulcer in 3 patients and was not plantigrade in 1. Only 1 of 4 feet that had an ulcer at the time of reconstruction had a successful result, compared with 10 of 11 feet without ulcerations. A total of 16 reconstructive procedures were performed. There were 3 complications: accelerated bone resorption and collapse in 2 patients and infection in 1.

Conclusion.—For patients with diabetic neuropathy, which causes uncontrollable deformities of the feet after a fracture, reconstructive surgery can allow a plantigrade foot and the use of a protective orthosis.

The results are better for patients without ulcerations at the time of reconstruction. Such surgery should be deferred until the ulcer has healed.

▶ The authors describe their experience with a very challenging patient population, patients with type I diabetes who also have neuropathic osteoarthropathy of the hindfoot. Soft bone secondary to hyperemia, altered bony anatomy secondary to bone collapse, and delayed healing all complicate attempted arthrodesis in these patients. Arthrodesis and/or osteotomy of the hindfoot is indicated in the face of uncontrollable deformity with a custommade ankle-foot orthrosis or recurrent skin breakdown.

They emphasize several important points. Osteotomies were liberally used to maximize bone apposition and an overall plantigrade foot. Large screws and staples were used exclusively to achieve internal fixation. External fixation arthrodesis favors pin tract infections in the diabetic population. Generally, an external fixator cannot be maintained long enough in patients with delayed bone healing. In cases in which neutral foot alignment is achieved with solid bony arthrodesis, the patient may become brace-free. However, the authors correctly point out that the vast majority of patients with significant hindfoot involvement will be brace-dependent indefinitely. For this reason, a very satisfactory result can be achieved, even with pseudarthrosis, provided the foot is plantigrade and long-term stability is achieved with the brace.

Perhaps one of the most challenging aspects of treating this population is early patient education. Patients must be aware that many months and even years of treatment are involved, sometimes with prolonged periods of non–weight-bearing. Defining the goals of treatment and reasonable expectations for outcome are essential elements in the patient education process of this unique population.—M.G. Wilson, M.D.

The Maisonneuve Fracture of the Fibula
Merrill KD (Univ of Missouri, Kansas City)
Clin Orthop 287:218–223, 1993   129-94-5–15

Background.—The Maisonneuve fracture of the fibula (MFF) has been considered a highly unstable ankle injury. However, little is known about the structures involved. The stability of an MFF was investigated to determine whether surgical intervention is routinely necessary.

Methods.—Eight of 9 patients with an MFF were treated with closed reduction and plaster casts; 1 underwent open reduction and internal fixation. Follow-up included subjective, objective, and functional evaluations, as well as stress roentgenograms, and ranged from 8 months to 4.5 years.

Results.—The outcome was excellent in 6 patients, good in 2, and fair in 1. Eight patients resumed preinjury activity levels; the remaining patient had a peroneal nerve palsy of unknown etiology. The range of motion in the injured ankle and subtalar joints was equal to that of the contralateral side in the 7 patients who were reexamined. Follow-up roentgenograms showed no increase in medial clear space or in the syndesmosis in 8 patients; 1 patient had a 1-mm increase in medial clear space. Only 1 patient had visible roentgenographic evidence of arthrosis.

Conclusion.—An MFF is often more stable than is generally assumed and often occurs with a partial syndesmotic diastasis. Injuries with partial syndesmotic disruption may be treated successfully without operation by internally rotating the foot to create an anatomical reduction.

▶ This small series of proximal fibula fractures associated with ankle injuries demonstrates that surgical repair of the syndesmosis is not necessarily required to provide long-term stability. Satisfactory stabilization of the mortise was provided with the use of cast immobilization in this series. Pankovich (1) pointed out that the MFF occurs as a result of lateral rotation force on the lateral malleolus, either in the supinated or, more commonly, in the pronated position. In fact, the high fracture of the fibula occurs because of pure rotation force along the axis of the fibula, whereas a lower fracture will occur when an additional force of abduction occurs. More often than not, the posteroinferior tibiofibular ligament is intact (grade III injury) and the ankle mortise will remain stable with closed treatment. Grade IV injuries, with rupture of the posterior ligament, will create problems of chronic instability and require internal repair.

The evaluation of ankle fractures and soft tissue injuries must be individualized. The importance of the lateral malleolus to the health of the mortise is clear. Indirect force injuries occurring at or above the syndesmosis should be evaluated for disruption either by preoperative stress radiography or intraoperative stress testing. Excessive shortening of the fibula must also be evaluated and corrected.—M.G. Wilson, M.D.

Reference

1. Pankovich AM: *J Bone Joint Surg (Am)* 58-A:337, 1976.

Early Mobilization of Operated on Ankle Fractures: Prospective, Controlled Study of 40 Bimalleolar Cases
Ahl T, Dalén N, Lundberg A, Bylund C (Danderyd Hosp, Sweden; Karolinska Hosp, Stockholm)
Acta Orthop Scand 64:95–99, 1993   129-94-5–16

Objective.—In a randomized study of patients operated on for displaced bimalleolar and trimalleolar ankle fractures, early and late weight-bearing and active ankle movements were compared.

Patients and Methods.—Thirty-seven patients were included in the study. Excluded were children and those with open fractures. Randomization after operation was to a dorsal splint group (no weight-bearing) or an orthosis group (weight-bearing). All patients were encouraged to move the ankle actively. The groups were identical in mean age (55 years) and had similar male/female ratios. Thirty-five cases involved fractures of the posterior tibial margin. All ankles were operated using cerclage wires, staples, and pins. Postoperative radiographic examinations were performed at 3 months and at a minimum of 18 months.

Results.—All fractures healed properly. Five minor complications—3 superficial wound infections, 1 local wound necrosis, and 1 skin irritation—occurred in the orthosis group; all healed with local treatment. At 18-month follow-up, all but 1 patient had a capacity of dorsiflexion exceeding 10 degrees and of plantar flexion exceeding 20 degrees. Arthrosis was observed in 3 ankles in each group. There was a small but significant increase in fracture instability in the early motion group. Early ankle movement was not associated with lasting superior clinical results.

Conclusion.—A plaster cast and late or no weight-bearing are still widely used after operations on ankle fractures. Others have advocated active ankle movements without weight-bearing during the entire period of rehabilitation. In the patients included in this study, early active ankle movements did not reveal lasting clinical advantages. Early postoperative weight-bearing in a walking cast is recommended because it aids rehabilitation.

▶ This very important and well-constructed prospective randomized study examines the role of early weight-bearing and early range of motion after surgical treatment of ankle fractures. Bimalleolar and trimalleolar fractures were included, and patients were well matched for age and Lauge-Hansen classification. Stereophotogrammetric analysis using implanted tantalum markers was used in approximately half of the group to detect any subtle shift in fracture fragments after fixation. In terms of pain relief, range of motion, and early radiographic analysis for arthrosis, all groups performed equally whether weight-bearing or range of motion was instituted early or not.

Certainly, allowing early weight-bearing in a cast would greatly facilitate postoperative rehabilitation, especially in the elderly population. However, it should be noted that when the authors added early motion, 1.2 mm of ankle mortise widening and 2.3 mm of angulation of the lateral malleolus were noted by their sensitive x-ray analysis. Even though this subset of patients did not display early arthrosis, further collaborative studies are indicated to demonstrate the safety of early motion combined with early weight-bearing. In the interim, the authors' recommendation of early weight-bearing with cast mobilization seems prudent. Of course, injuries that are not length-stable, such as plafond injuries, should have weight-bearing delayed during the initial 8–12 weeks.—M.G. Wilson, M.D.

Unilateral External Fixation for Severe Pilon Fractures

Bonar SK, Marsh JL (Univ of Iowa, Iowa City)
Foot Ankle 14:57–64, 1993   129-94-5–17

Introduction.—Although open reduction and rigid internal fixation are generally recommended for tibial plafond fractures, such treatment has a high complication rate in severe fractures. This rate could be reduced by some form of treatment that achieved articular alignment while stabilizing the fracture with minimal soft tissue disruption. The use of an external fixator to maintain alignment and length in severe plafond fractures, combined with limited internal fixation for articular reconstruction, was investigated.

Patients.—The retrospective study included the first 21 consecutive patients treated by external fixation. All patients had severe tibial plafond fractures. By the Ovadia and Beals classification, there were 9 type III, 4 type IV, and 8 type V fractures. By the methods of Rüedi and Allgöwer, there were 9 type II and 12 type III fractures. There were 7 open fractures. Three patients had associated vascular injuries, and 5 had permanent neurologic deficits. All patients were treated with unilateral, large screw external fixation in the talus and calcaneus. Limited external fixation was used when feasible to reconstruct the articular surface.

Results.—Severe comminution prohibited an attempt at articular reconstruction in 5 patients. Ankle arthrodeses were needed in 4 of these patients, and the remaining patient, who had a type IIIB fracture, required late amputation. In the remaining 16 patients, the articular surface was fixed with an average of 3 small fragment screws. Reduction of the articular surface was anatomical in 11 patients and fair in 5. Healing occurred in all these patients, with no wound infection, skin sloughing, or osteomyelitis.

Conclusion.—For patients with severe tibial plafond fractures, large screw external fixation can avoid the potentially disastrous complications associated with open reduction and internal fixation. The less-extensive tissue dissection in an area that is prone to wound complications may account for the low rates of infection, nonunion, and other serious problems. This technique provides safe and accurate reduction while allowing motion. A prospective multicenter trial of this method is underway.

Pilon Fractures: Treatment With Combined Internal and External Fixation

Tornetta P III, Weiner L, Bergman M, Watnik N, Steuer J, Kelley M, Yang E (Kings County Hosp Ctr, Brooklyn, NY; Mt Sinai Med Ctr, New York)
J Orthop Trauma 7:489–496, 1993   129-94-5–18

Background.—Fractures of the distal end of the tibia are difficult to treat. Nonoperative treatment gives poor results, and external fixation does not permit early motion of the joint. In a prospective study, the use of limited internal fixation with lag screws, combined with a hybrid external fixator that does not cross the ankle joint, was evaluated in the treatment of distal tibial fractures.

Patients and Methods.—The 26 patients had distal tibial fractures, all within 5 cm of the ankle joint. The average patient age was 32 years, and follow-up ranged from 8 to 36 months. Treatment consisted of limited internal fixation and the use of a hybrid external fixator as a neutralization device. This device included tensioned wires distally and 5-mm half-pins proximally attached to a semicircular frame without crossing the ankle joint. At operation, accurate reduction and fixation of the intra-articular component of the fracture were achieved via an incision based over the fracture site, followed by metaphyseal stabilization using the hybrid external fixator. In the series, there were 17 intra-articular, 9 extra-articular, and 6 open fractures. Bone grafting was required in 11 patients.

Results.—Healing occurred in an average of 4.2 months. Eighty-one percent of patients had good to excellent results, including 70.5% in patients with intra-articular fractures and 69% of those with Ruedi type III fractures. Two patients in the latter classification had poor results. Complications included 1 superficial and 1 deep infection, 3 pin tract infections, and 1 malunion in 10 degrees of varus.

Conclusion.—Combined internal and external fixation for patients with fractures of the distal end of the tibia produced good results in this study. The technique, which reduces the soft tissue dissection necessary for the placement of large plates, preserves the goals of early motion and fracture stability. The keys to the success of the procedure are careful placement of the incision over a major fracture line and the use of a hybrid external fixator to stabilize the methaphysis.

▶ There is practically no subcutaneous tissue at the level of the ankle and distal tibia. Swelling that occurs as a result of high-energy trauma occurs in a relatively noncompliant space. Soft tissue contusion and devascularization from extensive exposure combined with large metallic implants causes frequent wound breakdown and frank wound sepsis after traditional methods of rigid internal fixation for pilon fractures. Teeny et al. noted a 37% deep infection rate in a series of 60 patients treated with open reduction with internal fixation (1). The combination of deep sepsis and extensive bone devascularization requires either amputation or complicated bone reconstitution after radical débridement. There is currently a groundswell of interest in more indirect reduction techniques to lessen the implant loading of a wound and maintain fracture vascularity.

These 2 classic articles (Abstracts 129-94-5–17 and 129-94-5–18) describe the use of external fixation combined with minimal internal fixation of the articular surface. The 2 described techniques differ slightly in that the one described by Bonar and Marsh spans the ankle joint with a medial external fixator, whereas the one by Tornetta et al. contains all fixation within the tibia using the fixator at the metaphyseal level and encourages early postoperative ankle motion. The advantages of the latter technique can only be considered theoretical at this time. The authors do not directly report the range of motion obtained in their patients, and a true comparison to a matched subset spanning the ankle joint has yet to be performed. Furthermore, I believe that the second technique, using metaphyseal pin fixation, is suitable only for cases involving 2 or 3 main articular fragments (Ruedi type II) because the metaphyseal pins cannot truly buttress areas of large comminution. In more comminuted instances (Ruedi type III), I would prefer to span the ankle joint with the external fixator, thus neutralizing compressive forces. Tornetta et al. experienced 4 of 13 failures using the metaphyseal pin fixation in Ruedi type fractures.

Despite these variations in technique, both groups of authors succeeded in their main objective, gaining bony union and restoring function in the vast majority of patients with only 1 case of deep wound infection. Any surgeon considering treatment of high-energy pilon fractures should at least be aware of the technique of unilateral external fixation with minimal internal articular fixation.—M.G. Wilson, M.D.

Reference

1.   Teeny S, et al: *Orthop Trans* 14:265, 1990.

Analysis of Morphology and Gait Function After Intraarticular Calcaneal Fracture
Mittlmeier T, Morlock MM, Hertlein H, Fässler M, Mutschler W, Bauer G, Lob G (Universität München, Germany; Universität Ulm, Germany)
J Orthop Trauma 7:303–310, 1993   129-94-5–19

Background.—An increasing number of investigators are finding that open reduction and internal fixation is the preferred treatment for displaced intra-articular calcaneal fractures. Many surgeons, assuming that quasi-anatomical reduction coincides with adequate function, use morphological parameters to show the efficacy of surgery with optimum restoration of calcaneal geometry and joint surfaces. A prospective study was done to correlate morphological parameters and functional evaluation.

Methods.—Forty-five patients were assessed after surgical treatment of intra-articular calcaneal fractures. Standard radiographic and CT scores, clinical findings, and gait analysis were used. The mean follow-up after reconstruction was 23 months.

Findings.—Although clinical findings and gait function were well correlated, radiographic scores had only a poor-to-moderate correlation with functional assessment, which was probably the result of the missing analysis of soft tissue parameters. Comparison of clinical findings and gait parameters with individual radiographic parameters enabled an identification of factors with the greatest effect seen on functional prognosis.

Conclusion.—Morphological analysis after calcaneal reconstruction using radiographic techniques does not predict subsequent function or substitute for functional evaluation. However, it does enable clinicians to draw conclusions about surgical strategy in primary osseous reconstruction or secondary corrections.

▶ This study by Mittlmeier et al. comparing functional and radiographic outcome of surgically fixed calcaneal fractures may seem at face value to demonstrate how little we know about the natural history of these injuries. Overall, there was a general lack of correlation between the clinical result of surgery and the radiographic appearance of the calcaneus at follow-up. One surprising finding was the lack of correlation between the degree of articular congruence and the functional outcome. Other radiographic parameters such as the width of the calcaneus (which implies lateral soft tissue impingement) and the overall radiographic score better correlated with the functional outcome.

This reinforces the basic principle of calcaneal fixation that restoration of the subtalar joint surface is only one of the principal goals of treatment. Narrowing the heel, bringing the Achilles insertion down to a normal level, and correcting varus and valgus alignment are equally, if not more, important than the condition of the posterior facet. This paper attacks head-on a very critical question: Why do some patients' clinical performances not mirror the radiographic appearance of their hindfeet? One shortcoming of this study is that it relies on a historically obsolete preoperative classification that relies on plain radiography rather than CT scan.—M.G. Wilson, M.D.

Intraarticular Calcaneal Fractures: Results of Closed Treatment
Crosby LA, Fitzgibbons T (Creighton Univ, Omaha, Neb)
Clin Orthop 290:47–54, 1993   129-94-5–20

Introduction.—Closed treatment of extra-articular fractures of the calcaneus has yielded predictable and satisfactory results, but the proper management of intra-articular calcaneal fractures remains uncertain.

Series.—Twenty-seven patients were seen with 30 intra-articular fractures of the calcaneus in 1984–1988. Three of the patients had bilateral injuries. A majority of the fractures resulted from a fall. Half the patients had associated injuries. There were 30 type I fractures, which were slightly displaced or not displaced; 10 displaced type II fractures with at least 2 mm of either diastasis or depression of the fragments, or both; and 7 comminuted type III fractures. The average follow-up after treatment was 3 years.

Treatment and Results.—Most type I fractures were managed with a compression dressing and early motion, but 2 patients underwent closed reduction. Patients resumed weight-bearing an average of 8 weeks after injury. The outcome was excellent in 8 instances, good in 4, and fair in 1. Three of the 10 type II fractures were treated by compression with early motion, 5 by closed reduction and a plaster cast, and 2 by the Essex-Lopresti method of reduction. Two feet in this group had a good result, 4 a fair result, and 4 a poor outcome. The same methods were used to treat the 7 type III fractures, all of which had a poor outcome. In all, 47% of feet in this series had an excellent or good result, whereas 37% had a poor result. On multiple regression analysis, the type of fracture was the only significant prognostic factor.

Recommendations.—Closed treatment is appropriate for type I intra-articular calcaneal fractures. Patients with more severely displaced fractures may do better if the injury is anatomically reduced and securely fixed.

▶ Crosby and Fitzgibbons propose a very reasonable classification scheme of intra-articular calcaneal fractures based on coronal CT scans. Using closed treatment techniques, the vast majority of their patients with type I, nondisplaced fractures did well. Their 1 fair result may have been caused by extra-articular deformity. The remaining 12 excellent or good results in this group validate closed treatment for nondisplaced or minimally displaced fractures. The most significant clinical findings were in those patients with significant displacement of the articular surface but who had 2 or 3 major fracture fragments. These type II patients uniformly did poorly with closed treatment techniques, including 2 percutaneous pin manipulations. These are the specific fractures for which internal fixation is most gratifying, as accurate articular reconstruction is possible to a high degree. Clinically, the greatest tragedy is when this type of fracture is not even detected because early treatment is initiated based solely on plain radiographs. The patients with type III, comminuted articular fractures all did poorly with closed treatment. Although the articular surface in these injuries may not be reconstructible, these injuries also tend to have greater extra-articular deformity, which can often be successfully addressed by early surgery. Later fusion is also more straightforward, avoiding the need for challenging reconstruction techniques such as additional osteotomy or distraction bone blocks.—M.G. Wilson, M.D.

Operative Treatment in 120 Displaced Intraarticular Calcaneal Fractures: Results Using a Prognostic Computed Tomography Scan Classification
Sanders R, Fortin P, DiPasquale T, Walling A (Tampa Gen Hosp, Fla; Florida Orthopedic Inst, Tampa)
Clin Orthop 290:87–95, 1993   129-94-5–21

Background.—The diagnosis and treatment of displaced intra-articular fractures of the calcaneus may pose difficult problems. For several years, these fractures have been treated operatively, via a lateral approach with lag screws and side plate without bone grafting, at 1 institution.

Methods.—A classification of intra-articular calcaneal fractures by which to evaluate the results was developed. The classification used standardized coronal and transverse CT scans of both feet. Nondisplaced fractures, which were treated nonoperatively, were classified as type I. Two-part or split fractures were classified as type II, three-part or split depression fractures as type III, and four-part or highly comminuted articular fractures as type IV. The results of 120 fractures treated during 4 years were evaluated by means of the Maryland Foot Score and repeat CT scans. The mean follow-up was 29 months.

Results.—Despite the degree of preoperative displacement, radiographic evaluation showed complete restoration of heel height, width, and length in all patients. Anatomical radiographic joint reduction was achieved in 86% of the 79 type II fractures and 60% of the 30 type III fractures but in none of the 11 type IV fractures. Clinical results were good to excellent in more than 70% of type II and III fractures; the percentage of such results increased with time, from 27% in the first year to 84% in the fourth. However, the results for type IV fractures failed to improve, with only 9% being good or excellent.

Conclusion.—The classification of displaced intra-articular calcaneal fractures is a clinically useful one with prognostic significance. As the number of fragments increases the results deteriorate because of the difficulty of achieving anatomical reduction. Even with such a reduction, there is no guarantee of a good result. The surgeon's results will improve over time for type II and III fractures. Results are worse with type IV fractures, for which primary arthrodesis should be considered.

▶ This article by Sanders et al. is an absolute classic on the acute treatment of intra-articular calcaneal fractures. This large series of patients, treated consistently according to a logical operative protocol, were uniformly assessed by standard functional scoring but also, importantly, by follow-up CT scan evaluation to assess the quality of the reduction. In fractures with 2 or 3 main fragments, reproducibly good or excellent results were obtained by the described technique. This is precisely the group of patients that is helped so dramatically by internal fixation, in contrast to the dismal results of closed treatment in the same group, as described by Crosby and Fitzgibbons (Abstract 129-94-5-20).

Interestingly, those patients with multiple fracture fragments (type IV patients) received poor functional scores, which argues in favor of early fusion of the joint surface. Nevertheless, the positive effects of restoring the normal calcaneal anatomy was still believed to justify the reduction attempt in this comminuted subgroup. Most significantly, this study validates the classification scheme, as it demonstrates true prognostic value and guides the surgeon in patient selection. In my trauma practice, I rely exclusively on this classification scheme by Sanders and find it extremely useful.—M.G. Wilson, M.D.

Late Complications of Fractures of the Calcaneus
Myerson M, Quill GE Jr (Union Mem Hosp, Baltimore, Md; Louisville, Ky)
J Bone Joint Surg (Am) 75-A:331–341, 1993   129-94-5–22

Objective.—Because inadequate primary treatment of a calcaneal fracture can lead to persistent foot pain from a variety of possible sources, the operative results were reviewed in 42 patients having surgery for 43 calcaneal fractures in 1986–1988.

Injuries and Treatment.—The patients were seen with pain in the foot and/or ankle a mean of 26 months after injury. The 36 men and 6 women had a mean age of 36 years at the time of injury. Most injuries had resulted from a fall. Three patients had open fractures. All but 2 of 37 evaluable injuries were intra-articular fractures. Fifteen patients initially underwent an in situ subtalar arthrodesis, 14 had a subtalar distraction bone-block arthrodesis, and 5 had a triple arthrodesis. Seven patients underwent lateral calcaneal ostectomy, and 7 had transection with proximal transposition of the sural nerve. Five patients had release of the tibial nerve.

Findings.—Pain was relieved at least partly in 90% of patients and function improved in 83% of the group. Three fourths of patients returned to work or to their preinjury level of activity a mean of 8 months postoperatively. The interval tended to be longer as the time from injury to operation increased. Patients having a subtalar arthrodesis had the best outcome. There were 7 operative complications, including 2 malunions after a subtalar distraction bone-block arthrodesis. No patients had pseudarthrosis, skin necrosis, thrombophlebitis, or reflex sympathetic dystrophy.

Suggested Management.—Secondary surgery is indicated when primary treatment of a calcaneal fracture fails, because few patients can be expected to improve even with aggressive nonoperative management. Most patients will do well with a subtalar arthrodesis using an in situ or bone-block technique. If indicated, this may be supplemented by an ostectomy of the lateral calcaneal wall, but this procedure is not effective when used alone. Triple arthrodesis rarely is appropriate in these cases.

▶ This work by Myerson and Quill describes the difficulties in salvaging late complications of untreated or poorly treated calcaneal fractures. The authors compare, in a retrospective fashion, a spectrum of treatment options ranging from sural nerve decompression to distraction bone-block arthrodesis. The latter option provides the most predictable improvement in symptoms and is superior to in situ fusion of the subtalar joint. The addition of a bone block in the subtalar joint restores heel height and talar declination and thus decompresses the anterior ankle joint and adequately decompresses the lateral subfibular space. Distraction arthrodesis is the current gold standard for salvaging late calcaneal deformity, but it is a challenging procedure, particularly in the phase of marked varus deformity.—M.G. Wilson, M.D.

6 Orthopedic Oncology

Metastatic Carcinoma

▶↓ Metastatic carcinoma remains the most common malignant disease of the musculoskeletal system. In the usual situation, a patient with a known primary malignancy of the breast or lung has a painful lesion in a long bone and we, as orthopedic surgeons, are asked whether the patient should have a prophylactic fixation or whether the patient can be treated with irradiation alone. The time-honored criteria used as indications for prophylactic fixation as suggested by Fidler in 1973 (1) (pain, a radiolucent lesion larger than 2.5 cm, with greater than 50% of the cortex destroyed) have been questioned and are probably not adequate. Wilson Hayes, Ph.D., and his associates have been studying the strength-reducing effect of metastatic disease in an attempt to provide us with better criteria for prophylactic fixation.—D.S. Springfield, M.D.

Reference

1. Fidler M: *BMJ* 1:341, 1973.

Evaluation of Finite Element Analysis for Prediction of the Strength Reduction Due to Metastatic Lesions in the Femoral Neck
Cheal EJ, Hipp JA, Hayes WC (Harvard Med School, Boston)
J Biomech 26:251–264, 1993   129-94-6–1

Objective.—The frequency of bone metastasis requires clinicians to decide which patients require stabilization to prevent pathologic fracture. The ability of continuum finite element analysis to predict the fracture resistance of the proximal femur when a metastatic lesion is present in the femoral neck was investigated.

Methods.—Lesions were simulated in cadaver specimens by making 12.7-mm-diameter drill holes in the femoral neck, perpendicular to the axis of the neck and just distal to the subcapital line. The holes extended for 75% of the width of the femoral neck. A hole was drilled in the superolateral or inferomedial direction in the neck of 1 or both of 17 pairs of femurs, which then were loaded to failure. In vitro studies were done to quantify the decrease in strength associated with these defects. Two 3-dimensional finite element models were analyzed for each lesion and for the intact femur. A "global" model represented the entire proximal femur with a relatively coarse mesh, whereas a "local" model included only the femoral neck and lesion. Each analysis examined 5 different loading conditions.

Observations.—The fracture strength of a lesioned bone was about 45% less than that of the paired intact femur. The fracture strength of a bone with an inferomedial lesion was approximately 20% less than that of a bone with a superolateral lesion. The peak failure stresses predicted for axial loading were relatively constant for all finite element models. Directly comparing the strengths predicted by the finite element models with fracture strength values measured in vitro indicated that the models performed poorly. Nevertheless, the trends for gait and stair ascent loading for lesions at both sites were consistent with the in vitro findings. Incorporating anisotropic and asymmetric strength properties did not improve the performance of the models over that achieved using simpler octahedral shear stress and strain energy density criteria.

Conclusion.—The risk of fracture from femoral bone metastasis appears to be greatest when a lesion penetrates the inferomedial cortex of the femoral neck. A linear, macroscopic, continuum-based method of analysis does not accurately predict the fracture resistance of the proximal femur.

▶ The authors' complex mathematical model is beyond the understanding of the average orthopedic surgeon, but there is no need to struggle with the equations of finite element analysis. The authors are in the process of developing a model that can be used to assist us in predicting which lesion will lead to a fracture. In the future, we should be able to do a CT scan and feed the data into a finite element model that will provide a reliable risk factor for a pathologic fracture for the lesion in question. Designing the model has not been easy and the variables are greater than predicted, so to date we do not have an adequate model.

The orthopedic surgeon still must use clinical judgment in deciding which impending fractures to fix internally. I recommend prophylactic internal fixation for all painful lesions when a fracture would significantly increase the patient's morbidity. Humeral fractures are just about as easy to treat as an impending humeral fracture; therefore, I rarely fix a humerus prophylactically. On the other hand, a displaced pathologic fracture through the intertrochanteric area of the femur is much more difficult to treat than an impending fracture in this location, so I almost always treat these lesions when they are first discovered. We can look forward to the day when better methods of predicting will be available.—D.S. Springfield, M.D.

Strength Reductions From Trabecular Destruction Within Thoracic Vertebrae

McGowan DP, Hipp JA, Takeuchi T, White AA III, Hayes WC (Harvard Med

School, Boston)
J Spinal Disord 6:130–136, 1993

129-94-6-2

Introduction.—An in vitro model of metastasis in the thoracic vertebrae was used to show whether the extent of reduction in cross-sectional vertebal area may be used to predict the resultant reduction in strength.

Methods.—Trabecular defects were created in alternating vertebrae of fresh human thoracic spines. Most defects were made by passing an expanding reamer through the posterior vascular foramen. The lesioned vertebrae were tested to failure using a combined axial-flexion loading system. Linear regression analysis was used to relate the cross-sectional area of the superior end-plate to the load at failure for intact vertebrae.

Results.—The normalized strength of thoracic vertebrae bearing trabecular defects was linearly related to the reduction in cross-sectional diameter, with a correlation coefficient of .51. The mean failure load for intact vertebrae was significantly greater than that for vertebrae with defects. The fractures were similar in each instance, but more of the superior end-plate was involved when a defect was present, and, as a result, a larger part of the wall of the anterosuperior vertebral body buckled with the fracture.

Implications.—In contrast to a pathologic fracture in an extremity, fracture in the spine may result in impaction of trabecular bone and can even result in a strengthened vertebral body. The patient usually remains able to walk, and often pain decreases after a few weeks at rest. Secondary pain may result from the kyphotic deformity produced by pathologic fractures. Skin breakdown and neurologic deficit are also possible sequelae.

▶ Metastatic disease to vertebral bodies is common. These usually can be treated with irradiation; it is uncommon for the orthopedist to be faced with a decision about protecting an impending vertebral fracture, but with better management of patients with metastatic disease this may become an issue. It is clear that if we can prevent vertebral collapse, the quality of the patient's life will improve. The trabecular bone provides considerable strength to the vertebral body, and it is interesting that the reduction in strength of the body is directly related to the loss of trabecular bone. This should make us more attentive to the small lesion within the trabecular bone of a vertebral body, and we should at least recommend early irradiation and some protection (reduced activities or a brace) until the bone has a chance to heal. Prophylactic fixation of the spine is still controversial.—D.S. Springfield, M.D.

Spinal Instrumentation for Metastatic Disease: In Vitro Biomechanical Analysis

Heller JG, Zdeblick TA, Kunz DA, McCabe R, Cooke ME (Emory Univ, Atlanta, Ga; Univ of Wisconsin, Madison)
J Spinal Disord 6:17–22, 1993   129-94-6–3

Background.—The vertebral bodies are involved in 85% of patients with spinal metastases and, as a result, anterior surgical approaches are being increasingly used. Excellent visibility is possible, and tumors may be more completely resected than when using a posterior approach. Sublaminar wires have been used to provide segmental fixation at multiple spinal levels via a posterior approach. Both methyl methacrylate and cross-linking of rods have been used in an attempt to enhance mechanical stability.

Methods.—A complete corpectomy of the middle vertebra was performed in the calf spine. Biomechanical testing was done with a Bionix device modified to allow unconstrained motion under axial compression and pure moments of torsion and sagittal bending. The constructs tested included a Harms titanium cage; a cross-linked rectangular anterior Texas Scottish Rite Hospital (TSRH) construct; posterior Luque rods; cross-linked posterior Luque rods; and posterior Luque rods embedded in polymethylmethacrylate.

Findings.—The anterior TSRH construct, along or combined with posterior Luque rods, restored stability to the level seen with the intact spine on axial loading. On torsional testing, these constructs and cemented Luque rods provided a degree of stiffness equal to that of the intact spine. Cemented Luque rods were more effective in restoring sagittal stiffness on flexion/extension testing. Anterior TSRH instrumentation provided 5 times the sagittal stiffness of the intact specimen. A combination of anterior and posterior instrumentation yielded nearly 30 times the control stiffness.

Implications.—If the anterior and middle columns of the spine are incompetent, a condition that often results from metastatic disease, surgery is aimed at restoring spinal stability and decompressing the neural elements. Available forms of spinal instrumentation differ in their ability to restore axial, sagittal, and torsional stiffness.

▶ Patients with metastasis to the spine with destruction of the vertebral body, or in whom the vertebral body is removed, need a reconstruction that will provide sufficient strength to stabilize the spine so that they can be mobile and comfortable. These data from Heller and associates suggest that the spine that has lost its anterior and middle columns needs both an anterior and a posterior reconstruction. I think this is true for patients with metastatic disease, who are best treated with a method that provides immediate strength and for whom wearing a brace for a significant portion of their remaining life seems inappropriate. On the other hand, I have treated patients with only an anterior bone graft after having done a vertebrectomy when they could tolerate prolonged bracing. Patients who have lost some of their posterior stability, either from prior surgery or from bone destruction from the metastatic disease, should have posterior internal fixation in addition to the anterior procedure.—D.S. Springfield, M.D.

Osteosarcoma

Complications and Surgical Indications in 144 Cases of Nonmetastatic Osteosarcoma of the Extremities Treated With Neoadjuvant Chemotherapy

Ruggieri P, De Cristofaro R, Picci P, Bacci G, Biagini R, Casadei R, Ferraro A, Ferruzzi A, Fabbri N, Cazzola A, Campanacci M (Univ of Bologna, Italy)
Clin Orthop 295:226–238, 1993   129-94-6–4

Series.—One hundred forty-four patients (75 males and 69 females aged 3–41 years) were treated for localized osteosarcoma of the extremity from 1986 to 1989. Sixty-five of the patients were younger than 14 years of age. All of the patients had high-grade extracompartmental osteosarcoma without metastatic disease (stage IIB) when initially seen. Two thirds of the tumors were osteoblastic osteosarcomas.

Treatment.—All patients received preoperative chemotherapy and underwent surgery 3 weeks after completion of the second cycle of treatment, when the lesion was restaged. The goal was to obtain wide margins, but ablation was performed only when limb salvage procedures offered uncertain results. Limb salvage was possible in 122 patients; 13 patients had amputation, and 9 had rotationplasty. Chemotherapy was continued postoperatively. A modular cemented prosthesis, the Modular Resection Shoulder, was used for the proximal humerus, and the modular cementless Kotz Modular Femur Tibia Resection system was used in the lower extremity.

Results.—The surgical margins were classified as radical in 6% of cases, wide in 76%, marginal in 8%, intralesional in 5%, and wide but contaminated in 5%. When tumor necrosis exceeded 90%, the disease-free survival rate was 79%, compared with 72% for poor responders. Two of the 32 patients in whom lung or bone metastases developed also had local recurrences. The time to metastatic relapse averaged 22 months. Most limb salvage operations caused complications, but more than half of them yielded functional results exceeding 50% according to Enneking's new system.

Conclusion.—Limb salvage surgery is an effective approach to nonmetastatic osteosarcoma of the extremity when combined with neoadjuvant chemotherapy.

▶ During the past decade, limb salvage surgery for osteosarcoma has become the standard treatment and amputations are uncommon. Although we have assumed that limb salvage is better than an amputation, this has been difficult to demonstrate. In addition, the complications of limb salvage surgery are greater than those after an amputation. Only with long-term follow-up of results are we able to judge the place of limb salvage for patients with osteosarcoma. We have found that complications are more common than we had predicted, and these complications can have a dramatic effect on a patient's life.

Limb salvage is still the best treatment for the majority of patients with a limb osteosarcoma, but we must tell the patients and their families that the limb salvage operation is more difficult, the recovery is longer, and the risk of complication is higher than with an amputation. In addition, if a complication interferes with the administration of chemotherapy, it reduces the chance for cure, and it is better to accept an amputation than the increased chance of metastatic disease. We should not allow saving a limb to threaten the chance for cure.—D.S. Springfield, M.D.

Giant-Cell Tumor of Bone

▶↓ Giant-cell tumor (GCT) of bone is a common tumor of the musculoskeletal system. It usually arises in the epiphysis/metaphysis of a long bone in patients between 20 and 40 years of age. In the 1970s, resection of GCT of bone was common, either as the initial management or in the case of a recurrence, but now it is more popular to do an aggressive curettage. Giant-cell tumor of bone is a lesion with many characteristics of a malignant tumor but with little potential for taking a patient's life. It should provide an excellent model for studying the genetic defects that produce tumors but not the defects that allow a tumor to metastasize.—D.S. Springfield, M.D.

Monocyte-Macrophage Lineage of Giant Cell Tumor of Bone: Establishment of a Multinucleated Cell Line
Huang T-SW, Green AD, Beattie CW, Das Gupta TK (Univ of Illinois, Chicago; Humana Hosp Michael Reese, Chicago)
Cancer 71:1751–1760, 1993   129-94-6–5

Background.—Giant-cell tumor (GCT) of bone sometimes evolves into malignant GCTs possessing morphological features of bony sarcoma. This type of GCT of bone may be a variant of the pathogenic process of osteogenic sarcoma. However, the histogenesis of the tumor cells has not been determined. A new cell line, UISO-GCT-1, which maintains multinucleated cells, has been created to identify the putative origin of GCT lesions.

Methods.—The cell line was established from a histologic grade 1 GCT of the left proximal tibia in a man aged 18 years. Immunohistochemical, cytogenic, ultrastructural, and growth characteristics were analyzed.

Results.—The UISO-GCT-1 cells at passage 5 had a high plating efficiency, with a 76.8-hour doubling time. Cells with more than 4–6 nuclei persisted in culture at passage 17. In monolayer culture, mononuclear and multinucleated cells expressed vimentin and tartrate-resistant acid phosphatase and reacted with monoclonal antibodies for CD13 and CD68, which suggests a monocytic-macrophage origin. Mononuclear and multinuclear cells also selectively expressed high-molecular-weight cell membrane antigens specific to soft tissue sarcomas and osteosarcomas. The UISO-GCT-1 cells were hypodiploid, hypotetraploid, and multiploid; some cells contained more than 200 chromosomes per mitosis. Additional chromosomal aberrations included ring chromosomes, double minutes, translocations, multiple fragments, and multiradials.

Conclusion.—Karyotypically abnormal GCTs of bone arise from a line of monocyte-macrophages and express antigens similar to those of malignant mesenchymal tumors. The large number of chromosomal aberrations associated with the UISO-GCT-1 cell line correlates with the locally aggressive nature but not the tumorigenicity of GCT of bone.

▶ Recent analysis of the genetic material from the tumor cells has shown that many tumors are caused by similar alterations in their DNA. The same oncogenes have been found in a variety of different tumor types. We have found that the same oncogenes are often present in osteosarcoma, colon cancer, and breast cancer. There has been little examination of the genetic material of benign tumors. Giant-cell tumor of bone should be an excellent tumor for chromosomal and DNA analysis. Its local behavior is similar to that of a malignant tumor, but it rarely has the ability to metastasize.

The chromosomal and DNA alterations in GCT of bone should be those that produce an aggressive local tumor but not ones that permit metastatic spread. Chromosomal analysis has suggested that the origins of GCT of bone is monocyte-macrophage and not stromal as is the case with other bone tumors. This is just the beginning, and more detailed examinations will be necessary to find the oncogenes, including DNA analysis.—D.S. Springfield, M.D.

Solid Variant of Aneurysmal Bone Cyst
Bertoni F, Bacchini P, Capanna R, Ruggieri P, Biagini R, Ferruzzi A, Bettelli G, Picci P, Campanacci M (Ospedale Malpighi, Bologna, Italy; Istituto Ortopedico Rizzoli, Bologna, Italy)
Cancer 71:729–734, 1993   129-94-6–6

Background.—The aneurysmal bone cyst (ABC) apparently has a solid variant, which is characterized by fibrous proliferation with giant cell and bone production along with fibromyxoid areas and small aneurysmal spaces in the solid parts of the cyst. Lesions with these characteristics have also been called extragnathic, giant-cell reparative granulomas. The clinical, radiologic, and histologic appearances of solid ABC were analyzed to identify the morphological features that may differentiate it from malignant conditions.

Methods.—By using Sanerkin's criteria, 15 cases of solid variants of ABC were identified. Clinical information and histologic sections were reviewed for all cases; preoperative radiographs were reviewed for 14.

Results.—The metaphysis was involved in 8 of 11 lesions in long bones. The adjacent ABC did not cross the physis in the 5 patients with open physis. The preoperative radiographic appearances were nonspecific. In 7 patients the radiographs revealed stage 3 lesions, but in 3 cases a benign vs. malignant distinction could not be made. Microscopic examination revealed consistent spindle and oval cell proliferation of fibroblasts and fibrohistiocytes with mitoses in all cases. Scattered myxoid areas were present in 80% of cases. The presence of giant cells was another consistent feature; however, abundance and concentration varied. Marginal resection was performed in 3 patients with a diaphyseal location. The remaining patients underwent intralesional excision, followed by phenol therapy in 2 patients and by radiation therapy in 1. Twelve patients were followed for a mean of 59 months without recurrence.

Discussion.—A solid ABC is easily mistaken for a spindle cell neoplasm. The abundant mitoses suggest the reactivity of the lesion. The zonal diffusion indicates an injury and repair lesion. The higher cellular and mitotic activity distinguishes solid ABC from low-grade osteosarcoma, and a short clinical history of ABC is unlike the long history in well-differentiated osteosarcoma. The pattern of bone production in solid ABC differs from the type of bone associated with low- and high-grade osteosarcoma.

▶ Aneurysmal bone cyst is usually a blood-filled cavity with a thick lining composed of benign spindle cells, multinucleated giant cells, and, often, islands of osteoid. Some believe that ABC is not a neoplastic lesion but is secondary to another lesion or a reactive process. It is true that ABC-like areas are common in giant-cell tumor of bone, chondroblastoma, osteoblastoma, and osteosarcoma, but it is very uncommon for the primary lesion not to be obvious.

Whether there is a solid variant of ABC is controversial. It is hard to separate this lesion from giant-cell tumor of bone. This may not be important, as both should be treated with an aggressive curettage. Of more importance is the recognition that the histology of this lesion can be confused with an osteosarcoma, and we must be wary of that mistake. It is unlikely that you will put solid ABC on your prebiopsy differential diagnosis; however, if you find a solid lesion and the pathologist suggests that it is an atypical osteosarcoma, remember this lesion. Whether phenol should be used or whether it is necessary in the treatment of these lesions is not known. I do not use phenol.—D.S. Springfield, M.D.

▶↓ These next 2 articles discuss atypical giant-cell tumor (GCT) of bone. The first discusses GCTs of bone that are atypical because of the age of the patients and the second because of the location. Half of the nonepiphyseal lesions were in patients older than 20 years of age, indicating that this unusual location is not related to age.—D.S. Springfield, M.D.

Giant Cell Tumor in Children and Adolescents

Schütte HE, Taconis WK (Univ Hosp Rotterdam, The Netherlands; Onze Lieve Vrouwe Gasthuis, Amsterdam)
Skeletal Radiol 22:173–176, 1993   129-94-6-7

Background.—Although giant-cell tumors (GCTs) primarily occur in patients older than age 20 years, cases in children and adolescents younger than age 19 years have been reported. The characteristics of GCT in a population of children and adolescents were studied.

Methods.—The records and radiographs of 49 patients younger than age 19 years with a histologically confirmed diagnosis of GCT and adequate radiographs were reviewed. Most of the 31 female and 18 male patients were aged 15–18 years.

Results.—Thirty-four tumors were located in short and long tubular bones; all involved the proximal and distal metaphysis and the adjacent diaphysis. Metaphyseal lesions occurred in 3 patients with an average age of 11 years; metadiaphyseal lesions occurred in 6 patients with an average age of 13 years; epimetaphyseal lesions occurred in 10 patients with an average age of 17 years; and epimetadiaphyseal lesions occurred in 17 patients with an average age of 17 years. Lesions in tubular bones with open epiphyseal growth plates did not involve the epiphyses; possible exceptions were 2 epimetadiaphyseal lesions in which it was difficult to verify epiphyseal growth plate closure.

Conclusion.—Epiphyseal involvement of GTC appears to increase with patient age. A predominance of GCT in girls and female adolescents is also suggested.

► Giant-cell tumor of bone is a lesion that almost always occurs in patients with closed growth plates and is rarely included in the differential diagnosis of a lesion in a teenager. Osteosarcoma can look like a GCT of bone and is more likely in a teenager. If the lesion is a GCT of bone (be cautious accepting that diagnosis), it can be treated with a curettage as can other GCTs.—D.S. Springfield, M.D.

Nonepiphyseal Giant Cell Tumor of the Long Bones: Clinical, Radiologic, and Pathologic Study

Fain JS, Unni KK, Beabout JW, Rock MG (Mayo Clinic and Found, Rochester, Minn)
Cancer 71:3514–3519, 1993   129-94-6-8

Background.—Metaphyseal or diaphyseal giant-cell tumors (GCTs) without epiphyseal involvement are rare, and their clinical, histologic, and radiographic features have not been defined. Data from bone tumor surgical pathology files were reviewed to better characterize nonepiphyseal GCT.

Methods.—Fourteen cases of nonepiphyseal GCT were reviewed. Hematoxylin-eosin–stained tissue slides, clinical information including follow-up, and radiographs for all patients were studied.

Results.—The age at diagnosis ranged from 8 to 64 years; 5 patients were younger than age 15 years. Six cases involved the proximal tibia, 3 involved the distal radius, and 2 involved the fibula. The distal ulna, proximal humerus, and distal femur were each involved in 1 case. Ten GCTs were metaphyseal; 2 were metadiaphyseal; and 2 were diaphyseal, occurring in patients with closed epiphyses. Half the GCTs occurred in patients with open growth plates; 6 abutted the growth plate and the seventh was metadiaphyseal. The tumors had the typical histology of GCT of the bone: solid masses of plump, round-to-oval stromal cells intermingled with multinucleated osteoclast-type giant cells. Tumors recurred in 3 of 7 patients treated with curettage. Tumors excised en bloc did not recur.

Conclusion.—Although most GCTs occur in or near the epiphysis, GCT should also be suspected if the epiphysis is not involved. Exclusively metaphyseal or diaphyseal GCTs resemble epiphyseal GCTs in their biological aggressiveness and high recurrence rate after curettage; however, metaphyseal and diaphyseal GCTs tend to occur in younger patients, generally before epiphyseal growth plate closure. Radiographs are not diagnostic for this subset of GCT; histologic examination of the lesions is required in each case to differentiate nonepiphyseal GCT from more common bone metaphyseal and diaphyseal lesions.

▶ Giant-cell tumor of bone rarely occurs without epiphyseal involvement; most of the patients with nonepiphyseal GCTs are children. The diagnosis usually is not expected from the prebiopsy evaluation and pathologists should be questioned when they make this diagnosis in a nonepiphyseal lesion. It is unlikely that GCT of bone behaves more aggressively in this location, as suggested by these authors, but rather it probably is not curetted as aggressively. On the other hand, the consequence of a wide resection usually is not substantially greater than an aggressive curettage and, therefore, the treatment of choice in most of these lesions is a wide resection.—D.S. Springfield, M.D.

Giant Cell Tumor of the Sacrum
Turcotte RE, Sim FH, Unni KK (Mayo Clinic and Found, Rochester, Minn)
Clin Orthop 291:215–221, 1993   129-94-6–9

Background.—Giant-cell tumor (GCT) of the sacrum is rare; neverthe-less it accounted for 8% of all GCTs seen at 1 center during a 27-year period. The sacral location complicates treatment of these tumors, and treatment remains controversial. The records of all patients with sacral GCT treated from 1960 through 1986 were reviewed to evaluate treat-ment methods for this tumor.

Patients and Methods.—The charts, radiographs, and histologic slides of 26 patients with sacral GCT were reviewed. Sixteen cases involved ini-tial treatment; 10 involved local recurrences.

Results.—Patient age ranged from 15 to 77 years. The average dura-tion of follow-up was 7.8 years. Pain was generally located in the lower back, involving 1 of the buttocks and extending toward the posterior as-pect of the thigh. The average duration of pain was 8 months. Twenty-three patients (88%) experienced neurologic symptoms, generally neuro-genic bladder dysfunction, sphincter weakness, and perineal hypoesthe-sia. Twenty-one patients were treated surgically and 21 received radia-tion therapy. The local recurrence rate was 33% after curettage. Malignant transformation occurred in 3 patients after radiation therapy. Three benign tumors metastasized to the lungs. Four of 5 patients treated only with radiation were recurrence-free at follow-up ranging from 1 to 14 years. When this study was completed, 3 patients had died of tumor-related complications; 2 were alive with the disease.

Discussion.—Complete curettage is the principal treatment for sacral GCT. Wide resection, combining anterior and posterior approaches, compromises distal neurologic function and spinal stability and should be reserved for patients with exceptionally large tumors or malignant de-generation. Radiation therapy is not an alternative to surgical treatment and should be reserved for incomplete resection and local recurrence.

▶ Giant-cell tumor of the sacrum can be a difficult lesion to manage. When both S2 nerve roots and one S3 nerve root can be saved and the lesion re-sected, it should be treated with a resection. The patient will have a minimal risk of recurrence and will maintain normal bowel, bladder, and sexual func-tion. If a higher level of resection is needed, the risk of bowel, bladder, or sex-ual dysfunction is at least 50%. In the patients with more proximal lesions, the best management is a resection of the distal portion (below S3) of the tumor and curettage of the proximal component. I agree that irradiation should be reserved for patients with rapid recurrence who cannot be treated with a resection.—D.S. Springfield, M.D.

Giant-Cell Tumours of the Spine

Sanjay BKS, Sim FH, Unni KK, McLeod RA, Klassen RA (Mayo Clinic and Found, Rochester, Minn)

J Bone Joint Surg (Br) 75-B:148–154, 1993   129-94-6–10

Background.—Giant-cell tumors (GCTs) of the spine are rare, surgically challenging lesions. Treatment remains controversial, partly because of small patient numbers in published reports. This retrospective study represents the largest series of GCTs of the spine treated surgically at a single center.

Methods.—The records, imaging studies, and histologic slides of 24 patients with GCTs were reviewed. Follow-up included radiographic and clinical evaluation or evaluation by a community physician or a tumor registry letter.

Results.—Follow-up ranged from 1.5 to 29.6 years. All patients when first seen had pain, and half had a neurologic deficit. Tumors were equally distributed among the cervical, thoracic, and lumbar spines. Fourteen patients underwent 1-stage surgery, and 5 had local recurrence. The remaining 10 patients had 2-stage procedures, and 5 had local recurrence. Adjuvant radiation therapy was administered to the primary lesion in 1 patient and to recurrent lesions in 6. One of these patients subsequently had sarcoma. After surgery, improvement was seen in all but 1 of the patients who had been seen with radicular pain and in all patients who had had paraparesis.

Conclusion.—Giant-cell tumors of the spine should be completely removed. Because of their location, removal generally entails excision with an intralesional margin. To reduce risk for sarcomatous transformation, radiation therapy should be reserved for patients with incomplete excision or local recurrence.

► Giant-cell tumor of the spine is similar to that in the sacrum; whenever a resection can be done without neurologic deficit, it is better to do so, but a safe resection often cannot remove all of the tumor. In this case, a limited resection should be combined with a curettage and irradiation reserved for recurrent disease. It should be remembered that chordoma can occur in the spine at sites other than the sacrum and clivus. When it does, it is similar to GCT of the spine. The biopsy must be done carefully to reduce the risk of spreading the tumor cells unnecessarily.—D.S. Springfield, M.D.

The Treatment of Giant-Cell Tumors of the Distal Part of the Radius
Vander Griend RA, Funderburk CH (Univ of Florida, Gainesville)
J Bone Joint Surg (Am) 75-A:899–908, 1993   129-94-6–11

Background.—Among the possible treatments for giant-cell tumors (GCTs) of the distal part of the radius, curettage with subsequent bone grafting has been associated with a high rate of recurrence. The recurrence rate is lower for resection with arthroplastic reconstruction or arthrodesis. Although the overall effectiveness of each method has been analyzed, the indications for choice of treatment have not been clearly defined. The outcomes of patients treated for GCT of the distal part of the radius were reviewed to identify criteria that would guide treatment selection.

Patients and Methods.—The records of 23 patients diagnosed as having benign GCT of the distal part of the radius were reviewed; 7 cases involved local recurrence. Treatment was based on the extent of the tumor as shown on preoperative radiographs.

Results.—Five patients underwent extended curettage followed by packing of the cavity with methyl methacrylate. There was no local recurrence in these patients during an average follow-up of 6 years, and neither functional impairment nor degenerative changes were apparent. In the 18 remaining patients, the tumor exhibited extraosseous extension. Seventeen underwent resection of the distal part of the radius; the remaining patient had a below-the-elbow amputation. Resection followed by radiocarpal arthrodesis and use of an intercalary bone graft that was stabilized with a long plate provided the best functional result. Among the patients treated with resection and reconstruction, there was no local recurrence in 2 to 19 years of follow-up.

Discussion.—Curettage and packing has been considered the treatment of choice for GCTs; nevertheless, resection was more frequently used in this series of distal tumors of the radius. Three factors supported this treatment choice: extensive tumor involvement, which precluded curettage and the use of cement; the availability of several function-sparing resection and reconstruction options; and concerns regarding treatment difficulties and functional consequences of aggressive local recurrence after unsuccessful curettage.

▶ The distal radius is a common site of GCT of bone. It seems to have a higher risk of recurrence, probably because of the difficulty we have in doing an adequate curettage. Despite this, an aggressive curettage is the treatment of choice and should be done whenever possible. For those patients with recurrence, a repeat curettage can be done if it is technically possible; if it is not, a distal radial resection is indicated. The reconstruction options are numerous, and deciding which to use should be influenced by the patient's demands. The strongest reconstruction is an arthrodesis, but if the patient needs or wants more motion and does not need full strength, a transposition of the proximal fibula or an osteoarticular allograft can be done.—D.S. Springfield, M.D.

Giant Cell Tumour of Bone: A Surgical Approach to Grade III Tumours

Rooney RJ, Asirvatham R, Lifeso RM, Ali MA, Parikh S (King Faisal Specialist Hosp and Research Centre, Riyadh, Saudi Arabia)

Int Orthop 17:87–92, 1993   129-94-6–12

Background.—In Saudi Arabia, intralesional excision and bone grafting or cement is the standard treatment for benign giant-cell tumor (GCT) of bone, regardless of tumor extent, because cultural and religious habits necessitate preservation of knee function. This method is the accepted treatment for Campanacci grade I and grade II benign GCT; treatment of Campanacci grade III lesions has remained controversial. Records of patients with benign GCT of bone were reviewed to determine the appropriateness of intralesional excision with subsequent bone grafting or cement in Campanacci grade III lesions.

Methods.—The study included 31 skeletally mature patients with benign GCT of bone diagnosed by radiograph and histology. Radiographs were graded by using Campanacci's system. Patients underwent intralesional excision, marginal excision, wide excision, or radical excision, followed by cement packing or bone grafting.

Results.—Twenty-nine benign GCTs were Campanacci grade III; 2 were grade II. Eighteen grade III lesions and both grade II lesions were treated with intralesional excision, followed by cement packing or cancellous grafting. Among the patients treated with intralesional excision, 3 local soft tissue lesions and 2 local bone lesions recurred within 36 months of treatment. Only 1 of the 11 patients treated with marginal or wide excision had a recurrence. All recurrences were in grade III lesions.

Conclusion.—Grade III benign GCT may be treated by modified intralesional excision as long as the articular surfaces and part of the metaphysis are intact.

▶ The behavior of GCT of bone is unpredictable. Campanacci suggested a grading system based on the clinical presentation and plain radiograph, which were supposed to predict the behavior of the tumor. This grading system has not worked. Grade III lesions can be aggressive and can recur after a curettage or they may be permanently controlled with a curettage. We have not used Campanacci's grading system to decide how to treat a patient with GCT. We recommend an aggressive curettage of all GCTs as the initial treatment whenever possible. Resection should be reserved for recurrent lesions that cannot be curetted again or for the initial lesion if it has destroyed too much bone for a curettage.—D.S. Springfield, M.D.

Cementation in the Treatment of Giant Cell Tumor of Bone
Komiya S, Inoue A (Kurume Univ, Japan)
Arch Orthop Trauma Surg 112:51–55, 1993   129-94-6–13

Background.—The generally recommended treatment for giant-cell tumor (GCT) of bone is excision of the main bulk of the tumor with curettage of the peripheral portion to preserve function in the adjacent joint. Cementation may kill residual tumor cells after curettage, but the biological basis has not been determined. Cases of GCT of bone treated with cementation were reviewed to determine the effect of hyperthermia on GCT cells.

Methods.—Eleven patients with GCT of bone were treated by tumor excision and cementation with polymethyl methacrylate. A cell line of GCT containing only mononuclear cells was subcultured, and the cellular response to temperatures up to 60°C for as long as 10 minutes was examined. The surviving cells were counted, and flow cytometry was used to analyze the surface antigen expression and DNA distribution at the various temperatures.

Results.—All patients had excellent results without tumor recurrence, cement loosening, or osteoarthrosis. Hyperthermia caused a fair number of cells to fall into S phase with an unusually low tetraploid value. Cell survival and monocytic phenotype expression were inversely related to temperature and time. The rate of monocyte antigen expression fell from 97.3% in control cells to 74.1% in heated cells. No cells survived after heating at 60°C for 10 minutes.

Conclusion.—The tumoricidal effect of polymethyl methacrylate cementation in GCT is the result of hyperthermia resulting from polymerization. Excision plus cementation is a simple treatment for GCT of bone and procduces few complications. This procedure should gain acceptance in the treatment of benign aggressive bone tumors.

▶ The use of polymethyl methacrylate (PMMA) to fill the cavity left after an aggressive curettage of a GCT of bone is an accepted treatment and is thought to play a role in the reduction of recurrences. Whether there is actually a reduction in local recurrence has not been proven, and what role PMMA plays in this reduction is debatable. I suspect the more aggressive techniques of curettage are more important than is the PMMA. It is also not clear that the temperature of the bone and tumor cells adjacent to the PMMA gets to the 60°C that seems to be needed to produce significant necrosis. The advantage of PMMA is, I believe, its ability to immediately stabilize a large defect adjacent to the articular cartilage. I use PMMA in the treatment of GCT for its strength, not its heat.—D.S. Springfield, M.D.

Radiation Therapy for Giant Cell Tumor of Bone

Bennett CJ Jr, Marcus RB Jr, Million RR, Enneking WF (Univ of Florida, Gainesville)
Int J Radiat Oncol Biol Phys 26:299–304, 1993   129-94-6–14

Background.—Giant-cell tumor (GCT) of bone is a locally aggressive growth that frequently recurs locally but has a low potential for metastasizing. There has been concern that irradiating low-grade lesions may lead to "malignant transformation." Traditionally, GCTs have been managed by surgery only, but simple curettage is followed by local recurrence in as many as 60% of patients.

Series.—The results of radiotherapy were examined in 16 patients with histologically confirmed monostotic GCT of bone. Ten patients had not been previously treated, whereas 6 were seen with recurrent tumor. Soft tissue extension was present in 11 patients. Radiotherapy was delivered at various energy levels to a total tumor dose of 35 to 54 Gy, the mean dose being 43 Gy. Patients were followed for at least 32 months; 63% were followed for 5 years or longer, and 44% for 10 years or more.

Results.—Local control was achieved in three fourths of the patients, including 4 of the 6 patients who were treated for recurrent disease. All failures were at sites of irradiation. All 4 failures were in women, a trend seen in previous reports. Nine of the 11 tumors with soft tissue extension were controlled. There were no serious complications, and there has been no development of sarcoma within the radiation field.

Recommendations.—Curettage or wide resection is indicated if serious loss of function will not ensue. Radiotherapy should be considered if gross disease remains or if the lesion has recurred. Presently, a tumor dose of at least 40 Gy is recommended. Giant-cell tumor of bone is not a radioresistant lesion.

▶ Giant-cell tumor of bone can be treated with irradiation, but the risk of malignant degeneration makes this not the ideal treatment. It is difficult to know whether the new techniques used by the radiotherapist will reduce the risk of secondary malignancy as suggested, and it will be some years before we know the answer. Certainly, irradiation is a useful treatment for the patient with a recurrent GCT that cannot be resected or can only be resected with an amputation.—D.S. Springfield, M.D.

Ewing's Sarcoma

▶↓ Ewing's sarcoma is an uncommon malignant tumor of childhood. There was a time when all but a few patients died of this malignant tumor. The advances in our understanding and treatment of this disease have improved dramatically in the past decade.—D.S. Springfield, M.D.

Cytogenetic and Pathologic Aspects of Ewing's Sarcoma and Neuroectodermal Tumors
Stephenson CF, Bridge JA, Sandberg AA (Cancer Ctr of Southwest Biomedical Research Inst and Genetrix, Inc, Scottsdale, Ariz; Univ of Nebraska, Omaha)
Hum Pathol 23:1270–1277, 1992   129-94-6–15

Cytogenetic Comparison.—In Ewing's sarcoma, the reciprocal translocation t(11;22)(q24;q12) is a consistent primary chromosomal alteration. It may occur as a simple translocation, a complex one involving chromosomes in addition to 11 and 22, or a variant involving chromosome 22 and 1 or more others besides 11. The breakpoints are consistently q24 on chromosome 11 and q12 on chromosome 22. Secondary numerical and structural chromosomal changes, including trisomy 8, are common in Ewing's sarcoma. The basic translocation seen in Ewing's sarcoma is also described in various primitive neuroectodermal tumors. Some of these tumors, including those found in the posterior fossa, are associated with various numeric and structural arrangements but not t(11;22).

Histogenetic Observations.—It has generally been thought that Ewing's sarcoma arises from a noncommitted primitive mesenchymal cell, but there is some evidence supporting a neuroectodermal origin. Occasional examples of Ewing's sarcoma are positive for neuron-specific enolase, possess pseudorosette-like structures, and have ultrastructural characteristics similar to those of neuroblastoma. The morphological and histochemical differences among Ewing's sarcoma, peripheral neuroepithelioma, and Askin's tumor are quite subtle. The translocation t(11;22) is common to all these tumor types. Some Ewing's sarcoma cell lines exhibit only neuroectodermal markers.

Clinical Implications.—The translocation t(11;22)(q24;q12) is found in more than 90% of cases of Ewing's sarcoma and primitive neuroectodermal tumor. Both Askin's tumor and neuroepithelioma have been thought of as atypical neuroblastomas but have proved resistant to treatment. Because these lesions appear to be more closely related to Ewing's sarcoma, they should be treated as such.

▶ Genetic alterations in tumor cells that probably occur during reproduction of their DNA seem to be the cause of a cell becoming malignant and producing a sarcoma. These genetic alterations have been found with increasing frequency during the past few years. With this new knowledge we should be able to understand these sarcomas better and, with any luck, be able to treat the patient better. It is possible that in the future, patients who have tumors will be able to have the genetic defect repaired, the function lost because of the genetic alterations replaced, and their tumors cured.—D.S. Springfield, M.D.

Ewing's Sarcoma: Long-Term Follow-Up in 49 Patients Treated From 1967 to 1989

Mameghan H, Fisher RJ, O'Gorman-Hughes D, Bates EH, Huckstep RL, Mameghan J (Prince of Wales Children's Hosp, Randwick, NSW, Australia; Prince of Wales Hosp, Randwick, NSW, Australia)
Int J Radiat Oncol Biol Phys 25:431–438, 1993   129-94-6–16

Objective.—The results of treatment for Ewing's sarcoma of bone and soft tissues were reviewed in 49 patients seen from 1967 to 1989. The patients, with a median age of 16 years, were available for follow-up for an average of 12 years.

Management.—Treatment was individualized. Either amputation or definitive resection was done primarily if disease could be totally removed. Otherwise, patients underwent resection after receiving chemotherapy and/or radiotherapy to minimize the mutilating effects of surgery. The primary tumor was irradiated with a margin of normal tissue. New cytotoxic drugs were used as they became available.

Results.—Fifeen patients remain alive without disease; 2 others died of treatment-related complications without evidence of Ewing's sarcoma. Thirty-two patients, 8 of whom had metastatic disease when initially seen, have died of disease. The 5-year actuarial survival rate was 33% and the rate at 10, 15, and 20 years was 30%. Younger patients and those with localized disease at the time of diagnosis had the best outlook. Both local and distant failure during follow-up strongly predicted a shortened survival. Local control was achieved in three fourths of patients. Severe or fatal complications developed in nearly one third of patients within 10 years. They included 1 case of postradiation sarcoma.

Conclusion.—Approximately one third of these patients were cured of Ewing's sarcoma. Older patients and those with metastases when initially seen have a relatively poor outlook. Most severe treatment-related complications are correctable.

▶ The treatment of Ewing's sarcoma has changed dramatically during the period covered by this review. In 1967, patients were treated with irradiation alone and had a less than 10% chance of being cured. By 1987, all patients were receiving adjuvant chemotherapy with the primary tumor either resected or irradiated. The predicted survival of patients with Ewing's sarcoma diagnosed in 1994 is at least 60%. The increased survival rate is welcomed but will bring an increased incidence of complications. Recent interest in trying to reduce the late complications has produced a reevaluation of the treatment of Ewing's sarcoma. Increasingly, surgical resection is used for the management of the primary tumor. One of the reasons is to reduce the risk of a secondary sarcoma after irradiation. It will be years before we know whether this is the correct management.—D.S. Springfield, M.D.

The Role of Surgical Therapy in Patients With Nonmetastatic Ewing's Sarcoma of the Limbs
Toni A, Neff JR, Sudanese A, Ciaroni D, Bacci G, Picci P, Barbieri E, Campanacci M, Giunti A (Istituto Rizzoli, Bologna, Italy; Univ of Kansas, Kansas City; Istituto del Radio "L Galvani" Policlinico S Orsola, Bologna, Italy)
Clin Orthop 286:225–240, 1993   129-94-6–17

Background.—Traditionally, Ewing's sarcoma has been treated with radiation therapy, with amputation being reserved for lesions of the extremities. However, late recurrence after irradiation is a growing concern. The effects of surgery, surgery plus radiation therapy, and radiation therapy alone in providing relapse-free local control were reviewed in patients with nonmetastatic primary lesions of Ewing's sarcoma of the extremities.

Methods.—Patient charts, histopathology slides, and radiographic data for 131 patients with Ewing's sarcoma were reviewed. Patients still being actively followed were examined to evaluate the overall functional status of the involved extremity.

Results.—Amputation or resection was performed in 69 patients. Fifty-six were local resections and in 31 of these cases adjuvant radiation therapy was required. In 38 patients, surgery with wide margins was the only method of local tumor management. There were 12 conventional amputations and 1 ray amputation of the foot. Extremity-sparing procedures were performed in 25 patients; 23 of these surgeries were preceded by 3 cycles of chemotherapy. Local recurrence was reported in 2 patients treated with surgery alone; both specimens had had disease-free margins. Thirty-one patients underwent surgical resection followed by radiation therapy; only 1 recurrence was reported in this group. Radiation therapy was the only treatment in 62 patients; all had extremity primary lesions. Local recurrence was reported in 21 of these patients; however, there was no local failure in 6 who had undergone 3 cycles of chemotherapy before radiation. According to actuarial projections, surgery with or without radiation therapy significantly improved local disease-free survival compared with radiation alone. However, the risk for distant metastasis was similar among the 3 treatment groups.

Conclusion.—Although this study involved 3 separate populations, the results suggest that surgery improves disease-free survival compared with radiation therapy alone. In future studies, patients should be randomized to receive preoperative chemotherapy before local surgical treatment or radiation therapy.

▶ Surgical resection of Ewing's sarcoma involving an expendable bone (e.g., a proximal fibula, rib, or clavicle) seems obviously appropriate if it can reduce the need for irradiation. There are increasing data—although they are all retrospective—suggesting that surgical resection improves overall survival of patients with Ewing's sarcoma. The incidence of local recurrence with irradiation alone is difficult to determine. The bone remains abnormal and many of the patients die before a local recurrent disease is manifest. Suffice it to say that irradiation has a local recurrence rate greater than surgical resection and the risk of late secondary sarcoma. I recommend surgical resection whenever it is possible.—D.S. Springfield, M.D.

Ewing Sarcoma of the Pelvis: Clinicopathological Features and Treatment

Frassica FJ, Frassica DA, Pritchard DJ, Schomberg PJ, Wold LE, Sim FH
(Mayo Clinic and Found, Rochester, Minn)

J Bone Joint Surg (Am) 75-A:1457–1465, 1993   129-94-6–18

Series.—The treatment results were reviewed for 27 patients seen from 1973 to 1988 with Ewing's sarcoma of the pelvis. Multidrug chemotherapy was routinely used during this period. The average patient age at the time of initial treatment was 19 years. Six patients had metastatic disease at diagnosis. All but 2 of the surviving patients were followed for 5 years or longer.

Results.—Five of the 6 patients with metastasis at the time of diagnosis received radiotherapy in addition to chemotherapy, but none of these patients lived 5 years. Five of the 6 patients died at a median of 1 year after treatment. Thirteen patients with localized disease received both radiotherapy and chemotherapy, in most cases simultaneously. The actuarial survival rates at 3 and 5 years were 34% and 25%, respectively. Eight other patients with localized disease underwent resection and received chemotherapy, and 4 of them also received external-beam irradiation. Patients undergoing local resection retained their hip joints and had excellent function. The 3- and 5-year actuarial survival rates for this group were both 75%. The combined 5-year actuarial survival rate of all patients seen initially with localized disease was 45%.

Conclusion.—Resection of pelvic Ewing's sarcoma provided excellent control in this series. External-beam irradiation should be considered if the adequacy of the margins is in doubt. Patients given radiotherapy and multidrug chemotherapy are at risk of postradiation sarcoma all their lives, but resection of involved bone may lessen the risk.

▶ Ewing's sarcoma has a poor prognosis no matter where it arises, but when it starts in the pelvis it is particularly dangerous. This may be the result of a later diagnosis, resulting in the pelvic lesion being larger than an extremity lesion, or it may be the result of its anatomical location. Surgical resection is difficult and is associated with some morbidity, but it seems to improve the chance of survival and will, we hope, reduce the incidence of irradiation-associated sarcomas in the patients who survive. The most aggressive treatment is indicated.—D.S. Springfield, M.D.

7 Hand

Introduction

After years of difficulty in selecting from an enormous publication reservoir for the interests of the "hand surgeon," it is even more intimidating to attempt to drastically winnow that same material for the "orthopedic surgeon." Nor is it likely that the increasing pressure to generalize and prioritize primary care will afford relief from this agony and ecstasy, because so much of hand surgery comes from frontline trench warfare with the environment and will confront any primary care warrior who still survives. Does that mean that the YEAR BOOKS OF EMERGENCY MEDICINE, OCCUPATIONAL AND ENVIRONMENTAL MEDICINE, SPORTS MEDICINE, and FAMILY PRACTICE will need similar material. Yes, it does!

With apologies for the great mass of material left out, and a not so subtle reminder that there is a YEAR BOOK OF HAND SURGERY for those who can tolerate more, your selections for this year fall into the categories of wrist problems at the distal radius level (no orthopedist can escape this most common of environmental defeats by gravity); wrist problems of the carpus; trauma and residua of both hard and soft tissues, with solutions that now often involve microsurgery; and a potpourri of problems, evaluations, and solutions that do not involve acute trauma.

In recent years, much has been made of the degrees of joint surface comminution and displacement in distal radius fractures; even more recently, there has been a renewed emphasis on the association of these fractures with ligament damage and instability of the carpus. Nevertheless, long-term review of Colles' fractures continues to focus on the residual deformity of the radius and the distal ulna as being the major factors in persistent symptoms, although it continues to be comforting that most of these complaints subside with time. Nor have we come to terms with the simplest of all treatments for the residual Colles' problems (i.e., removal of the distal ulna). It is also interesting to note that the spate of new diagnoses and new operations for carpal problems have not displaced such old faithfuls as radial styloidectomy, proximal row carpectomy, forearm leveling osteotomies, the Matti-Russe procedure, and wrist fusion; in fact, many of these are staging comebacks. However, interest in the wrist remains at peak level, and good investigative work is being done at many institutions.

Other areas of special interest have found their niche in orthopedics and will maintain or enlarge their scope. Although orthopedists have not become as active in microsurgery as was hoped, microsurgery has become quite prevalent in orthopedics and its indications and accomplishments must be reviewed. The same is true of arthroscopy, endoscopy, external fixation in its various modes, and many other special techniques that surface from time to time in one of the many orthopedic subspecialties. Each year, we will cull the pertinent contributions and offer them to you. However, please remember that this is a two-way street, and your suggestions to the editor, the section editors, or the publisher will improve the information that you receive.

James H. Dobyns, M.D.

Wrist

DISTAL RADIUS

The Distal Radio-Ulnar Joint in Colles' Fractures
Roysam GS (St George's Hosp, London)
J Bone Joint Surg (Br) 75-B:58–60, 1993   129-94-7–1

Background.—The importance of distal radioulnar joint (DRUJ) involvement in Colles' fractures is only now being appreciated. To date, there have been no controlled prospective studies of the effect of DRUJ involvement in Colles' fractures.

Methods and Findings.—Follow-up of 170 patients with Colles' fractures was conducted for 1 year after their casts were removed. Eighty-one patients had DRUJ involvement and 89 did not. At all stages of follow-up, patients with DRUJ involvement had a significantly weaker grip than patients with no DRUJ involvement. The former group also had a significantly higher incidence of pain and tenderness over the joint at all stages. The range of supination was poorer in patients with DRUJ involvement at 6 months and 1 year. Functional outcomes were unrelated to the presence or absence of an ulnar styloid fracture.

Conclusion.—Colles' fractures that extend into the DRUJ are associated with a worse prognosis than those that do not. Patients with DRUJ involvement are likely to have decreased grip strength and a restricted range of supination. They may also have chronic pain around the head of the ulna.

▶ At least in the short term, ulnar wrist pain in general and DRUJ pain in particular are common residua of distal radius fractures. Instability of the distal ulna, ulnocarpal impingement, and instability of the ulnar carpus are all known causes, but the author further implicates articular damage, fracture involvement, or both. Preventive treatment measures for this problem are not routine, nor is the importance of this short-term problem (manifested by decreased grip strength and some limitation of supination) documented as a long-term problem.—J.H. Dobyns, M.D.

Poor Results of Darrach's Procedure After Wrist Injuries

Field J, Majkowski RJ, Leslie IJ (Bristol Royal Infirmary, England)
J Bone Joint Surg (Br) 75-B:53–57, 1993   129-94-7-2

Study Design.—Thirty-six patients who had undergone Darrach's procedure for post-traumatic dysfunction of the distal radioulnar joint were studied, with a mean follow-up of 6 years.

Outcome.—Only 50% of patients achieved satisfactory results using the modified Gartland and Werley criteria. Nine patients had ulnar impingement syndrome, and 9 patients had radiographic evidence of carpal collapse. All patients had ulnar translation of the carpus as measured by the carpal/ulnar distance ratio of Youm et al., but only 22 had this deformity when the carpal/radial distance ratio was used. Compared with patients with satisfactory results, the unsatisfactory group had significantly more cosmetic deformities, reduced grip strength, and decreased wrist movements. Furthermore, unsatisfactory results were significantly associated with short ulnar segment, osteoarthritis of the wrist, and occurrence of algodystrophy. Carpal instability, carpal collapse, and ulnar translation did not correlate with the clinical result.

Conclusion.—These results of the Darrach's procedure for post-traumatic symptoms in the distal radioulnar joint are much worse than those previously reported. Osteoarthritis, algodystrophy, and short ulnar segment are associated with poor results.

▶ It is frustrating that one of the simplest, most straightforward operations in all of orthopedics—excision of the distal ulna—remains controversial because good results are not dependable. When the results are good they are very, very good, but when they are bad they are horrid. The literature is abundant, both ways, but there is an emerging consensus that: Darrach's procedure works better for weak wrists (such as rheumatoid arthritis) than for strong wrists (post-trauma osteoarthritis, etc.); with excision of an ulnar segment longer than 2 cm, the incidence of problems increases; maintaining **some** stability by means of a soft tissue column from distal ulnar stump to carpal ligament complex may help; and in addition to the short ulna and the unstable ulna, bad results correlate with deformity, algodystrophy ("pain dysfunction syndrome" or "reflex sympathetic dystrophy" in the United States), and osteoarthritis. Reluctance to give up a simple solution to this common problem has led to many modified methods that are undergoing their own controversial reviews. This problem will not go away!—J.H. Dobyns, M.D.

Fractures of the Distal End of the Radius in Young Adults: A 30-Year Follow-Up

Kopylov P, Johnell O, Redlund-Johnell I, Bengner U (Univ of Lund, Malmö, Sweden)
J Hand Surg (Br) 18-B:45–49, 1993   129-94-7–3

Objective.—The long-term outcome was examined in 76 patients evaluated clinically and radiologically as many as 36 years after a distal radial fracture. The patients had an average age of 31 years when injured and 63 years at follow-up. The prognostic influence of articular fracture was examined in the 47 patients affected.

Functional Results.—In 81% of patients there was no difference between the injured and uninjured sides. More than one third of patients had minimal complaints, but none had to change work or leisure activities. Flexion and grip strength were consistently decreased on the injured side, but there were no differences in pronation and supination or ulnar deviation. Minor degenerative changes correlated with increased axial compression but not with a higher frequency of complaints.

Articular Fracture.—Only 13% of patients with joint fracture had a difference between the injured and uninjured sides. There was significantly less flexion and grip strength on the injured side but no difference in the clinical outcome of intra-articular and extra-articular fractures. More degenerative change was seen in the radiocarpal joint in patients with articular fractures. The chief factor related to degenerative change was incongruity of the joint surface.

Recommendations.—Treatment of articular fractures of the distal radius in younger patients should attempt to minimize axial compression and to eliminate incongruity at the radiocarpal and distal radioulnar joints, by open reduction if necessary. Symptomatic osteoarthritis is infrequent, and conservative management generally is adequate.

▶ Long-term follow-up is of great value to musculoskeletal practitioners and is comforting when the findings, as in this study, suggest that the long-term result of fractures of the distal radius may be better than the short-term results. In 81% of patients with an average follow-up of 32 years, no clinical difference between the injured and the uninjured wrists and hands was noted. Thirty-seven percent had complaints, which were said to be minimal, that had not resulted in occupational or avocational alterations.

In this study, instabilities of the carpus or of the distal ulna were not specifically addressed, nor was provocative testing done. The study did confirm the relationship of persistent complaints and progressive arthritis to axial compression deformity (short radius with ulna plus) and to intra-articular deformity. Although instant return to normal function and appearance is often the expectation of the modern patient and doctor, reassurance that our forebears did satisfactorily with less dramatic and perhaps less risky management may reopen a lost perspective for some.—J.H. Dobyns, M.D.

Moving?

I'd like to receive my *Year Book of Orthopedics* without interruption.
Please note the following change of address, effective:

Name: ____

New Address: ______________________________________

____

City: ____________________ State: ________ Zip: ________

Old Address: _______________________________________

____

City: ____________________ State: ________ Zip: ________

Reservation Card

Yes, I would like my own copy of *Year Book of Orthopedics*. Please begin my subscription with the current edition according to the terms described below.* I understand that I will have 30 days to examine each annual edition. If satisfied, I will pay just $72.00 plus sales tax, postage and handling (price subject to change without notice).

Name: ____

Address: ____

City: ____________________ State: ________ Zip: ________

Method of Payment
O Visa   O Mastercard   O AmEx   O Bill me   O Check (in US dollars, payable to Mosby, Inc.)

Card number: _______________________ Exp date: ____________

Signature: ____

LS-0909

**Your Year Book* Service Guarantee:

When you subscribe to the *Year Book*, we'll send you an advance notice of future volumes about two months before they publish. This automatic notice system is designed to take up as little of your time as possible. If you do not want the *Year Book*, the advance notice makes it quick and easy for you to let us know your decision, and you will always have at least 20 days to decide. If we don't hear from you, we'll send you the new volume as soon as it's available. And, of course, the *Year Book* is yours to examine free of charge for 30 days (postage, handling and applicable sales tax are added to each shipment.).

BUSINESS REPLY MAIL
FIRST CLASS MAIL   PERMIT No. 762   CHICAGO, IL

POSTAGE WILL BE PAID BY ADDRESSEE

Chris Hughes
Mosby-Year Book, Inc.
200 N. LaSalle Street
Suite 2600
Chicago, IL 60601-9981

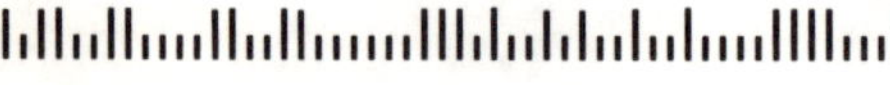

BUSINESS REPLY MAIL
FIRST CLASS MAIL   PERMIT No. 762   CHICAGO, IL

POSTAGE WILL BE PAID BY ADDRESSEE

Chris Hughes
Mosby-Year Book, Inc.
200 N. LaSalle Street
Suite 2600
Chicago, IL 60601-9981

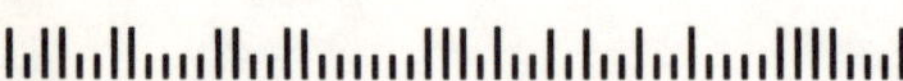

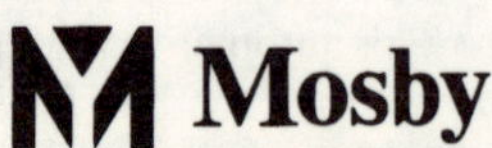

Mosby

Dedicated to publishing excellence

Severe Fractures of the Distal Radius: Effect of Amount and Duration of External Fixator Distraction on Outcome

Kaempffe FA, Wheeler DR, Peimer CA, Hvisdak KS, Ceravolo J, Senall J
(State Univ of New York, Buffalo)

J Hand Surg (Am) 18A:33–41, 1993   129-94-7–4

Introduction.—Closed reduction and external immobilization may be inadequate in patients with severely comminuted and markedly displaced fractures of the distal radius. In some cases, external fixation and simultaneous percutaneous pinning or open reduction must also be used to obtain good results. A retrospective review was designed to determine the amount and duration of fixator distraction required to maximize outcome.

Methods.—Twenty-six of 44 consecutive patients treated during a 5-year period with external fixation for unilateral severe distal radius fractures were available for complete follow-up. There were 20 cases of Frykman class VII and VIII fractures. The average delay from time of injury to surgery was 4 days. External fixation was maintained for an average of 7 weeks. All patients were evaluated by chart review, questionnaire, radiography, and physical examination an average of 104 weeks after the injury. The carpal height index (CHI) was used to determine objectively the amount of distraction used.

Results.—At follow-up, two thirds of patients reported no restrictions in their daily activities; an equal proportion were free of pain during those activities. Average wrist extension was 39 degrees and average flexion was 55 degrees. Both extension and flexion were three fourths of that on the unaffected side. Radius length was restored to within an average of 1.4 mm of the uninvolved side. The distraction used to achieve reduction corresponded to an average CHI of .58, and worse outcome was associated with an increasing CHI. Outcome, particularly motion, was adversely affected as the duration of distraction increased. Overall, 85% of patients achieved New York Orthopedic Hospital grades of good or excellent.

Conclusion.—Findings show that an increase in distraction (CHI) within the range of .49 to .71 may improve reduction and radiographic scores but is associated with decreasing scores for function, pain, grip strength, and motion. This is the first study to reveal potentially negative effects of increased distraction and prolonged fixation.

▶ In the United States, external fixator support of unstable distal radius fractures has become a standard treatment, with or without percutaneous or open accessory procedures. Like all other methods, it has its advantages and its disadvantages. One of the more subtle of the disadvantages is the effect of persistent distraction. There has been a general awareness of distraction as a probable cause of pain, stiffness, and fibrosis for some time, but a more precise indication of how much traction is too much has been lacking until now.—J.H. Dobyns, M.D.

The Ulnar Impaction Syndrome: Follow-Up of Ulnar Shortening Osteotomy

Chun S, Palmer AK (State Univ of New York, Syracuse)
J Hand Surg (Am) 18A:46–53, 1993   129-94-7–5

Background.—Ulnar impaction syndrome results from the ulnar head impinging against the triangular fibrocartilage complex and the ulnar carpus. Progressive trauma results, including a torn triangular fibrocartilage complex, chondromalacia, and ulnocarpal osteoarthritis. The syndrome may result from congenital positive ulnar variance, radial shortening from any cause, or dynamic ulnar positive variance secondary to pronation of the wrist and a forceful grip. Operative management is based on mechanical decompression of the distal ulnocarpal articulation.

Patients.—An ulnar shortening osteotomy was performed in 30 wrists of 27 patients with ulnar impaction syndrome, including 16 males and 11 females (average age, 28 years). Traumatic injuries were most frequent. All the patients had pain in the ulnar region of the wrist, and some had clicking, a decreased range of motion, and a weak grip as well. Conservative measures were tried for an average of 6 months, and 19 patients were available for follow-up at an average of 51 months.

Technique.—An incision is made on the subcutaneous border of the forearm. A 6-hole, 3.5-mm AO plate is placed on the dorsal ulnar surface, and a distal screw is inserted. After marking the osteotomy site on the ulna, the plate is swung away and an oblique cut is made through 70% of the bone. A second cut follows, with the goal of achieving a final ulnar variance of 0 or −1 mm. The ulna then is reduced, the plate is swung into place, and an independent interfragmentary screw is placed 90 degrees to the plate. A short-arm cast is applied for 2–4 weeks.

Results.—The mean ulnar variance was reduced from 2.5 to .9 mm postoperatively. Postoperatively, the state of the wrist was regarded as excellent in 24 wrists, good in 4, fair in 1, and poor in 1. The subjective range-of-motion scores nearly doubled, but objective improvement was less marked. Pain scores improved substantially, and functional scores more than doubled. Complications were rare, and no patient had ulnar nonunion.

Conclusion.—The distal ulnar shortening osteotomy is an excellent operative treatment for ulnar impaction syndrome.

▶ First mentioned in 1941 but seldom used until it was reintroduced in 1985, shortening of the distal ulna to decompress impaction from any cause between the distal ulnar head, interposed soft tissues, and adjacent carpus has proven to be one of the most useful procedures for ulnar wrist pain. Even when such impaction is not the sole cause of pain, it is often the most significant factor. Much current literature has focused on control and fixation of the ulnar osteotomy; it is good to see an article that emphasizes the results.—J.H. Dobyns, M.D.

Function Ten Years After Colles' Fracture

Warwick D, Field J, Prothero D, Gibson A, Bannister GC (Southmead Hosp, Bristol, England)
Clin Orthop 295:270–274, 1993   129-94-7–6

Purpose.—Long-term functional outcome data after displaced distal radial fractures are not available; the longest follow-up to date is 6 years. The 10-year outcome after Colles' fracture was examined in 100 patients.

Methods.—The study sample included 86 women and 14 men (average age, 61.7 years). All fractures were treated by manipulation using regional analgesia and then by cast immobilization for 6 weeks. Each patient was examined 3 months after cast removal and recalled 10 years later. The follow-up examination included radiographic assessment.

Findings.—At 10 years, 35 patients with Colles' fractures had died, and 10 were lost to follow-up. Of those who were reexamined after 10 years, 27 had excellent wrist function, 20 were rated good, 6 fair, and 2 had poor functional outcomes. Overall, 85% of the surviving patients had satisfactory functional outcomes. During the 10-year interval, 19 of the 38 patients with good function at 3 months improved to excellent and 6 deteriorated to fair. Radial shortening and finger stiffness at 3 months were significantly associated with long-term functional outcome. Extreme dorsal angulation was associated with early unsatisfactory function but not with long-term functional outcome. Nineteen of 51 patients (37%) whose wrists were radiographed at the 10-year follow-up visit had signs of osteoarthrosis, but only 7 patients (4%) had degenerative changes attributable to Colles' fracture. Functional deterioration was significantly associated with the development of algodystrophy.

Conclusion.—The long-term outcome of displaced Colles' fractures is relatively benign. Deterioration and unsatisfactory functional outcome are predicted by extreme radial shortening, intra-articular fracture, and early finger stiffness.

▶ Long-term follow-up is indispensable to those concerned about the musculoskeletal system, but such follow-up is surprisingly difficult to obtain. This baseline study of Colles' fractures treated by closed reduction and shortarm cast support is deficient in categorizing the 100 fractures reviewed. Nevertheless, 51% of patients had intra-articular fractures, 55 of whom had follow-up for 10 years or more. It is encouraging that the ratio of those who had improvement between the 3-month check and the 10-year check vs. those who had deterioration was 3:1.

The early deleterious effects of dorsal angulation usually disappeared with time, but other anticipated factors in diminished results held constant. These were excessive shortening (> 1/2 of 1 SD from the mean, ± 2 mm of shortening); algodystrophy (joint tenderness, digit stiffness, vasomotor instability); and osteoarthritis (7 of 19 with articular fractures had greater arthritis on the injured side). Shortening is responsive to external, internal, or combined fixation. Algodystrophy ("reflex sympathetic dystrophy" or "pain dysfunction syndrome" in American terminology) and osteoarthritis ("post-traumatic arthritis" in American terminology) reflect the degree of injury to the tissues, and both can be modified to some extent by early treatment. Our goal is to raise the authors' 85% satisfactory rate, using the treatments of 2 and 3 decades ago, to a 95% satisfactory rate.—J.H. Dobyns, M.D.

Biomechanical Evaluation of Distal Radioulnar Reconstructions
Petersen MS, Adams BD (Univ of Arkansas, Little Rock; Univ of Vermont, Burlington)
J Hand Surg (Am) 18A:328–334, 1993   129-94-7-7

Background.—Chronic instability of the distal radioulnar joint (DRUJ) can produce significant disability. Three basic types of reconstruction have been used to repair this instability. However, objective information on the mechanical performance of the joint after repair has not been available. Therefore, the ability of several surgical reconstructive procedures to restore stability was compared.

Methods.—Six upper extremity fresh-frozen cadaveric specimens from young adults were analyzed in a jig designed to rigidly hold the upper extremity while allowing for variable forearm rotation. After baseline measurements were performed, instability was created in the DRUJ and then 4 soft tissue reconstructions were performed sequentially: Eliason, Fulkerson-Watson, Boyes-Bunnell and Hui-Linscheid. Instability was created in the resected distal ulna (RDU) and repaired sequentially with the Bunnell and the Breen and Jupiter procedures.

Results.—None of the reconstructive procedures examined in this study restored the natural stability of the joint. A radioulnar sling design was much more effective than either tenodesis or ulnar collateral ligament reconstruction procedures.

Conclusion.—On the basis of tests with cadavers, none of the current reconstructions restore the DRUJ to its natural level of stability. The development of other treatment approaches and improved reconstruction design will be necessary to restore full stability to this joint.

▶ One of the most common post-traumatic problems at the human wrist is that of instability of the distal ulna. Although static testing with only axial loading is hardly representative of the vivacious in vivo performance required of the distal ulna, it is sufficient to indicate that most (perhaps all) of our reconstructive techniques do not stabilize the distal ulna; some, in fact, may result in increased instability. It may be time to come "out of the closet" with my long-time favorite procedure for distal ulna instability, wherein there is a satisfactory distal radioulnar joint. A simple, snug repair of all the torn or lax support tissues of the distal ulna is much more difficult when the distal ulna has been excised. However, even in that situation, surprisingly good soft tissue stability can be accomplished.—J.H. Dobyns, M.D.

CARPUS

Complications and Results of Scapho-Trapezio-Trapezoid Arthrodesis
Ishida O, Tsai T-M (Univ of Louisville, Ky)
Clin Orthop 287:125–130, 1993   129-94-7–8

Background.—Scapho-trapezio-trapezoid (STT) arthrodesis is widely used. However, there have been reports of high complication rates. The complications and outcomes of STT arthrodesis in 1 series of patients were analyzed.

Patients and Findings.—Forty patients undergoing STT arthrodesis were included. Indications included rotatory subluxation of the scaphoid in 30 patients and STT arthrosis in 10. Mean follow-up was 41 months. Ten patients needed a total of 13 additional procedures. Nonsurgical complications included pin tract infection, sympathetic dystrophy, delayed union treated with brace, and radial nerve irritation. The overall complication rate was 53%. Some patients had more than 1 complication. In 5 patients, degenerative arthritis at joints around the STT mass was suspected. Fifty-eight percent of the patients became free of pain or had minimal pain with a limited arc of motion. Twenty of 34 patients resumed their regular work. Sixty-eight percent of the patients believed that the results of the procedure were good or excellent.

Complications.—Complications are common in patients undergoing STT arthrodesis. In most patients, the procedure results in a pain-free wrist with a limited arc of motion. However, of 40 patients, nonunion occurred in 9.

▶ One of the most popular of the limited carpal fusions continues to record many complications in the hands of some of its users. The most common problems, delayed union and nonunion, are technique-related and thus amenable to correction, as is the problem of styloscaphoid impingement. There is no likelihood of restoring radiolunate stress bearing without significant alteration of the technique to stabilize the lunate, a feature not considered necessary by the prime proponents of STT fusion. Neither singular nor group experience can yet predict the incidence of periarthritis changes developing about the radial metacarpal, which are produced by STT fusion.—J.H. Dobyns, M.D.

Dorsal Approach to Scaphoid Nonunion

Watson HK, Pitts EC, Ashmead D IV, Makhlouf MV, Kauer J (Univ of Connecticut, Hartford; Yale Univ, New Haven, Conn; Univ of Massachusetts, Worcester)
J Hand Surg (Am) 18A:359–365, 1993　　　　　　　　129-94-7-9

Background.—The surgical treatment of scaphoid nonunion typically involves various combinations of screws and Kirschner wires with or without bone grafts. The results of dorsal-approach bone grafting procedures for scaphoid nonunion in which the distal radius was used as the donor site for cancellous graft material and Kirschner wires were used for fixation were evaluated.

Patients.—Thirty-six patients aged 9–65 years with scaphoid nonunions were treated between 1975 and 1991. The interval between initial fracture and bone grafting ranged from 3 months to 20 years (mean, 3 years). Sixty-one percent of patients had some form of treatment during this time. The mean follow-up was 5 years.

Outcomes.—In 89% of patients, union was achieved. Flexion and extension averaged 76% of that in the opposite wrist. Grip strength was 88% of that in the opposite hand. Ninety-one percent of patients who were employed returned to their original jobs.

Conclusion.—The dorsal approach preserves the anterior ligaments and provides excellent exposure of the scaphoid and surrounding structures. The use of 2 parallel Kirschner wires combined with cast immobilization enables adequate fracture fixation, resulting in good union rates and functional outcomes.

▶ The concept is certainly not new and has never been completely dropped from the armamentarium of certain surgeons or from the pages of certain texts. Nevertheless, it has become "politically correct" over the past decade to declare and practice the palmar approach to scaphoid injuries for a variety of reasons that have never been proven. Perhaps the fashions, never stable in any one configuration, are swinging back, and those not familiar with the simpler and safer dorsal and dorsoradial approaches to the scaphoid will rediscover the usefulness of these approaches.—J.H. Dobyns, M.D.

Scaphocapitolunate Arthrodesis

Rotman MB, Manske PR, Pruitt DL, Szerzinski J (Washington Univ, St Louis, Mo)
J Hand Surg (Am) 18A:26–33, 1993　　　　　　　　129-94-7-10

Background.—Scaphocapitolunate (SCL) arthrodesis has been used to treat a variety of painful wrist conditions, including Kienböck's disease, carpal instabilities, and scaphoid nonunion. In previously reported cases, results of this operative procedure have been favorable. Experience with SCL arthrodesis at 1 institution was reported.

Patients and Methods.—A total of 21 patients with either chronic incompetence of the scapholunate ligament or a scaphoid nonunion have undergone SCL arthrodesis since 1985. At operation, the average patient age was 31 years. Follow-up was performed at an average of 29 months. Preoperatively, all patients reported disabling wrist pain, with an average score of 4.5 on a 5-point scale, with 5 representing pain with wrist motion.

Technique.—A dorsal wrist oblique skin incision extending from the ulnar aspect of the distal radius to the distal pole of the scaphoid is used. In the interval between the third and fourth dorsal compartments, the wrist capsule is exposed and opened in an inverted-T fashion, thus exposing the adjoining articular surfaces of the scaphoid, capitate, and lunate. Rongeurs and curettes are used to remove articular cartilage and subchondral bone. The articular spaces are preserved and filled with cancellous bone graft taken from the distal radius in 14 patients and the iliac crest in 7 patients. The arthrodesis is fixed with 4–5 intercarpal Kirschner wires after any noted instability patterns are reduced. Wrists are immobilized in a long arm thumb spica cast for 4 weeks after the procedure. Subsequently, a short arm cast is used until fusion is demonstrated via radiographs at approximately 4–6 weeks. A removable thumb spica splint is then applied, and range-of-motion and strengthening exercises are begun. By 3 months, the Kirschner wires are removed.

Results.—After the primary procedure, 81% of the patients healed. One patient experienced a major infection. In 80%, a significant reduction in pain was achieved. Average range of motion included 35 degrees of extension, 30 degrees of flexion, 10 degrees of radial deviation, and 20 degrees of ulnar deviation. An average 70% grip strength of the uninvolved side was also noted. Sixteen patients were able to return to work. At final follow-up, radiographic examination revealed mild degenerative changes at the radiocarpal joint in 2 patients.

Conclusion.—Although SCL arthrodesis does not entirely relieve all symptoms, it can provide a significant reduction in pain and maintenance of adequate motion for daily activities in the majority of patients.

▶ Those whose only exposure to limited carpal arthrodesis began and ended with the radial and central midcarpal fusion of Graner et al. (circa 1966) may breathe again. This old technique is revisited by the authors, who find that it has some advantages (*not* including range of motion) over the more popular and newer techniques. So many of these cases involved salvage of other, earlier failed methods of treating scaphoid nonunion and scapholunate dissociation that they finally saw the light and began treating such problems initially by this method.

The principal advantage of this treatment over total wrist fusion is that it preserves some motion. Its presumed advantage over scapho-trapezio-trapezoidal fusion is that load bearing is shared between the radioscaphoid and the radiolunate joints rather than at the radioscaphoid joint only. Such sharing between joints of disparate shape and arc of motion may not be an advantage; more time and more evaluation of both procedures will be needed.—J.H. Dobyns, M.D.

Proximal Row Carpectomy: A Multicenter Study
Culp RW, McGuigan FX, Turner MA, Lichtman DM, Osterman AL, McCarroll HR (Naval Hosp, Oakland, Calif)
J Hand Surg (Am) 18A:19–25, 1993   129-94-7–11

Patients.—The effectiveness of proximal row carpectomy in treating patients who have wrist pain and decreased function from radiocarpal and intercarpal arthritis was examined in 20 such patients treated in 1980–1988, 13 men and 7 women with a mean age of 47 years. The dominant hand was involved in 15 of the 20 patients. The patients were seen with chronic pain and decreased function, and they expressed a wish to retain wrist motion. The most common diagnoses were Kienböck's disease, scaphoid nonunion, and chronic scapholunate dissociation. Nonoperative measures had been tried in all patients.

Management.—A longitudinal or transverse dorsal incision was used. About half of the 17 patients with nonrheumatoid conditions had the radiocapitate articulation pinned. Radial styloidectomy was done in 50% of patients when trapezial impingement was seen during radial deviation. One of the 3 patients with rheumatoid disease also underwent radial styloidectomy. Postoperative immobilization lasted 2–6 weeks.

Results.—During a mean follow-up of $3\frac{1}{2}$ years in the patients with nonrheumatoid involvement, motion in all planes decreased slightly to about half that on the normal side. Grip strength improved by 22% but was only 67% of that on the unaffected side. Three fourths of the patients had little or no pain at follow-up, but 18% had marked pain. About half of the patients were able to easily perform all activities of daily living. More than 80% of the patients believed that they were improved, but few laborers returned to their work. Moderate or severe degenerative change on preoperative x-ray films predicted a poor outcome. Two patients had pin track infection. Two required further surgery but did well after wrist arthrodesis. Surgery failed in all 3 patients with rheumatoid arthritis. Two of them successfully underwent total wrist arthroplasty, whereas 1 had arthrodesis.

Conclusions.—Proximal row carpectomy is an effective means of relieving pain in patients with radiocarpal or intercarpal arthritis of nonrheumatoid origin. Laborers should be selected carefully for this operation.

▶ Multicenter studies are not as controlled, but they compensate for this by better reflecting the at-large experience of the profession. More numbers need to be gathered, but I believe that the authors' conclusions are more indicative of the broad cross-section of experience with proximal row carpectomy than many of the papers on the subject. Their conclusions are: that proximal row carpectomy is usually a salvage treatment for chronic wrist pain; that the procedure is appropriate with mild but not moderate, severe, or systemic arthritis of the critical lunate sulcus of the radius or the proximal pole of the capitate; that residual motion is one half normal, grip is two thirds normal, comfort is improved in four fifths, and return to work is more likely in nonlaborers; and that failure of proximal row carpectomy can be salvaged simply and effectively by total wrist fusion. In summary, proximal row carpectomy is too good to abandon but not good enough to use indiscriminately.—J.H. Dobyns, M.D.

Palmar Midcarpal Instability: Results of Surgical Reconstruction
Lichtman DM, Bruckner JD, Culp RW, Alexander CE (Natl Naval Med Ctr, Bethesda, Md; Naval Hosp, Oakland, Calif)
J Hand Surg [Am] 18-A:307–315, 1993   129-94-7–12

Background.—There have been few reports on the surgical management of palmar midcarpal instability (MCI). Most patients with this condition respond well to nonsurgical treatment; however, there are occasions when surgery is required. The results of a number of surgical procedures for refractory palmar MCI were examined and some general observations about the nonoperative treatment of this condition were reported.

Patients and Methods.—The records of 15 operations (in 13 patients) for palmar MCI were reviewed. The initial complaints of all patients were a painful clunking of the wrist with activity and difficulty participating in work and sports. No incidence of severe trauma was reported before symptoms, although most patients had experienced mild wrist sprains in the past. All patients had undergone unsuccessful conservative therapy, including splinting, anti-inflammatory medication, and rest. Six patients had a limited midcarpal arthrodesis, and 9 patients had 1 of 4 different soft tissue reconstructive procedures. Surgery was considered successful if it eliminated the painful midcarpal clunk and allowed the patient to return to work. Follow-up consisted of clinical examination and assessment of grip strength, along with interviews with the patient to evaluate the success of treatment.

Results.—All 6 midcarpal arthrodeses were successful. Three of the 9 soft tissue procedures were successful, but 6 failed. Five of these 6 patients experienced a return of the wrist clunk. However, 1 procedure, a distal advancement of the ulnar arm of the arcuate ligament combined with a dorsal capsulodesis, restored stability in 3 of 5 patients. Patients who underwent arthrodesis experienced a 28% loss in motion, but they had a 3% increase in grip strength. Those who had soft tissue reconstruction lost 27% of motion along with a 2% loss in grip strength. All patients who underwent limited midcarpal arthrodesis returned to work, whereas only 33% of the patients who had soft tissue reconstruction were able to return to work.

Conclusion.—The midcarpal joint is potentially unstable and is subject to chronic problems under the influence of a variety of factors. Nonsurgical management of palmar MCI includes splinting and may be successful. However, in some patients surgical intervention is necessary. Soft tissue procedures for restoring ligamentous stability were relatively unsuccessful in treating palmar MCI. However, limited midcarpal arthrodesis showed a 100% success rate and should, therefore, be considered the preferred method of surgical treatment for this condition.

▶ We are still discovering features about all the carpal instabilities, but our understanding of this entity is more primitive than that of the others. The very name, "palmar midcarpal instability," blinds us at the outset. The entire proximal carpal row is an intercalated segment, is easily destabilized, and may be affected (speaking only of ligament injuries at this time) by dorsal or ventral (ventral to preserve the time-honored acronym "VISI," rather than substituting the wretched "PISI") lesions, by radiocarpal or midcarpal lesions, or by any combination thereof. These protean possibilities for the inadequate soft tissue support have made identification and specific repair and reconstruction of ligaments both challenging and unrewarding to date. Therefore, temporarily, the recommendation to fuse the midcarpal joint when surgery is needed for these patients is appropriate. However, be warned: some of these proximal carpal row instabilities are sufficiently unstable at the radiocarpal level that the entire fusion mass may deform, more often ulnar than dorsal or ventral. Investigators are still searching for the specific soft tissue lesions in the hope of early and appropriate repair.—J.H. Dobyns, M.D.

Trauma and Residua

Free Toe Transfer for Thumb and Finger Reconstruction in 300 Cases
Yu-dong G, Gao-Meng Z, De-Shong C, Ji-Geng Y, Xiao-ming C (Shanghai Med Univ, China)
Plast Reconstr Surg 91:693–700, 1993   129-94-7–13

Background.—Free toe transfer for thumb reconstruction was first successfully performed by microsurgical techniques in 1966. The outcomes of procedures done since that time were reviewed.

Patients and Findings.—The outcome in 300 patients aged 5–58 years was reviewed. Two hundred twenty-five patients were male. Finger defects were caused by trauma in 296 patients. In 248 patients, the thumb was reconstructed. There were 286 survivals and 14 failures, for a total survival rate of 95.6%. At a follow-up of 2–23 years, movement and sensation of the reconstructed thumbs and fingers were satisfactory in all

286 patients. The main indications for surgery were defect of the thumb at the plane of the metacarpophalangeal joint and defects of the second to fifth fingers. Special attention was given to atraumatic isolation of the second toe, microsurgical suturing technique, intraoperative vascular variations, providing the double arterial blood supply system if needed, and identifying and managing postoperative circulatory crises.

Conclusion.—The total survival rate in this series of patients undergoing free toe transfer for thumb and finger reconstruction was 95.6%. Movement and sensation of the reconstructed thumbs and fingers in the surviving digits were satisfactory in all patients.

▶ Microsurgery techniques for both emergency and reconstructive surgery of the extremities are now widely available, widely used, and widely accepted. Nevertheless, reassurance that this is indeed the valuable resource that we believe it to be is always useful. This paper, which reports on a large number of flexor tendon transfers for digit reconstruction, is reassuring with regard to survival (> 95%) and function (return to some work of slightly more than half of the patients; change of work in the rest) of the hands and of the donor feet (some problems in 12% in the early years, declining to 8% at > 5 years). The details of sensory motor function are not as precise as might be wished, but the discussion of anatomical and technique variations to maximize survival and function are valuable adjuncts to the presentation.—J.H. Dobyns, M.D.

Microsurgical Reconstruction of Distal Digits Following Mutilating Hand Injuries: Results in 121 Patients
Wei FC, Epstein MD, Chen HC, Chuang CC, Chen HT (Chang Gung Mem Hosp, Taipei, Taiwan)
Br J Plast Surg 46:181–186, 1993   129-94-7–14

Background.—Replanting amputated distal digits is now common practice. Reconstructing nonreplantable distal digits with like-tissue transfers from the feet also has many similar advantages. The results of microsurgical reconstruction of distal digits after mutilating injuries were examined.

Methods and Findings.—One hundred fifty-two mutilated distal digits were reconstructed with microsurgical foot tissue transfers in 121 patients between 1982 and 1989. Foot tissues used included wrap-around flaps or pulp from the big toe, second toe, or third toe, as well as partial toe, nail, web space skin, and other parts of the foot. Reconstructions were primary in 78 patients and secondary in 74. The procedure was successful in 98% in the short term. Most patients were satisfied with the aesthetic and functional result.

Conclusion.—Foot-tissue transplantation provides a useful reconstructive alternative for distal digits that cannot be replanted. Functional and aesthetic outcomes are better than those obtained with conventional methods.

▶ Free vascularized, wraparound flaps of pulp or partial toe segments, including nails, webs, and joints, are all available and routinely used both primarily and secondarily in the repair of mutilated hand segments when replantation is not required. An immediate viability success rate of 98% is almost matched by the long-term functional and cosmetic results. These are never perfect but they are routinely more satisfactory than alternative techniques; residual and functional foot problems were avoided because of the limited donor tissue used.—J.H. Dobyns, M.D.

Open Hand Fractures: An Analysis of the Recovery of Active Motion and of Complications

Duncan RW, Freeland AE, Jabaley ME, Meydrech EF (Univ of Mississippi, Jackson)
J Hand Surg (Am) 18A:387–394, 1993   129-94-7–15

Background.—Several factors are known to affect the recovery of active range of motion and the severity of complications in hand fractures. An end-result analysis of open hand fractures treated with internal fixation was done to determine which factors predict outcome and complications.

Methods.—Of 104 patients undergoing surgical fixation of open hand fractures, 75 were reassessed 6 months to 7 years after injury. One hundred forty fractures involving 125 fingers had occurred.

Findings.—The results, evidenced by total active range of digital motion at final follow-up, strongly correlated with the severity of soft tissue injury. In a comparison of open fractures of comparable severity in groups that did and did not need further extension by incision for acceptable reduction and stabilization, some additional loss of active range of motion was noted in the group treated surgically. Significantly better outcomes were associated with metacarpal fractures compared with phalangeal fractures. The poorest prognosis was seen with fractures of the proximal phalanx or proximal interphalangeal joint, particularly when associated with tendon injury. Significant complications occurred in 13 fingers, with infection and subsequent amputation related to wound severity.

Conclusion.—The damage caused by the original injury strongly correlated with final outcome in this series. A significantly greater proportion of good and excellent outcomes was associated with less severe open fractures than with more severe wounds.

▶ This article is a good review of open hand wounds with fractures, excepting devascularized or amputated digits. Its conclusions are the expected ones. The highest correlate with final result was the severity of the soft tissue injury. The site of fracture is a significant factor, with proximal phalanx, proximal interphalangeal joint, and middle phalanx injuries more likely to give poor results. Systematic disease was not a significant factor except with regard to deep infection. Finally, wound extension for surgical fixation purposes affects results adversely but mildly compared with other factors. Early wound care, fracture stabilization with a minimum of invasive exposure and apparatus, special precautions for the combination of category IIIB or greater wounds plus systemic problems, and early, appropriate rehabilitation are the important treatment factors.—J.H. Dobyns, M.D.

Extremity Transplantation: A Review of Its Current State of Development
Nolan LM, Bowen V (Univ of Toronto)
J Hand Surg (Am) 18A:153–159, 1993   129-94-7-16

Introduction.—The discovery of the immunosuppressant cyclosporin A and the development of microsurgical free-tissue transfer techniques have brought extremity allograft transplantation closer to realization. The history of experimental extremity allograft transplantation and the problems that still need to be resolved before extremity transplant procedures can become a clinical reality were reviewed.

Review.—Immunologic incompatibility is the major problem facing limb allograft transplantation, as microsurgical techniques to accomplish these operations are already available. Before the discovery of cyclosporin A in 1976, extremity transplantation in laboratory animals was carried out with agents such as azathioprine, 6-mercaptopurine, and prednisolone and procedures such as splenectomy and exchange transfusion. Although those early experiments were interesting and successful, they had no clinical application. Cyclosporin A is much less toxic than the earlier immunosuppressants, but serious side effects such as acute renal failure, hypertension, and increased susceptibility to serious bacterial and viral infections preclude its routine use. The future of limb transplantation rests with the discovery of immunosuppressive techniques that will be less toxic but as effective as cyclosporin A. The immunosuppressant FK-506 has already been used for experimental allograft transplantation in rats. Although preliminary results have been encouraging, many of the rats receiving long-term FK-506 subsequently had *Pneumocystis carinii* infection.

Conclusion.—Although limb allograft transplantation is feasible and is expected to become a reality in the near future, the procedure is currently on hold for clinical use until an immunosuppressive agent with an acceptable side effect profile becomes available.

▶ Current risks are acceptable for the transplantation of vital organs, but the routine use of well-known techniques for the transplantation of extremities (in part or in whole) awaits only the development and testing of a less toxic immunosuppressant agent than cyclosporin A.—J.H. Dobyns, M.D.

High-Pressure Injection Injuries of the Hand: Review of 25 Patients Managed by Open Wound Technique
Pinto MR, Turkula-Pinto LD, Cooney WP, Wood MB, Dobyns JH (Mayo Clinic and Found, Rochester, Minn)
J Hand Surg (Am) 18A:125–130, 1993   129-94-7–17

Introduction.—High-pressure injection injuries of the hand can have devastating effects, particularly when oil-based solvents are involved. Amputation rates as high as 48% have been reported. Often the importance of the injury is not obvious and definitive treatment is delayed. However, these hands may be salvaged by wide débridement with drainage and delayed closure.

Patients.—Twenty-five patients with high-pressure injection injuries of the hand were managed by the open wound technique in 1975–1990 and were followed for a mean of 10 months. The materials most frequently injected were hydraulic fluid, paint, grease, and paint thinner.

Management.—A Bruner type of incision was made to expose the injury widely, and all devitalized tissue and injected material were débrided. Pulsed lavage irrigation aided the procedure. The wound was packed open, and further débridement was done after 24–72 hours as needed. Either the wound was closed later or closure by secondary intention was allowed. Patients received a broad-spectrum antibiotic but not steroids. Intensive physical therapy stressing active motion was begun as soon as it was tolerated.

Results.—The index finger and then the thumb were the most commonly affected sites. Treatment was delayed for as long as 8 days. Infection was confirmed in 15 patients; 5 were polymicrobial in origin. All patients responded to operative treatment combined with systemic antibiotic therapy. Only 4 patients required amputation. The final flexion lag exceeded 2.5 cm in 9 patients. All patients were able to resume work, most of them at their previous jobs.

Conclusion.—Early and aggressive operative treatment of high-pressure injection injuries of the hand using the open wound technique can be expected to improve outcome. Patients should be immediately referred to an experienced hand surgeon.

▶ The amount and toxicity of the agent is critical in high-pressure injection injury but not under the control of the medical manager. What the management system can and must do for these patients is: recognize that serious hidden damage that increases geometrically with time is present; arrange immediately for inspection débridement and cleansing; and make subsequent débridement simple and diminished pain rehabilitation easier through use of the open wound technique. Not all digits can be saved, but many can be, and those salvaged digits can be maximally rehabilitated by this method.—J.H. Dobyns, M.D.

Microsurgical Neurolysis: Its Anatomical and Physiological Basis and Its Classification

Millesi H, Rath T, Reihsner R, Zoch G (Univ of Vienna; Ludwig-Boltzmann-Inst for Experimental Plastic Surgery, Vienna)
Microsurgery 14:430–439, 1993   129-94-7-18

Introduction.—Neurolysis is indicated if a peripheral nerve ceases to glide normally and adhesions and fibrosis develop as a result. External neurolysis is an accepted peripheral nerve operation, but internal neurolysis remains controversial. Just as the paraneurium provides for movement between the nerve and surrounding tissues, the interfascicular epineurium allows movement within the nerve. Internal neurolysis is in order if the epifascicular epineurium is completely transected.

Technique.—Neurolysis is a stepped procedure that attempts to decompress the fascicles. Once this is achieved, the operation is terminated. One or more longitudinal incisions may be needed to decompress the entire nerve. If the interfascicular epineurium is involved and 1 or 2 simple epineuriotomies will not decompress all the fascicles, an epifascicular epineuriectomy is carried out, removing fibrotic epineurial tissue over the entire circumference of the nerve. If fibrosis extends between the fascicles, an interfascicular epineuriectomy is necessary. It is not necessary to excise all the interfascicular tissue, merely enough of them to allow the nerve to expand.

Results.—External neurolysis usually is clinically successful if it is possible to remove the causative agent. However, the results of internal neurolysis are difficult to evaluate. Satisfactory recovery cannot be expected if local damage is so marked that neurolysis fails to solve the local pathologic problem. Resection with nerve grafting is a better choice in such patients.

Complications.—Manipulating the nerve trunk during neurolysis may lead to paralysis and a sensory deficit. In addition, a pain syndrome may develop, particularly after intraneural procedures. The very symptoms that led to neurolysis may recur and be worse than before if conditions in general have not changed.

▶ Neurolysis is a common requirement, but recognition of the variable pathology as a guide to selecting the appropriate surgical technique is an uncommon bolus of knowledge. There are few with as much experience in evaluation and treatment of nerve scarring and none with greater insight into the pathophysiology of the scarred nerve than Dr. Hanno Millesi. This abstract can give you some of the flavor of this review of one of the fundamental problems in hand surgery, but those with real interest or real need should read the entire article and keep a copy of it available.—J.H. Dobyns, M.D.

Mesovascularized Island Flexor Tendon: New Concepts and Techniques for Flexor Tendon Salvage Surgery

Guimberteau JC, Panconi B, Boileau R (Bordeaux, France)
Plast Reconstr Surg 92:888–903, 1993   129-94-7–19

Purpose.—Although a number of operative techniques are satisfactory for isolated, simple reconstruction of the flexor tendons of the hand, they may be unsuitable for severe salvage cases. Avoiding adhesions is always a consideration in flexor tendon repair. A single-stage operation using flexor tendons with perfect mesotendon blood supply and an inherent gliding mechanism to minimize adhesions during tendon healing was described.

Methods.—The new technique views the tendon not as a simple string transmission but as a living organ, dependent on its intrinsic blood supply for optimal healing. The technique, inspired by reversed ulnar island forearm transfers, uses the flexor superficialis tendon of the ring finger. This tendon's blood supply comes from a vascular mesotendon emerging from the ulnar pedicle just before Guyon's canal. The use of mesovascularized flexor tendon ensures a perfect blood supply, a favorable environment for suturing, and, subsequently, good digital excursion. The common carpal sheath, mesotendon, and paratendon constitute a single gliding unit. Preservation of this unit allows transfer of a true digital flexor tendon, with a combination of firmness and flexibility.

Experience.—Superior results have been achieved with the mesovascular tendon island technique, and now it is used as standard procedure for patients in Boyes class III or IV. The vascularized tendon island avoids adhesions and improves the vascularity of the surrounding tissues. The transferred tendon retains the flexibility, pliability, and resistance of real flexor tendon. About 18–20 cm of tendon is available for transfer, allowing easy reconstruction of flexor tendon defects of all types, from the pulp to the carpal area. The main disadvantage of the procedure is the need to transect the ulnar pedicle, but thus far this has caused no long-term problems. Great improvement was seen in 9 of 12 patients undergoing flexor superficialis transfer and in 6 of 9 extreme salvage patients undergoing composite skin and flexor superficialis transfer.

Conclusion.—The technique of using islanded flexor tendon with its mesotendon vascular supply and gliding mechanism intact represents a major advance in avoiding adhesions in flexor tendon repair. The operation may be done in a single stage, allowing an earlier return to home and work. Ulnar vascularized tendon or tendon and skin transfers give good functional results in multiple applications.

Chronic Problems

Long-Term Follow-Up of Swanson's Silastic Arthroplasty of the Metacarpophalangeal Joints in Rheumatoid Arthritis
Wilson YG, Sykes PJ, Niranjan NS (South Wales Regional Centre for Plastic and Reconstructive Surgery, Chepstow)
J Hand Surg (Br) 18B:81–91, 1993   129-94-7–20

Background.—The Swanson silicone prosthesis is probably the most successful in arthroplasty. Most patients with implants have improved power and dexterity, pain relief, and a cosmetically acceptable result. Complications have included giant-cell reactive synovitis and lymphadenitis, apparently resulting from silicone particle shedding. However, silicone synovitis may not be as common as has been suggested. A long-term follow-up study was done of patients with rheumatoid arthritis undergoing Swanson's silastic arthroplasty of the metacarpophalangeal joint.

Methods.—Sixty-two women and 15 men underwent metacarpophalangeal joint arthroplasty on 375 joints between 1976 and 1985. Forty-eight were contacted by postal questionnaire. Thirty-five of these patients also had objective evaluations at 5- to 14-year intervals postoperatively.

Findings.—Most patients were satisfied with their outcomes, both early and late. The treatment provided pain relief, deformity correction, and improved range of motion. With time, some loss of mobility occurred; however, most patients retained functional improvements. There were no cases of silicone synovitis. Complication rates compared favorably with those of other reported series.

Conclusion.—Swanson's silastic arthroplasty provides lasting pain relief and enhances patients' sense of well-being. Moreover, it appears to be associated with few complications. There were no cases of silicone synovitis in this series of patients with rheumatoid arthritis.

▶ This article, despite some weaknesses, has many features of the quality control review that may soon be mandated. It analyzes the subjective and objective results of a standard reconstructive procedure, performed and rehabilitated in a standardized fashion. A suitable aliquot of patients underwent follow-up for a reasonable period (9.6 years). The results were acceptable to the physician and beneficial to the patient. Is this enough to validate a procedure for general and continued use? The authors think it is, and so do many other surgeons, both published and unpublished.

Nevertheless, there is a weakness in this review, and it is a common one, particularly when analyzing foreign materials that are implanted in the body. The visible (clinical and imaging) deformities of the materials and of the reconstructed body parts are often underreported, as they are in this article. The less visible manifestations, particulate reaction in this instance, are often said to be absent if gross clinical or imaging signs are not evident. Such reports are insufficient for validation!—J.H. Dobyns, M.D.

Total Collateral Ligament Excision for Contractures of the Proximal Interphalangeal Joint
Diao E, Eaton RG (Millard Fillmore Hosp, Buffalo, NY; St Luke's Roosevelt Hosp Ctr, New York)
J Hand Surg (Am) 18A:395–402, 1993   129-94-7–21

Introduction.—The proximal interphalangeal (PIP) joint is the chief determinant of useful finger motion. Its collateral ligament–palmar plate complex provides a stable joint while facilitating joint motion. Conventionally, it has been considered necessary to preserve at least part of this complex to avoid major instability.

Patient Population.—The effects of totally excising fibrosed PIP collateral ligaments were examined in 30 patients having joint release surgery in a 10-year period for primary joint contractures. In all patients, the collateral ligaments were totally removed. Most of the contractures resulted from PIP dislocation or fracture-dislocation. Sixteen patients (average age, 39 years) were operated on 18 months after injury. Average follow-up was 5½ years after operation. Most of the patients required excision of both collateral ligaments.

Results.—The average total active range of motion increased from 38 to 78 degrees after surgery. The joint was stable to active motion at 3 weeks, and subsequently to lateral stress as well. All patients had less than 5 degrees of radial and ulnar deviation at the PIP joint on maximal stress. All 9 patients whose dominant hand was operated on had greater grip strength than in the untreated hand. In 2 patients, PIP joint motion failed to improve postoperatively.

Conclusion.—A radical approach to contracted PIP joints that includes complete excision of the collateral ligaments can provide an improved range of motion without joint instability.

▶ It has been difficult for the profession to accept the concept that total excision of the collateral ligament systems at the PIP joints is a better method of contracture release than simple release or partial excision and that it will not result in a secondary instability. The authors make a convincing presentation. Count me among the converted.—J.H. Dobyns, M.D.

Tension Band Arthrodesis of Small Joints in the Hand
Stern PJ, Gates NT, Jones TB (Univ of Cincinnati, Ohio)
J Hand Surg (Am) 18A:194–197, 1993   129-94-7–22

Patients.—Tension band arthrodesis was performed on a total of 290 joints in 203 patients in the period 1979–1990. The 143 female and 60 male patients had an average age of 47 years. Most of the procedures involved the proximal interphalangeal (PIP) joints of the finger, but 60 thumb metacarpophalangeal joints and 17 finger metacarpophalangeal joints were fused. Arthrodesis was favored over arthroplasty if there was a history of sepsis, if gross instability was seen, or if bone stock was deficient. Inadequate soft tissue coverage or support also was an indication for arthrodesis.

Technique.—After releasing the central tendon from its insertion and detaching the collateral ligaments via a dorsal longitudinal incision, the joint surfaces are resected by parallel cuts in the desired degree of flexion. A transverse hole is made 5–10 mm distal to the fusion site using a .028-in. Kirschner pin just dorsal to the midaxial line, and a steel wire is threaded through it. Two parallel pins then are driven retrograde into the more proximal bone, exiting dorsally about 10–15 mm proximal to the fusion site. The cut surfaces are compressed, taking care to avoid malrotation, and the pins then are driven anterograde into the distal bone and seated in the palmar cortex. The pins should not engage the distal subchondral bone. The wire is looped about the pins in a figure-of-eight manner and the pins are folded over and clipped close to the bone. The digit is splinted for 3–5 days.

Results.—The fusion rate was 97%. Five of the 9 patients with nonunion were successfully re-treated, whereas 3 had painless fibrous ankylosis and 1 opted to have the little finger removed. In 3 cases of nonunion, a diastasis was present at the fusion site at the time of surgery but went unrecognized. Two other patients failed to comply with postoperative measures. Ten superficial wound infections occurred. Three joints were malpositioned but were easily re-fused into proper alignment. Hardware was removed in 9% of the patients when the wire penetrated the dorsal skin or a painful bursa developed.

Advantages.—Tension band arthrodesis is a simple and reliable means of fusing the small joints of the hand. The fusion is strong enough to permit early active motion, precluding the need for prolonged immobilization. No bulky splint is required to protect the PIP joint.

▶ Many successful methods of small joint fusion are known and practiced. The tension band method is particularly appealing because it is technically simple and uses common, readily available materials; it uses low-profile, minimally irritating fixation material that seldom has to be removed; and it is sufficiently effective biomechanically that external support is seldom necessary and early rehabilitation is feasible.—J.H. Dobyns, M.D.

Carpal Tunnel Release: A Prospective, Randomized Assessment of Open and Endoscopic Methods

Brown RA, Gelberman RH, Seiler JG III, Abrahamsson S-O, Weiland AJ, Urbaniak JR, Schoenfeld DA, Furcolo D (Massachusetts Gen Hosp, Boston; Univ of Lund, Malmö, Sweden; Hosp for Special Surgery, New York; et al)
J Bone Joint Surg (Am) 75-A:1265–1274, 1993   129-94-7–23

Background.—Some researchers have attempted endoscopic release of the carpal tunnel as an alternative to open carpal tunnel release in the hope of decreasing the prevalence of complications associated with open release. The role of 2-portal endoscopic carpal tunnel release in the treatment of median nerve compression at the wrist was investigated.

Methods.—One hundred forty-five patients with 169 affected hands were enrolled in a prospective, randomized, multicenter study. All had clinical features consistent with carpal tunnel syndrome, had not responded to or had refused nonsurgical treatment, and had electrodiagnostic investigations consistent with carpal tunnel syndrome. The patients underwent open or endoscopic carpal tunnel release. Follow-up examinations were done at 21, 42, and 84 days.

Findings.—At the end of follow-up, both open and endoscopic techniques had relieved pain and paresthesias. Numbness and paresthesias were alleviated in 98% of 82 hands in the group treated by open-release and in 99% of the 78 hands in the group treated by endoscopic release. Patient satisfaction, rated on a scale of 0% to 100%, was a mean 84% in the open-release group and 89% in the endoscopic release group. The open technique was associated with more scar tenderness than the endoscopic method. The open method also resulted in a longer time to return to work. Four complications occurred in hands undergoing the endoscopic technique: 1 partial transection of the superficial palmar arch, 1 digital nerve contusion, 1 ulnar nerve neurapraxia, and 1 wound hematoma.

Conclusion.—The endoscopic release method achieves functional outcomes more quickly than the open-release technique. However, endoscopic release is associated with a higher rate of complications, indicating that intraoperative safety must be improved before this method can be used on a widespread basis.

▶ Skilled surgeons at respected institutions have given us a useful biopsy of current, state-of-the-art surgical management of carpal tunnel syndrome. There are fewer secondary wound problems after endoscopic release and fewer secondary problems resulting from damage of deep structures after open release. Also, the rivalry between proponents of the 2 techniques has galvanized the development of procedures in an area that had become almost static. The tools and techniques of open and endoscopic methods are still being altered. Both are acceptable methods in the hands of those trained to use them, but patients must be alerted to the possibile neurovascular damage and/or rsidual problems. In endoscopic release, both patient and team must be ready to convert to an open technique for many reasons.—J.H. Dobyns, M.D.

Hand Function After Digital Amputation

Chow SP, Ng C (Hong Kong Society for Surgery of the Hand)
J Hand Surg (Br) 18-B:125–128, 1993   129-94-7–24

Background.—A previous study by Murray et al. of hand strength in patients with transmetacarpal amputation of the index finger indicated that hyperesthesia of the new web reduced hand strength. However, other possible factors may include residual length and stiffness of the remaining stump, which digits and how many of them are involved, and the levels of the amputations. These factors were considered in a prospective assessment of hand function in patients with digital amputation at 6 centers.

Method.—A total of 127 patients with traumatic amputation of fingers and thumbs between the level of the distal interphalangeal joint and the metacarpophalangeal joint were admitted. The first hand function assessment was carried out on discharge from the rehabilitation program. Further tests were carried out after 2 months, 6 months, and 1 year. The following measurements were made at each visit: range of movement of the joint just proximal to amputation, stiffness of the other joints in the hand, power grip by using a Jaymar dynamometer, key pinch between the thumb and the patient's preferred finger using a Preston pinch gauge, and pronation and supination power using a machine designed by the engineering workshop. After familiarization with the procedure, 3 tests were taken at intervals of 1 minute for each parameter, and the highest value was recorded. The strength of the uninjured hand was measured as a control. To correct for differences in strength between the dominant and nondominant hands, 50 normal individuals were also assessed, and the ratio between dominant and nondominant strength was calculated. Preinjury strength was estimated by multiplying the strength of the good hand with a correction factor according to the study in the 50 normal participants. The percentage of recovery in all powers was then compared with the estimated preinjury strength and called the "corrected percentage recovery."

Results.—Sensory disturbances decreased rapidly, although numbness of the amputation stump was still seen in 50% of patients after 1 year. The range of movement proximal to the amputation level was regained early, within 2 or 3 months of injury, along with pronation and supination. However, it took a year to regain 70% of power grip and key pinch. Further analysis revealed that patients with multiple digit amputations experienced the most difficulty with power grip. Power grip was worse in patients who had lost the thumb or the middle finger through the proximal phalanx. Almost all patients were equally impaired for key pinch to a level of 50% to 60%. Multiple finger amputees had decreased pronation, whereas thumb amputees experienced decreased supination. A total of 8.7% of the group had to change their hand dominance as a result of the injury; 23.6% had to change their job; and 19.7% requested a cosmetic prosthesis.

Conclusion.—When the results of ray amputation of the index finger in Murray's study are compared with those of index finger amputees in this series of patients who retained a stump, no great difference was seen in power grip. Key pinch was weaker when a stump is left, but pronation was stronger because of the larger effective span of the hand. These findings support Murray's findings that with sensory disturbances, key pinch and supination power are weaker; however, contrary to Murray's findings, these findings indicate that power grip and pronation were not affected.

▶ Giving a meaningful and statistical prognosis to those individuals who have lost digits of the hand has been difficult because we had few facts. The standard formulas for disability after hand digit amputation do not provide good guidance about the specifics of the residual disability. Even with this study, the heterogeneity of the sample and the small number in most subgroups tell us that larger sampling is needed. Nevertheless, we have more facts for our patients than we did before, including the welcome news that fewer than 10% require a change of job unless multiple digits are amputated.—J.H. Dobyns, M.D.

Motion After Metacarpophalangeal Joint Reconstruction in Rheumatoid Disease
El-Gammal TA, Blair WF (Univ of Iowa, Iowa City)
J Hand Surg (Am) 18A:504–511, 1993   129-94-7–25

Background.—Swanson implant arthroplasty and the crossed intrinsic transfer procedure are used to treat rheumatoid metacarpophalangeal (MP) joints. The long-term outcome in terms of active finger motion after these procedures has not previously been compared.

Patients.—Fifty-eight patients with rheumatoid MP joint reconstructions in 70 hands were examined. Crossed intrinsic transfer was performed in 21 hands of 19 patients and Swanson implant arthroplasty in 49 hands of 39 patients. The average follow-up was 6 years for crossed intrinsic transfer and 21 months for implant arthroplasty. Average postoperative extension, flexion, and active range of motion of the MP, proximal interphalangeal (PIP), and distal interphalangeal joints were measured at each follow-up visit.

Results.—After crossed intrinsic transfer the overall average MP active range of motion decreased by 18 degrees compared with preoperative values, but average PIP and distal interphalangeal active range-of-motion values were significantly increased during the first 5 years. After implant arthroplasty the overall average MP active range of motion had increased by 8 degrees, and it increased still more during the first 2 postoperative years. However, thereafter, the average MP active range of motion gradually declined, probably as a result of disease progression. The PIP active range of motion was also significantly increased during the first 2 years.

Conclusion.—Performing crossed intrinsic transfer early appears to prevent progressive joint deformity and destruction and to postpone the need for Swanson arthroplasty.

▶ It is too easy for both the patient and physician to wait until the rheumatoid hand can barely function before proceeding with the salvage operation of MP arthroplasty, which includes synovectomy, extensor tendon realignment, intrinsic release, and perhaps other procedures. This is a good salvage procedure but it is not as good as an early soft tissue procedure, if one has the option.

The standard soft tissue procedure is called "crossed intrinsic transfer" in this paper, but similar procedures without crossed intrinsic transfer are often used. The cluster of procedures common to this approach are synovectomy of the MP joint; release and rebalancing of the extensor mechanism; intrinsic release (with or without crossed intrinsic transfer), and occasionally other procedures such as rebalancing of the collateral ligaments and flexor tenosynovectomy.

I agree with the authors that these soft tissue procedures, done at a stage before serious joint damage is present, can mechanically realign and, therefore, protect the joints for a longer period ($\pm$ 5 years on average in this study) than can arthroplasty procedures carried out at a later stage of the disease. Neither of these procedures protect against the progression of disease.—J.H. Dobyns, M.D.

The Continuous Elongation Treatment by the TEC Device for Severe Dupuytren's Contracture of the Fingers
Messina A, Messina J (Traumatologic and Orthopaedic Hosp, Turin, Italy)
Plast Reconstr Surg 92:84–90, 1993   129-94-7-26

Background.—As part of a clinical investigation of Dupuytren's contracture of the hand, an apparatus for the continuous atraumatic lengthening of the retracted fingers was built. The TEC (technique of continual extension) device is used before excision of the pathologic palmar fascia.

Technique.—With the use of locoregional anesthesia, 2 self-drilling pins are inserted transversely through the proximal and distal metaphyses of the fourth and fifth metacarpal bones. A Kirschner wire is inserted through the phalanx metaphysis of the retracted finger and formed into a loop. The TEC device is secured to the 2 self-drilling pins by a rod. The Kirschner wire loop is attached to the TEC device. Continuous lengthening is performed by the patient at home at a rate of 2 mm per day.

Patients.—Since 1986, 85 fingers flexed by Dupuytren's contracture have been treated with the TEC device. In 1986 and 1987, 23 contracted fingers were treated with the TEC device only. From 1988 to 1991, 62 flexed fingers were treated with the TEC device before limited fasciectomy.

Results.—Fingers treated with the TEC device alone retracted an average of 3 months after completion of the continuous elongation treatment, although to a lesser flexed position than before treatment. Disease progression was halted in most hands treated with the TEC device and subsequently with limited fasciectomy.

Conclusion.—Bringing a finger flexed by Dupuytren's contracture back to its initial position with the use of the TEC device eliminates the need for plastic surgery to correct digital or palmar skin loss and avoids the necrosis, loss of vascularity, and bad functional results often seen after classic operations.

▶ The application of techniques that are newly developed or are newly revised to a higher level of usefulness is not consistent in all areas and may lag noticeably until some investigator matches the new application to an old problem. The use of skeletal external fixator-distractor units for skeletal problems has been widely applied, but the technique has been sparingly applied to primary soft tissue problems. If the experience of these investigators is confirmed, many types of contracture may be similarly tested. Any help will be welcome with these difficult problems, but it will be particularly interesting if there is a different response depending on the type of contracture.—J.H. Dobyns, M.D.

Long-Term Results of Carpal Tunnel Decompression: Assessment of 60 Cases
Haupt WF, Wintzer G, Schop A, Löttgen J, Pawlik G (Univ of Cologne, Germany)
J Hand Surg (Br) 18B:471–474, 1993   129-94-7-28

Background.—In carpal tunnel syndrome, compression of the median nerve beneath the flexor retinaculum is caused by increased tissue volume in the compartment, which is tightly enclosed by the retinaculum above and the carpal bones below, allowing little tissue expansion. Surgical division of the flexor retinaculum is the treatment of choice. Most published reports with a follow-up of as long as 2 years emphasize the favorable prognosis of surgery. The long-term prognosis after surgery and the effect of potential prognostic factors were investigated.

Method.—Sixty patients undergoing surgery for carpal tunnel syndrome were assessed preoperatively and followed a median of 5.5 years after surgery. Preoperative and postoperative assessment used a standardized grading system to analyze motor, sensory, trophic, and electrodiagnostic findings and to assess pain.

Findings.—Postoperatively, the surgical results were considered favorable in 86% of patients. Pain was the most prominent preoperative finding. The greatest clinical changes postoperatively were in pain relief, with 86% of the hands pain-free after surgery. The improvements in motor and sensory findings were similar, with the smallest change reported for trophic alterations. Patients with diabetes mellitus had less pain relief than nondiabetic patients. Pain relief was somewhat greater in patients having early operation. Pain lasting more than 5 years before surgery indicated a poor prognosis.

▶ Given adequate diagnostic criteria, the results of carpal tunnel release should be good and should remain so. This study, with a median follow-up of more than 5 years, reassures us that this is so. The level of good results decreases somewhat, as is expected, in certain groups such as patients with greater than 5 years of symptoms before surgery and patients with additional causes of peripheral neuropathy (mostly diabetes mellitus). The medical world already believes the premise that adequate decompression of the median nerve for carpal tunnel syndrome is good treatment but is concerned about a current tendency to overdiagnose the condition or to make it the sole or major component of multifactorial problems, as often seen in pain-dysfunction syndromes of the upper limb in occupational or sports-related conditions.—J.H. Dobyns, M.D.

8 Trauma and Amputation

Introduction

It is with a great deal of pleasure that I join Dr. Sledge's editorial team for the YEAR BOOK OF ORTHOPEDICS and accept the baton from my partner and mentor, Sigvard T. Hansen, Jr., one of the giants and founding fathers in the field of musculoskeletal traumatology.

This year's crop of trauma and amputation articles shows a distinct move toward improvement in basic research design. The basic science articles are especially sound in their design and methodology. Imaging techniques are coming under increased scrutiny in terms of efficacy. In this particular field, cost-effectiveness issues deserve an increased amount of attention in the future. We have cause to be encouraged about the ongoing assessments of new technologies. We see some blinded studies appearing in the literature. One particularly well-designed clinical study assessing the efficacy of CAD CAM technology for below-the-knee amputees is included (Abstract 129-94-8–13). Unfortunately, this was the only substantive article in the field of amputation surgery this year.

Tibial fractures continue to be a great stimulus for clinical research. It is in this field of research that design continues to be a bit backward. This year's batch of articles pose many more questions than they answer, but the ones selected are worthy of our attention. The danger of using standardized fracture classification systems without appropriate methodology or consensus classification is pointed out in two articles (Abstracts 129-94-8–22 and 129-94-8–23).

We have a particularly timely and important group of articles under the heading of clinical dilemmas. Questions about what to do with the dropped bone graft in the operating room (Abstract 129-94-8–28); about techniques for minimizing tension on wound closure (Abstract 129-94-8–26), and about what to do about implant removal (Abstract 129-94-8–24) are nicely addressed.

Compartmental syndrome remains the most common cause of legal action against an orthopedic surgeon. Three articles are included that advance our clinical understanding of the phenomenon (Abstracts 129-94-8–30 through 129-94-8–32).

We continue to be fascinated with the operative techniques for fixing pelvic and acetabular fractures. There are some good techniques to review this year. However, at some point in the future, we are going to have to come to grips with the question of whether anatomical reduction relates to functional outcome. Dr. Matta continues to provide tools to assess the appropriateness of operative intervention for acetabular fractures (Abstract 129-94-8-36). The question of anatomicity of the reduction vs. functional outcome needs to be addressed here as well.

The Hannover group (Abstract 129-94-8-37) has been at the forefront of indicating that there may be a significant problem with the reaming of femoral shaft fractures in the face of pulmonary injury. We have a particularly good series of articles that address this whole topic of adult respiratory distress syndrome, the effects of reaming, how to monitor patients after injury, etc. There will clearly be several more years of ongoing debate in this arena.

Finally, I am particularly pleased to point out two studies (Abstracts 129-94-8-42 and 129-94-8-43) that use general health-related quality-of-life instruments to address issues of musculoskeletal traumatology. They are very helpful and serve as a model for future clinical research. The use of these types of instruments combined with progress in clinical and experimental design give me reason to be optimistic about the future of the scientific platform of our subspecialty.

Marc F. Swiontkowski, M.D.

Basic Science

Healing and Remodeling of Articular Incongruities in a Rabbit Fracture Model

Llinas A, McKellop HA, Marshall GJ, Sharpe F, Lu B, Kirchen M, Sarmiento A
(Univ of Southern California, Los Angeles)
J Bone Joint Surg (Am) 75-A:1508–1523, 1993   129-94-8-1

Introduction.—An optimum method has yet to be defined for the restoration of normal anatomy in intra-articular fractures, and residual incongruity of the joint remains common. An incongruity model was developed using fractures in rabbits to study the healing pattern of articular step-offs to determine the potential for adaptation of cartilage and subchondral bone to incongruity and to determine the effects of the size of the step-off and the method of treatment on the quality of repair.

Methods.—Fifty-four adult New Zealand White rabbits were prepared with .5 or 1-mm step-off defects associated with displaced intra-articular fractures of the medial femoral condyle. The animals were treated with immobilization for 3 weeks, intermittent active motion, or continuous passive motion for 7 days. Twelve weeks after the fracture was created, the healing and remodeling of the step-off defects were examined with the use of contact-pressure maps on pressure-sensitive film, light microscopy, and scanning electron microscopy.

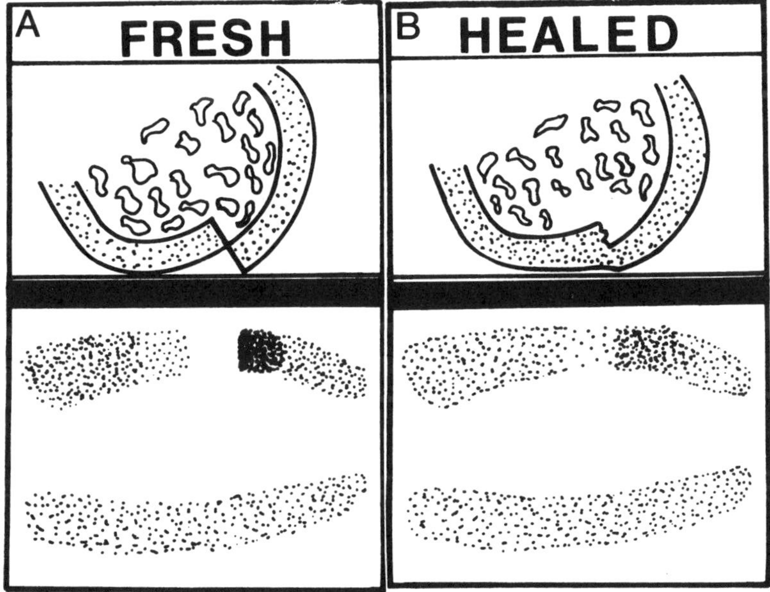

Fig 8–1.—Illustrations of the relationship of the pressure tracks between regions of the step-off and the condyle in a fresh (acute) specimen (**A**) and in a healed specimen (**B**). (Courtesy of Llinas A, McKellop HA, Marshall GJ, et al: *J Bone Joint Surg (Am)* 75-A:1508–1523, 1993.)

Results.—The .5-mm step-offs had rounded off to the point that the incongruity was imperceptible to touch, whereas the 1-mm step-offs were still palpable. With acute defects, contact-pressure patterns showed the gap of the unloaded area to be about 3 times the height of the step-off. In healed specimens, the unloaded gap averaged .35 mm for the .5-mm step-offs and 2.5 mm for the 1-mm step-offs (Fig 8–1). When examined by light microscopy, the cartilage on the elevated side of the healed step-offs had decreased in thickness and was displaced toward the defect. In contrast, the cartilage on the depressed side had thickened and failed to establish continuity between the sides of the defect (Fig 8–2). A marked increase in the subchondral vascular bed was observed, as well as reestablishment of the subchondral plate. Scanning electron microscopy showed that the .5-mm step-offs had healing at the extremes of the osteotomy site, mild fibrillation of the cartilage on the central portion of the condyle on the elevated side, and no synovial invasion or exposure of subchondral bone. However, the 1-mm step-offs, had severe fibrillation of the cartilage on the central portion of the condyle on the elevated side, peripheral synovial invasion, and exposure of subchondral bone.

Conclusion.—In step-off defects, cartilage and subchondral bone adapt to the surface incongruity by modifying their structure in healing. This adaptation was independent of the 3 methods of treatment used but was more successful in restoring the transmission of pressure across

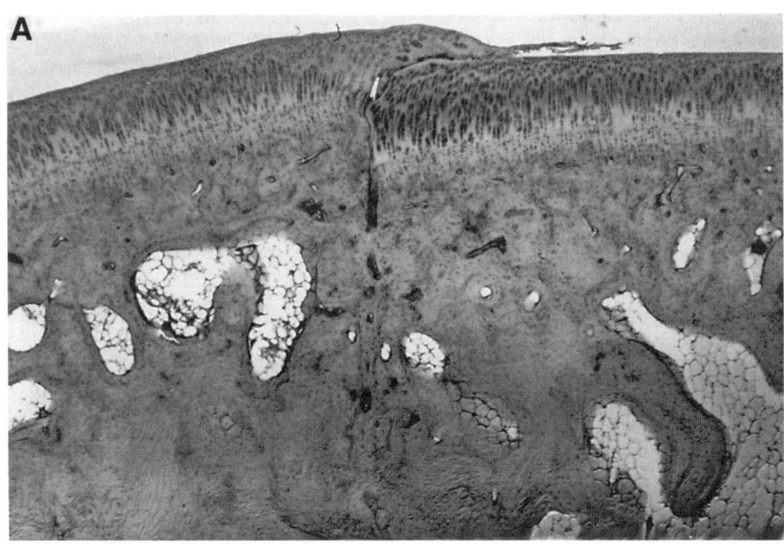

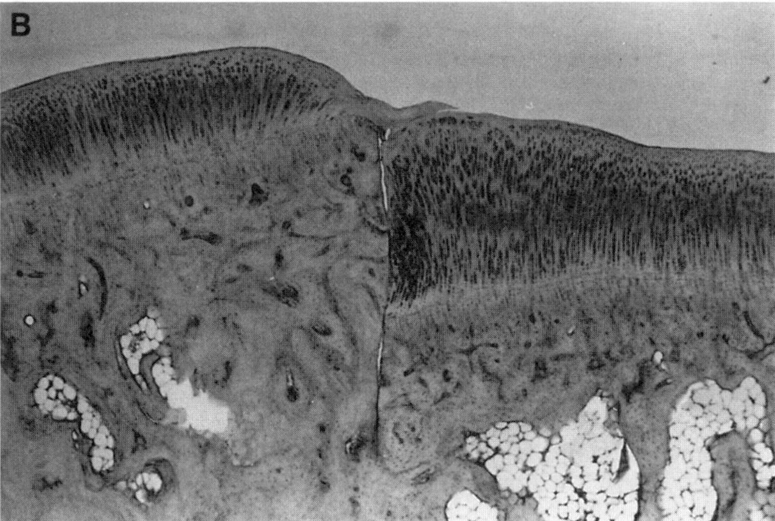

Fig 8–2.—A, photomicrograph of a .5-mm step-off. There is a flow of cartilage on the high side and an increase in thickness on the low side of the lesion. Hematoxylin-eosin; original magnification, ×130. **B,** photomicrograph of a 1-mm step-off. The cartilage on the low side has roughly duplicated its height. There is increased thickness of the subchondral bone on the high side. Hematoxylin-eosin; original magnification, ×130. (Courtesy of Llinas A, McKellop HA, Marshall GJ, et al: *J Bone Joint Surg (Am)* 75-A:1508–1523, 1993.)

the unloaded cartilage with the .5-mm step-offs than with the 1-mm step-offs. In this animal model, the healing and remodeling patterns of step-offs differed substantially from those reported for full-thickness lesions. Thus, continuous passive motion did not appear to improve healing or remodeling, particularly for large step-off defects.

▶ In this superb, well-controlled animal study, the authors demonstrate that articular step-offs substantially increase contact pressure on the high side and extend an unloaded zone on the depressed side. Histologically, .5-mm step-offs were reasonably well tolerated, with only mild fibrillation being demonstrated at 12 weeks. The 1-mm step-offs revealed severe fibrillation and exposure of subchondral bone. Continuous passive motion did not alter this effect. The take-home message is that, when fixing articular fractures, anatomical reduction provides the patient with the best potential for healing, and continuous passive motion does not provide a substitute for anatomical reduction.—M.F. Swiontkowski, M.D.

The Effect of Systemic Antibiotic and Antibiotic-Impregnated Polymethylmethacrylate Beads on the Bacterial Clearance in Wounds Containing Contaminated Dead Bone
Chen NT, Hong H-Z, Hooper DC, May JW Jr (Massachusetts Gen Hosp, Boston; Harvard Med School, Boston)
Plast Reconstr Surg 92:1305–1313, 1993   129-94-8–2

Introduction.—Antibiotic-impregnated acrylic bone cement, introduced in 1970, has proven effective in decreasing infection in major joint replacements. A more recent prophylactic technique has placed antibiotic-impregnated polymethyl methacrylate beads in the osteomyelitic cavity after débridement of infected and devitalized bone. Whether the beads provide additional bacterial clearance in contaminated wounds was investigated. Also evaluated was the role of tobramycin beads as an adjunct to systemic cefazolin and tobramycin administration with the muscle flap in treating contaminated bony wounds.

Methods.—A dorsal muscular wound model was used in 40 adult New Zealand White rabbits. Devitalized iliac crest bone preincubated with *Staphylococcus aureus* was implanted in each wound with or without tobramycin-impregnated polymethylmethacrylate beads. Half the rabbits received systemic tobramycin and half received systemic cefazolin for 7 days. The animals were killed at 7 and 14 days.

Results.—One animal died in each of 4 groups: 7-day tobramycin, 7-day cefazolin, 14-day tobramycin, and 14-day cefazolin. In each of these groups, the wounds containing tobramycin beads had significantly fewer bacteria than those without antibiotic beads. The decrease in bacteria associated with the beads did not differ significantly with respect to the concurrent systemic antibiotics or the duration of treatment. However, groups treated with cefazolin had significantly decreased bacterial counts in the wounds.

Conclusion.—Incomplete débridement of infected dead bone may lead to recurrent osteomyelitis. In this animal model, the use of tobramycin-impregnated polymethyl methacrylate beads as a wound spacer delivered high local concentrations of the antibiotic. The bactericidal effect of the beads was independent of and additive to the systemic antibiotic delivered to the wounds by well-perfused muscles.

▶ In this controlled rabbit study, the authors demonstrate the efficacy of tobramycin-impregnated polymethyl methacrylate beads. The effects of this locally delivered antibiotic are additive to systemic effects of intravenous antibiotics. This article must be interpreted with caution. These were not traumatized muscle beds but rather wounds inflicted with sharp surgical instruments. It is incumbent on the treating surgeons to provide a well-vascularized residual bed for antibiotic delivery by an aggressive débridement of all marginal tissues. However, when planning delayed bone grafting, antibiotic-impregnated polymethyl methacrylate beads are an excellent way to hold open dead space while providing high local concentrations of antibiotics that will effectively decrease bacterial counts.—M.F. Swiontkowski, M.D.

Imaging

Subtle Orthopedic Fractures: Teleradiology Workstation Versus Film Interpretation
Scott WW Jr, Rosenbaum JE, Ackerman SJ, Reichle RL, Magid D, Weller JC, Gitlin JN (Johns Hopkins Med Insts, Baltimore, Md)
Radiology 187:811–815, 1993   129-94-8–3

Introduction.—An interhospital teleradiology system allows radiologic examinations to be performed when a radiologist is not available at the examination site. However, in some studies a loss of diagnostic accuracy has been noted with on-screen interpretation in comparison with film interpretation. Teleradiologic and film interpretations were compared in difficult orthopedic trauma cases.

Methods.—Cases reviewed for interpretation had abnormalities that were initially missed in the emergency room or were correctly diagnosed despite their potential difficulty. From the patients initially selected, 60 had subtle fractures or dislocations observed on the original radiographs and 60 had typical age-related degenerative changes but no fracture or dislocation. Seven senior radiology residents and 1 radiology fellow each interpreted 60 cases with the teleradiology system (1,280 × 1,024-pixel monitors) and 60 cases with the original radiographs. Interpreters assigned confidence ratings of low, moderate, or high to each of their diagnoses.

Results.—The overall accuracy of the readers was significantly better for film interpretations (80.6%) than for teleradiology screen readings

(59.6%). For individual readers, interpretation accuracy with plain radiographs ranged from 68% to 90%; the range with on-screen images was 52% to 62%. Sensitivity also was significantly higher for individual readers when interpreting film images, but specificity was similar when dealing with screen and film images. After data were pooled, film readings were significantly better in accuracy, sensitivity, and specificity. Receiver operating characteristic analysis favored film interpretation over on-screen interpretation. All but 1 of the 8 readers believed that accuracy of interpretation was less with digital images.

Conclusion.—Findings indicate the teleradiology system used is not satisfactory for the primary diagnosis of subtle orthopedic fractures. A higher degree of spatial resolution is probably required to avoid missed fracture cases.

▶ Medical center information systems visionaries have promised me that soon I will be able to sit at home and call up a digital image on my computer screen to recommend treatment for colleagues actively managing a patient in the hospital! Scott et al. have taken a hard look at the quality of such images and have concluded that, for subtle fractures and dislocation, plain films are superior for the purposes of diagnostic interpretation. It would have been interesting had the authors considered more severe trauma cases and CT images related to the spine and pelvis. The message here is one of continued assessment and evaluation of this technology as we all continue to move into this future of digital imaging.—M.F. Swiontkowski, M.D.

Refining the Indications for Arteriography in Penetrating Extremity Trauma: A Prospective Analysis
Schwartz MR, Weaver FA, Bauer M, Siegel A, Yellin AE (Univ of Southern California, Los Angeles)
J Vasc Surg 17:116–124, 1993
129-94-8–4

Background.—Arteriography classically is the preferred means of detecting arterial injury in individuals with penetrating extremity trauma. However, its invasive nature and cost, as well as the possible complications should limit its use to patients likely to have arterial injury.

Methods.—A prospective study of 514 patients with isolated upper or lower extremity penetrating injury was conducted. Excluding patients with limb-threatening ischemia and those who refused arteriography, 469 remained for risk classification. Patients at high risk had "hard" clinical findings (shotgun injury, pulse deficit, or neurologic deficit). An intermediate risk status consisted of 1 or more "soft" findings (hematoma, history of bleeding or hypotension, bruit, fracture, major soft tissue deficit, delayed capillary refill) as well as a minimum ankle/brachial (or wrist/brachial) index (MABI) of less than 1. Patients at low risk had neither hard nor soft signs and an MABI of 1 or higher.

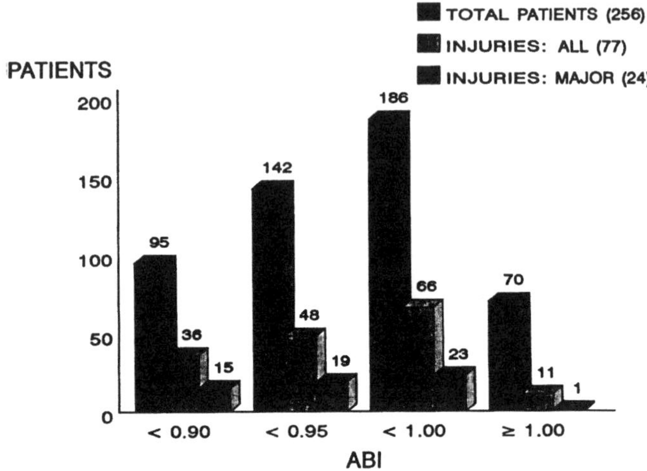

Fig 8–3.—Bar graph illustrates the number of arterial injuries and all major arterial injuries of 256 patients at high and intermediate risk within each MABI range. (Courtesy of Schwartz MR, Weaver FA, Bauer M, et al: *J Vasc Surg* 17:116–124, 1993.)

Results.—No delayed complications of arterial injury developed in 213 low-risk patients who were observed in the hospital for 24 hours. The remaining patients had arteriography, which disclosed 77 injuries, 24 of which threatened the extremity. Fourteen patients required transcatheter embolization or operative repair. Arterial injuries are related to the MABI in Fig 8-3. The only significant predictors of arterial injury were a pulse deficit and an MABI less than 1.

Conclusion.—Significant arterial injuries can be reliably detected by limiting arteriography to patients who have a pulse deficit or an MABI below 1, or both, in the injured extremity.

▶ In this large prospective clinical study defining the indication for arteriography with penetrating extremity trauma, clinical acumen is confirmed to have high value. Patients who had no "hard" clinical findings or "soft" findings, as noted above, can be safely observed clinically. Although diagnostic arteriography is not a quick or benign procedure, the authors' conclusions seem valid, and they have experience with 213 low-risk patients to back them up. Noninvasive duplex scans are on the increase and are becoming more cost-effective as the years roll by. This type of screening for patients with soft and hard findings lends a measure of expediency and accuracy without risk to the patient. I predict continued expansion of this technology in the emergency departments of trauma centers across the world (1).—M.F. Swiontkowski, M.D.

Reference

1. Johansen K, et al: *J Trauma* 31:515, 1991.

Bone Mineral Loss After Lower Extremity Trauma: 62 Cases Followed for 15–38 Years
Karlsson MK, Nilsson BE, Obrant KJ (Lund Univ, Malmö, Sweden)
Acta Orthop Scand 64:362–364, 1993   129-94-8-5

Objective.—Loss of bone mineral occurs in a limb after an injury, but whether this loss is permanent or reversible remains to be established. To address this, 62 patients who had been treated for tibial shaft fracture or knee ligament injury were reevaluated at 15–38 years (average, 21 years) after injury.

Methods.—Bone mineral density (BMD) in the total body, hips, femoral condyle, tibial condyle, and tibial diaphyses were measured using dual energy x-ray absorptiometry. Sixty-two age- and sex-matched individuals served as controls.

Outcome.—Bone mineral density differed between the injured and uninjured legs, and the differences were significant only in the femoral condyle. The same results were seen in patients with ligament injuries. Patients with tibial fractures of more than 28 years' duration retained their post-traumatic osteopenia in the ipsilateral femoral condyle. There was no correlation between early bone loss and late measurements. There was no difference in BMD in nonfractured regions between the injured patients and controls.

Conclusion.—Post-traumatic osteopenia is still evident in the injured leg decades after the injury.

▶ By means of dual-energy x-ray absorptiometry, these authors studied the effect of fractured tibia or knee ligament injuries on bone density 15–38 years after the fact. Using this reliable methodology, significant residual loss in bone mineral density was documented. Although the impact of this loss of BMD is unknown, this important finding deserves further follow-up. I question what the effect of early weight-bearing with similar injuries might be. Clearly, from these data, operative or nonoperative treatment did not alter the findings of decreased BMD. The role of early return to full weight-bearing and muscular activity warrants further study.—M.F. Swiontkowski, M.D.

Impairment of Blood Supply to the Head of the Femur After Fracture of the Neck
Takeuchi T, Shidou T (Nishio Municipal Hosp, Japan; Hamamatsu Med Centre, Japan)
Int Orthop 17:325–329, 1993   129-94-8-6

Introduction.—Internal fixation of fractures of the neck of the femoral head is associated with a high rate of complications. Impairment of the blood supply to the femoral head appears to be the cause of problems such as nonunion and segmental collapse. In an investigation of

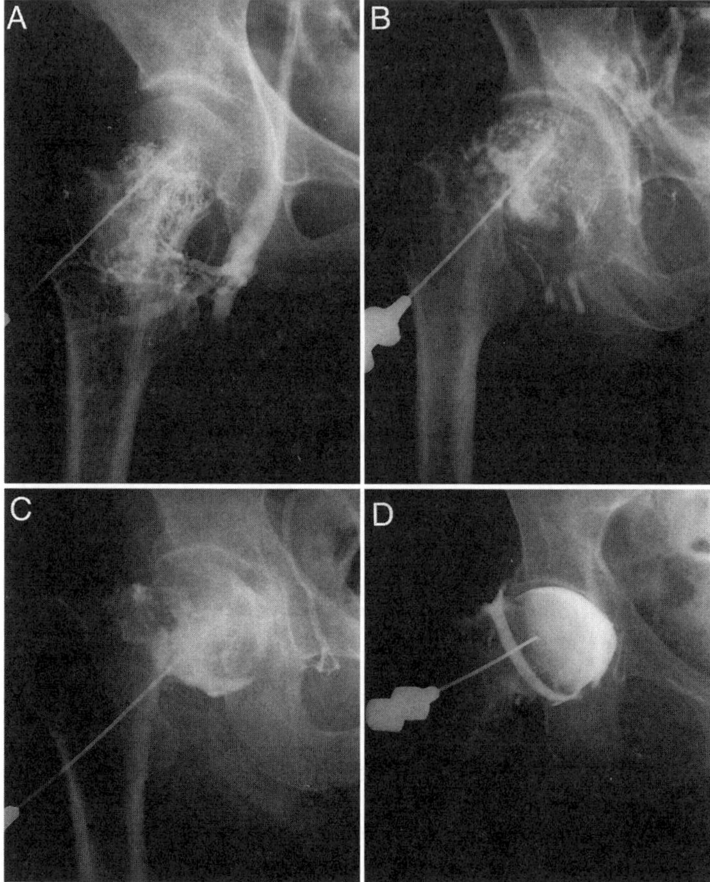

Fig 8–4.—Radiographs illustrating Shidou's classification of femoral neck fractures by intraosseous phlebography. **A,** type A, the inferior retinacular and some of the intramedullary vessels are patent; **B,** type B, the inferior retinacular and some of the ligamentous vessels are patent; **C,** type C, only the ligamentous vessels are patent; **D,** type D, the femoral head is avascular. (Courtesy of Takeuchi T, Shidou T: *Int Orthop* 17:325–329, 1993.)

103 patients with fractures of the femoral neck, the prognostic merits of intraosseous phlebography, scintimetry, and Garden's classification were compared.

Patients and Methods.—The patient group had a mean age of 72 years; 84 were women and 19 were men. All underwent intraosseous phlebography and ^{99m}Tc-methylene diphosphonate scintimetry within 2 weeks of the injury. Two anteroposterior radiographs were obtained with intraosseous phlebography and the films classified by Shidou's scheme (Fig 8–4) according to degree of vascularity as good (type A), fair (type B), insufficient (type C), or none (type D). The scintimetric uptake ratio (H-H) was calculated for each patient. Garden's classification,

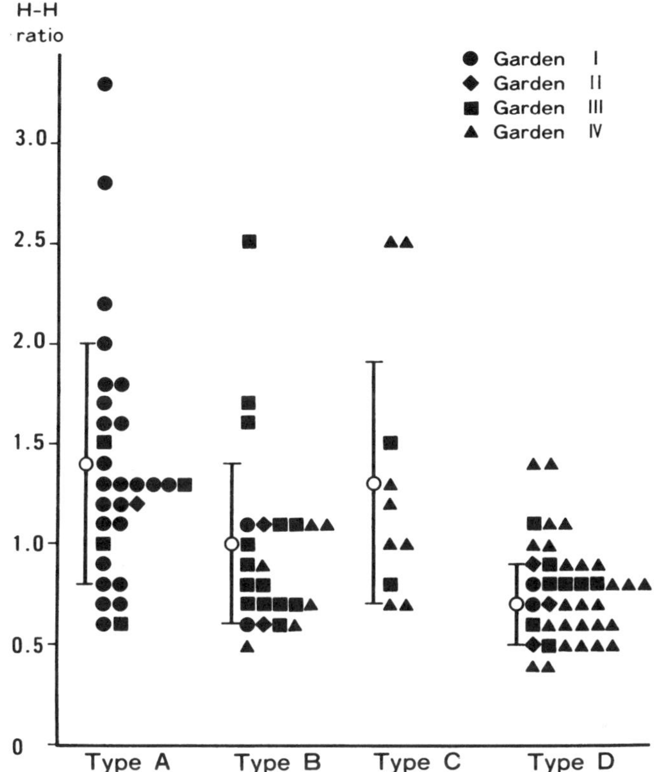

Fig 8–5.—Distribution of H-H ratio and Garden's classification in 103 patients against Shidou's classification by intraosseous phlebography. (Courtesy of Takeuchi T, Shidou T: *Int Orthop* 17:325–329, 1993.)

based on degree of displacement of the fracture, was applied by 3 or 4 orthopedic surgeons after assessment of preoperative radiographs. Patients were selected for osteosynthesis largely on the basis of Garden's classification. Internal fixation was used in 30 patients with undisplaced fractures and in 6 with displaced fractures.

Results.—The mean H-H ratios for types A, B, C, and D were 1.38, .97, 1.32, and .76, respectively. There were significant differences between types A and D and types C and D, but not between types B and D (Fig 8–5). The mean H-H ratios for patients in Garden's stages I, II, III, and IV were 1.34, .83, .99, and .89, respectively. There was a significant difference between the 35 patients with undisplaced fractures and the 68 with displaced fractures. Twenty-five with Garden's stages I and II were type A, but 5 were type D.

Conclusion.—Garden's classification did not accurately reflect the circulatory status after fracture. Scintimetry is not altogether reliable either; in this series H-H ratios below 1 were seen in 7 patients with nonunion and late segmental collapse, but in 2 with uneventful healing. Intraosseous phlebography was the most useful of the 3 methods for evaluating circulation of the femoral head after fractures of the femoral neck.

Periarticular Bone Sites Associated With Traumatic Injury: False-Positive Findings With In-111–Labeled White Blood Cell and Tc-99m MDP Scintigraphy

Seabold JE, Ferlic RJ, Marsh JL, Nepola JV (Univ of Iowa, Iowa City)
Radiology 186:845–849, 1993   129-94-8–7

Introduction.—The radiographic findings are often nonspecific in patients with bone and joint infection. The reliability of combined ^{111}In-labeled white blood cell (WBC) and ^{99m}Tc-methylene diphosphonate (MDP) scintigraphy for the detection of periarticular osteomyelitis in patients with radiographic evidence of adjacent traumatic arthropathy was evaluated in a retrospective study.

Patients and Methods.—In a review of the records of more than 200 orthopedic patients who underwent ^{111}In-WBC–[99m]Tc-MDP scintigraphy during a 7-year period, 38 patients with evidence of traumatic arthropathy at or adjacent to a potential site of osteomyelitis were identified. In 32, the results of bone-biopsy cultures were available for analysis. The ankle was the involved joint site in 23 patients. Twenty-eight patients had a history of traumatic intra-articular injury and 4 had malunion or nonunion of a periarticular fracture.

Results.—Fourteen of the 32 ^{111}In-WBC–[99m]Tc-MDP scans were interpreted as positive for osteomyelitis (Fig 8–6) and 18 were interpreted as negative. There were 27 negative and 5 positive intraoperative bone-bi-

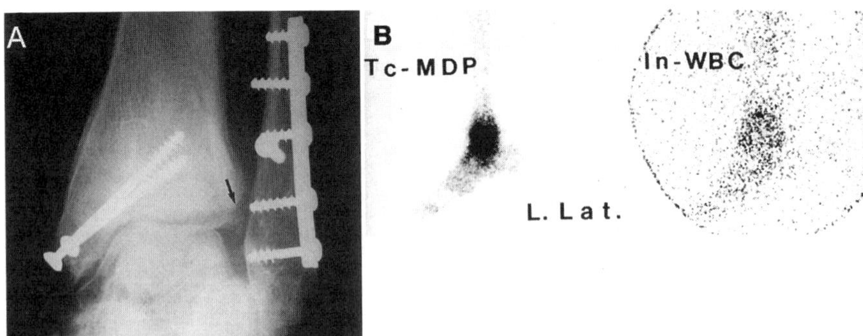

Fig 8–6.—Nonunion of left ankle 10 months after open reduction and fixation of a bimalleolar fracture with wound infection in a woman aged 55 years. **A,** plain radiograph shows nonunion of left lateral malleolus (*arrow*) with mild narrowing (grade 3 traumatic changes) of the joint. **B,** [111]In WBC–[99m]TC MDP images show abnormal WBC localization at culture-negative nonunion site (false positive study). *Abbreviation. L. Lat.,* left lateral. (Courtesy of Seabold JE, Ferlic RJ, Marsh JL, et al: *Radiology* 186:845–849, 1993.)

opsy cultures. Thus, the scan interpretations had a negative predictive value of 94% and a positive predictive value of only 28%.

Conclusions.—Because a high prevalence of false positive ^{111}In-WBC-^{99m}Tc-MDP scans may occur at periarticular sites of patients with associated traumatic arthropathy, positive scans must be confirmed by bone-biopsy culture. However, a negative scan has a high correlation with negative culture results, making osteomyelitis very unlikely. False positive findings are probably the result of ongoing consequences of the injury.

▶ In this retrospective study of more than 200 patients, the authors assessed the value of the two technologies of In-labeled WBC scans and MDP scans. With a positive predictive value of only 28%, the use of these technologies in the diagnosis of osteomyelitis is questionable at best. One would suspect that in centers where there is less volume of this type of work being done, the positive predictive value would be even less. Osteomyelitis in the adult is most often a surgical disease, and the diagnosis can and should be confirmed at the time of the débridement procedure, with reliance on débridement of nonviable bone and the consideration of antibiotics as only an adjunct and not the cure.—M.F. Swiontkowski, M.D.

New Technologies

Patient-Controlled Epidural Analgesia Following Post-Traumatic Pelvic Reconstruction: A Comparison With Continuous Epidural Analgesia

Nolan JP, Dow AAC, Parr MJA, Dauphinee K, Kalish M (Maryland Inst for Emergency Med Services Systems (MIEMSS) Shock Trauma Ctr, Baltimore)
Anaesthesia 47:1037–1041, 1992   129-94-8-8

Objective.—Patient-controlled epidural analgesia (PCEA) and continuous infusion epidural analgesia (CIEA) were compared for the treatment

| | Visual Analogue Pain Scores | | |
	PCEA (*n* = 10)	**CIEA** (*n* = 11)	**p***
Day 0**	2.0 (0.1–5.7)	1.4 (0–7.8)	NS
Day 1	2.6 (0.4–7.2)	1.4 (0.2–8.4)	NS
Day 2	1.5 (0–3.2)	2.1 (0.2–4.8)	NS
Day 3	1.3 (0–5.9)	1.1 (0–4.8)	NS

Note: Results are expressed as median (range).
* All analyses by Wilcoxon rank sum test. NS, not significant.
** Just before leaving the recovery area.
(Courtesy of Nolan JP, Dow AAC, Parr MJA, et al: *Anaesthesia* 47:1037–1041, 1992.)

of pain after post-traumatic pelvic reconstruction in a randomized, single-blind trial.

Treatment.—All patients received a loading dose of fentanyl, 50 μg, in 10 mL of bupivacaine .125% via the epidural catheter. In a randomized fashion, 11 patients received a background infusion of 4 mL/hr and 3–6 mL bolus doses, self-administered as required, with a lockout interval of 15 minutes. Twelve patients received a continuous infusion of 10 mL/hr to a maximum of 25 mL/hr as adjusted by the anesthetist, with the demand button deactivated. Pain scores, side effects, and the volumes of the drug infused during the first 3 postoperative days were compared between the 2 treatment groups.

Outcome.—One patient from each group was withdrawn because of catheter-related problems. Median pain scores on the visual analogue scale were similar in the group receiving PCEA and the group receiving CIEA (table). Although the PCEA group required less of the drug solution than the CIEA group, the difference did not reach statistical significance. The incidence of nausea, vomiting, and pruritus was similarly low in both groups, and none of the patients experienced respiratory depression or hypotension. Patient satisfaction was equal and very good in both groups.

Conclusion.—Patient-controlled epidural analgesia with bupivacaine .125% with fentanyl 1 μg per mL provides effective pain relief after post-traumatic pelvic reconstruction, similar to that provided by CIEA. However, PCEA does not decrease the analgesic dose required to achieve a comparable level of analgesia.

▶ A recent phenomenon in our hospitals has been the introduction of patient-controlled analgesia. These authors go the next step and critically study PCEA. In a randomized, single-blind trial, PCEA provided effective pain relief after post-traumatic pelvic surgery when compared with CIEA. Postsurgical epidural analgesia has been highly efficacious in our center, and this new concept may advance the usefulness of this approach further.—M.F. Swiontkowski, M.D.

The Role of Local Antibiotic Therapy in the Management of Compound Fractures
Ostermann PAW, Henry SL, Seligson D (Univ of Louisville, Ky)
Clin Orthop 295:102–111, 1993   124-94-8–9

Background.—Adjuvant local antibiotic solutions and crystals have long been used to control bacterial growth in compound fractures. Antimicrobial delivery from polymethyl methacrylate bead chains effectively controls deep infection in total hip arthroplasty and chronic osteomyelitis. This retrospective study evaluated the anti-infective efficacy of antibi-

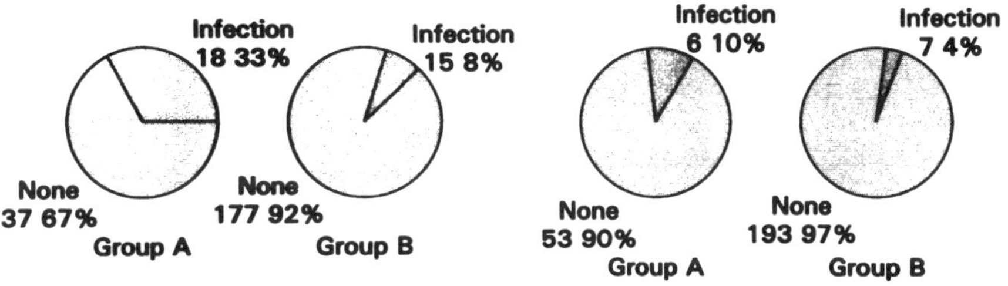

Fig 8–7.—The additional prophylactic use of the antibiotic beads (group B) led to a reduced infection rate in grade II and grade III open fractures. A statistically significant decrease was only evaluated for the grade III category. (Courtesy of Ostermann PAW, Henry SL, Seligson D: *Clin Orthop* 295:102–111, 1993.)

otic-impregnated bead chains as an adjuvant to systemic antibiotic prophylaxis in compound extremity fractures.

Methods.—After timely irrigation, débridement, and skeletal stabilization of their compound fractures, 157 patients received systemic cefazolin, tobramycin, and penicillin (group A), and 547 patients underwent local administration of bead chains impregnated with tobramycin in addition to systemic antibiotic prophylaxis (group B). Hospital charts and clinical records were reviewed to determine acute wound and bone infection rates.

Results.—The infection rate was 17% for group A and 4% for group B. Between-group differences were significant and pervaded all fracture grades (Fig 8–7). In acute wound infections, 2 or more pathogens were cultured in 67% of group A fractures and 46% of group B fractures. In chronic osteomyelitis, 33% of patients in group A had single-organism growth compared with 80% of those in group B. However, none of the group B osteomyelitis cultures grew 3 or more organisms, compared with 27% of those in group A. The most prevalent organism cultured in chronic osteomyelitis in both groups was *Staphylococcus aureus* (Fig 8–8). However, in group A, pseudomonads and serratiae were as prevalent as *S. aureus.* Pseudomonads were also significant pathogens in group B.

Conclusion.—Adjuvant local administration of bead chains impregnated with tobramycin prevents infections in compound fractures with

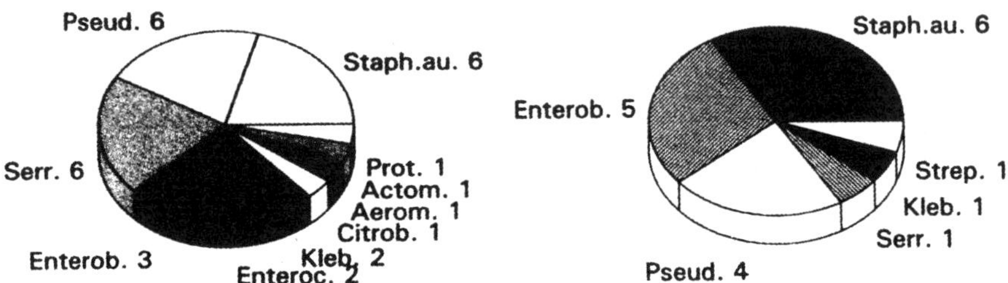

Fig 8–8.—*Staphylococcus aureus* was the most common cultured organism in chronic osteomyelitis in both groups. (Courtesy of Ostermann PAW, Henry SL, Seligson D: *Clin Orthop* 295:102–111, 1993.)

contaminated wounds, particularly those with a high grade of compounding. Further investigation is warranted in a prospective multicenter trial.

▶ Antibiotic-impregnated polymethyl methacrylate beads have proven to be a real advance in treatment for musculoskeletal trauma patients with open fractures and bone loss. This group from Louisville has been on the cutting edge of advancing this clinical research. In this retrospective report, 547 patients received tobramycin bead chains in addition to systemic antibiotic prophylaxis. They demonstrated a decrease in infection rate from 17% to 4%. Caution must be observed to prevent overinterpreting this work because it was not prospective or randomized and was uncontrolled for injury severity. However, this approach has certainly been beneficial for patients, especially as a method for holding open soft tissue planes for delayed bone grafting once contused muscle has recovered its optimum vascularity.—M.F. Swiontkowski, M.D.

Elderly Patients With Hip Fractures: Improved Outcome With the Use of Care Maps With High-Quality Medical and Nursing Protocols

Ogilvie-Harris DJ, Botsford DJ, Hawker RW (Univ of Toronto)
J Orthop Trauma 7:428–437, 1993   129-94-8–10

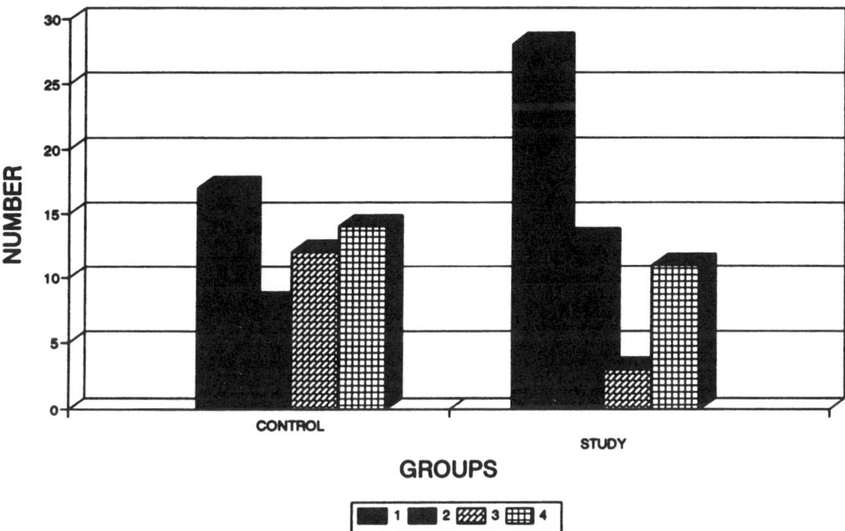

Fig 8–9.—Final outcome in the control and study group ($P = .036$). Group 1, patients who returned to previous level of ambulation and accommodation; group 2, loss of 1 level of ambulation *or* accommodation; group 3, loss of 1 level of ambulation *and* accommodation; group 4, loss of more than 1 level of ambulation *and* accommodation. (Courtesy of Ogilvie-Harris DJ, Botsford DJ, Hawker RW: *J Orthop Trauma* 7:428–437, 1993.)

Introduction.—Elderly patients who sustain hip fractures often have a poor prognosis. However, with changes in their care, the mortality rate can be decreased and ambulatory status can be maintained. In a prospective cohort study, outcome after standard nursing and medical treatment was compared with that after high-quality medical and nursing protocols in geriatric patients with hip fractures.

Patients and Methods.—A total of 106 patients enrolled, 51 in the control group and 55 in the intervention group. Eighty-four patients were women and 22 were men. Twenty were aged 65–75 years, 40 were aged 75–85 years, and 42 were older than 85 years of age. During the 6-month period after the controls were treated, the high-quality nursing and medical care protocols were introduced. The intervention group was cared for after this 6-month run-in period. Postoperative follow-up was 6 months for both groups. The care map used in the new protocol covered a 14-day period ending at postoperative day 12. Each day had specific orders regarding consultations, tests, treatments, medications, diet, activity, patient education, and discharge planning.

Results.—The control and intervention groups were similar in preoperative variables. Patients in the intervention group had a significantly lower rate of complications than controls. However, the in-hospital death rate was similar for the 2 groups. Excluding patients who were hospitalized for more than 28 days, the average length of stay was 15.3 days in the control group and 13.6 in the intervention group. Overall outcome was described in 4 grades (Fig 8–9) and was statistically different for the 2 groups. Twenty-eight patients in the intervention group but only 17 in the control group returned to their prefracture status in regard to ambulation and accommodation.

Conclusion.—The high-quality, more active medical and nursing protocols laid out in the care map can significantly improve outcome in geriatric patients with hip fracture. Complication rates and length of hospital stay were decreased, and overall outcome was enhanced. With hip fractures in this population becoming a serious and increasing problem, the improved protocols can also prove cost-effective.

▶ Care maps represent one attempt to decrease variation in patient management, thus improving the efficiency of care delivery. There is no better place to initially apply them than in patients with hip fracture, a public health problem that is rapidly increasing in proportion. The Toronto group showed a decreased rate of complications (e.g., urinary tract infection, deep venous thrombosis, etc.) after the institution of a care map, as well as a decrease in mortality. The reader must be cautioned that with 51 patients in the treatment group and 55 in the control group, the power of these statistics is relatively low. However, it is clear that with a substantial decrease in the length of stay of almost 2 days and improved independence of ambulation, this concept is worthy of further study and wide adoption.—M.F. Swiontkowski, M.D.

Intramedullary Supracondylar Nailing of Femoral Fractures: A Preliminary Report of the GSH Supracondylar Nail
Lucas SE, Seligson D, Henry SL (Univ of Louisville, Ky)
Clin Orthop 296:200–206, 1993   129-94-8–11

Introduction.—Open reduction with internal fixation consistently achieves better results than nonoperative management in patients with supracondylar femoral fractures. A new intramedullary nail has been developed for use in treating such fractures.

Patients and Methods.—Thirty-three patients with 34 acute supracondylar femoral fractures were treated operatively using a genucephalic intramedullary nail. Twenty-four patients (25 fractures) were available for follow-up evaluation. The group had an average age of 39 years; 79% had been injured in motor vehicle or motorcycle accidents. Sixteen patients had sustained multiple injuries and 8 had ipsilateral-associated knee injuries. There were no associated vascular injuries. The basic strategy of the operation was to assemble a condylar block and then fix it to the femoral shaft with the nail. The interlocking closed-section intramedullary nail was inserted retrograde into the femur through the intercondylar notch.

Results.—The average operative time was 156 minutes, and the average estimated blood loss was 224 mL. Follow-up ranged from 5 months to 50 months. All fractures had healed clinically and radiographically at the time of the most recent examination. Type C fractures (using the Comprehensive Classification of Fractures) had a better range of motion than did type A fractures. No patient had severe pain, and only 1 had significant shortening (3 cm). Seven patients had removal of either a distal blocking screw or a condylar screw for local pain symptoms. All treatment-related complications were successfully resolved. At the latest evaluation the average arc motion was 100 degrees.

Conclusion.—The genucephalic intramedullary nail is a good treatment for supracondylar femoral fractures. Further improvement in results should be obtained with increased use of the less traumatic percutaneous insertion technique and smaller locking holes (5 mm) to strengthen the implant.

▶ Two of the inventors of the GSH supracondylar nail report on 34 fractures treated with this device. They demonstrate good results with reasonable range of knee motion and a limited degree of shortening of the limb. The perceived advantages of this technique include less surgical exposure, less operative time, and less blood loss. Of course, these will be patient- and surgeon-dependent, but the technique seems to offer an advantage, particularly in elderly, debilitated patients with osteoporosis. Further improvements in the design of the implant have been carried out.—M.F. Swiontkowski, M.D.

The Role of Arthroscopy in the Assessment and Treatment of Tibial Plateau Fractures
Fowble CD, Zimmer JW, Schepsis AA (Boston City Hosp)
Arthroscopy 9:584–590, 1993   129-94-8-12

Background.—Tibial plateau fractures are relatively common injuries, but deciding on a specific plan of treatment is difficult. The results of arthroscopic treatment of tibial plateau fractures were compared with those of traditional open methods.

Methods.—Forty patients with tibial plateau fractures were seen from January 1989 to August 1992 at 1 center. Twenty-three patients with certain fracture patterns—local compression or split compression fractures—were included. A group of 12 patients were treated with arthroscopic reduction and percutaneous fixation (ARPF) (Fig 8–10), and a group of 11 had open reduction and internal fixation (ORIF).

Outcomes.—All reductions in the ARPF group were anatomical and remained fixed for at least 3 months after surgery. Only 55% of the ORIF group initially had anatomical reductions. In 1 patient in the ORIF group further loss of reduction was evident on follow-up radiography. Iliac crest bone graft was used in 2 patients in the ARPF group and in 10

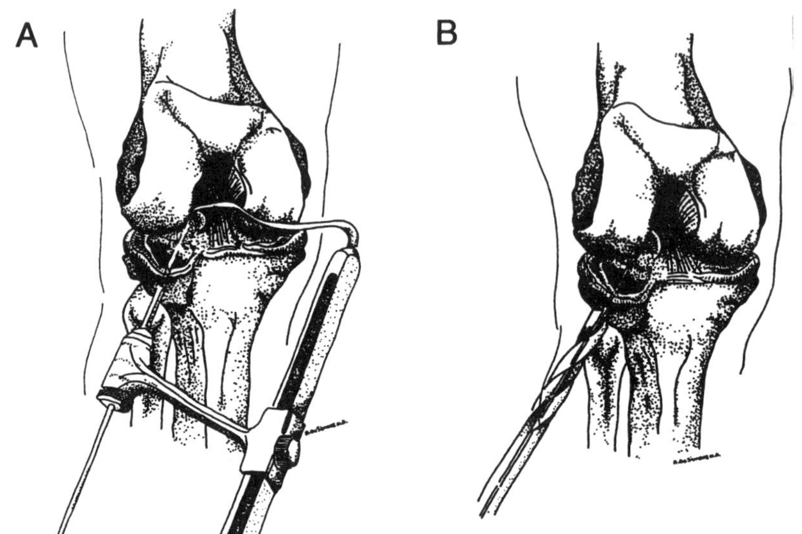

Fig 8–10.—A, an intra-articular guide placed into the fracture allows accurate placement of the anterior tibial tunnel; **B,** a cannulated drill bit is used to create the cortical window just beneath the level of the fracture. (Courtesy of Fowble CD, Zimmer JW, Schepsis AA: *Arthroscopy* 9:584–590, 1993.)

in the ORIF group. In the former group, the use of bone graft did not affect final outcome. Mean length of hospitalization after surgery was 5.4 days for patients with isolated tibial plateau fractures treated with ARPF and 10.3 days for those treated with ORIF. Mean time to full weight-bearing in the ARPF and ORIF groups was 9 and 12.3 weeks, respectively. None of the patients had medial collateral ligament repairs. None of those in the ARPF group had valgus laxity after surgery. One patient in the ORIF group had residual instability, and 1 needed a cane to walk. All concomitant knee abnormalities were addressed and treated arthroscopically in patients in the ARPF group. Open reduction and internal fixation was associated with more frequent and more severe complications.

Conclusion.—The outcomes of ARPF were superior to ORIF in this series. Length of hospitalization and time to full weight-bearing were shorter with ARPF. The ARPF procedure was more effective in achieving the goals of joint congruity, stability, and angular alignment. The rates of anatomical reductions in the ARPF and ORIF groups were 100% and 55%, respectively. Thus, in selected tibial plateau fractures, ARPF should be the treatment of choice.

Clinical Evaluation of Trans-Tibial Prosthesis Sockets: A Comparison Between CAD CAM and Conventionally Produced Sockets

Öberg T, Lilja M, Johansson T, Karsznia A (Univ College of Health Sciences,

Jönköping, Sweden)
Prosthet Orthot Int 17:164–171, 1993   129-94-8-13

Introduction.—The CAD CAM technique was introduced in the field of orthopedic technology in the mid-1980s. In prosthetic and orthotic applications, the form of the amputation stump is fed into a computer and the prosthetic form required is transferred to a computer-controlled carving machine. In contrast, traditional techniques depend on hand casting, which carries a risk for the uncontrolled deformation of the soft tissues. Patients' views of transtibial prostheses made with a CAD CAM technique (the CAPOD system) and those made by conventional methods were compared.

Patients and Methods.—The patients were 17 men (mean age, 61.5 years) and 5 women (mean age, 70.2 years). All had undergone unilateral transtibial amputation; none had experienced prolonged healing or ulcerations. Each patient tried 2 prosthetic sockets: 1 made by the CAD CAM and 1 by conventional techniques. Both sockets were used for 1 month in a single-blind study design. The patients were interviewed at the end of each 1-month period and examined by an independent prosthetist and physiotherapist.

Results.—A total of 175 variables were examined. Subjective evaluations of the patients did not favor 1 socket type over the other. The only difference noted was a smaller number of terry cloth stockings used in the CAPOD socket. Objective evaluation of gait parameters showed no significant difference between conventional and CAPOD sockets (Table 1). The 2 types of sockets fared equally when prosthetists and physiotherapists evaluated the patients' functional abilities (Table 2).

TABLE 1.—Gait Parameters Analyzed for Differences Between Conventional Socket and CAPOD Socket

Variable	Examiner: Prosthetist
Walking distance, metres	N.S.
Gait speed	N.S.
Gait frequency	N.S.
Step length	N.S.
Step length/leg length	N.S.
Duration of gait cycle	N.S.
Duration of stance phase	N.S.

Abbreviation: N.S., no significant difference found. Analysis by Student's *t*-test.

(Courtesy of Öberg T, Lilja M, Johansson T, et al: *Prosthet Orthot Int* 17:164-171, 1993.)

TABLE 2.—Activities of Daily Living and Social
Functions Analyzed for Differences Between
Conventional Socket and CAPOD Socket

Variable	Examiner	
	Prosthetist	Physiotherapist
Need of help from other person	N.S.	N.S.
Ability to take on/off the prosthesis	N.S.	N.S.
Ability to walk indoors with the prosthesis	N.S.	N.S.
Ability to rise from a chair with the prosthesis	N.S.	N.S.
Ability to sit down on a chair with the prosthesis	N.S.	N.S.
Ability of stair climbing with the prosthesis	N.S.	N.S.
Ability to walk outdoors with the prosthesis	N.S.	N.S.
Ability to enter a car with the prosthesis	N.S.	N.S.
Ability to enter a bus with the prosthesis	N.S.	N.S.
Ability to enter a train with the prosthesis	N.S.	N.S.
Degree of usage (Couch *et al.*, 1977)	N.S.	N.S.

Abbreviation: N.S., no significant difference found. Analysis
with χ^2 test.
(Courtesy of Öberg T, Lilja M, Johansson T, et al: *Prosthet
Orthot Int* 17:164–171, 1993.)

Conclusion.—The goal of prosthesis fitting is the rehabilitation of the
patient to an active life. Except for the number of terry cloth stockings,
none of the 175 subjective variables, objective measurements, or social
variables differed for conventionally produced and CAD CAM sockets.
Sweden has a high standard of conventional prosthetics, and the goal of
this study—to achieve the same quality using CAD CAM sockets—was
attained. With use of CAD CAM techniques, it may be possible to perform simulations before the final socket is made for the patient.

Tibial Fractures, Open and Closed

**Treatment of Complex Tibial Shaft Fractures: Arguments for Early
Secondary Intramedullary Nailing**
Siebenrock KA, Schillig B, Jakob RP (Univ of Bern, Switzerland)
Clin Orthop 290:269–274, 1993   129-94-8–14

Background.—There is no consensus regarding the optimal management of complex open tibial shaft fractures. The results of 3 different approaches to the management of these fractures were reviewed.

Patients.—The 3 approaches involved 135 patients, primarily with open tibial shaft fractures, who were initially treated with débridement, fasciotomy as needed, and external fixation. Fifty-four percent continued with external fixation until union; 28% underwent secondary plate fixation at an average of 13.1 weeks after injury; and 18% underwent delayed intramedullary nail fixation at an average of 6.4 weeks after injury. Reasons for secondary fixation included instability, displacement, and delayed union.

Results.—Primary external fixation and delayed intramedullary nailing resulted in the lowest rates of malunion and nonunion, the shortest healing time, and the lowest bone infection rates. The results in patients who underwent secondary plate fixation were similar to those in patients treated with external fixation alone.

Conclusion.—Sequential treatment of severe, open tibial shaft fractures using external fixation and then intramedullary nailing as soon as the soft tissues are healed is effective and has the least complications.

Comparison of Reamed and Nonreamed Solid Core Nailing of the Tibial Diaphysis After External Fixation: A Preliminary Report

Riemer BL, Butterfield SL (Allegheny Gen Hosp, Pittsburgh, Pa)
J Orthop Trauma 7:279–285, 1993   129-94-8–15

Objective.—Open tibial fractures are initially treated with external fixation. Intramedullary nailing is used as a secondary treatment when the fracture fails to unite. High infection rates have been reported when reamed solid core nails were used. The results and complications with secondary intramedullary nailing using either reamed or nonreamed solid core nails were compared.

Patients.—Thirty-two patients with open tibial diaphyseal fractures that had not united with external fixation alone were included. After removal of the external fixator, the nonunited tibia of 16 patients was reconstructed with a reamed solid core nail. The other 16 patients had a nonreamed nail inserted. Indications for secondary intramedullary nailing included atrophic nonunion, planned conversion, and inadequate external fixation caused by head injury. All patients but 1 had at least 1 year of follow-up.

Results.—In 7 patients whose tibia was reconstructed with reamed nails, postoperative infections developed. These required a total of 12 débridements and 2 operations to achieve union. None of the patients had clinical evidence of active pin infection or wound sepsis at the time of nail insertion. Postoperative infections developed in 2 patients with pin tract infections that had healed before intramedullary nailing. The mean interval between removal of the external fixator and intramedullary nailing was 18 weeks, and the average time from intramedullary nailing to union was 26 weeks. In contrast, postnail infection developed in only 1 of the 16 patients treated with nonreamed nails; 2 débridement procedures were required. The mean interval between removal of the fixator and intramedullary nailing was also 18 weeks, but the average time from intramedullary nail insertion to union was only 14 weeks. Three patients had prenail pin tract infections that resolved before intramedullary nailing, but postnail infections did not develop in any.

Conclusion.—The use of nonreamed solid core nails for intramedullary nailing after external fixation provides faster bone union with a lower infection rate and requires fewer débridement operations in comparison to reamed core nails.

▶ With a mean time to union of seven months or more after severe open tibial fractures, the clinical dilemma of what to do with an unhealed tibial fracture after an external fixator has been in place frequently rears its ugly head. Previously, this has been brought to our attention through deep infection rates of up to 44% when reamed nailing was used subsequent to external fixation, especially when a clinical pin tract infection was seen (1). Clearly, it is safest to convert early from external fixation to intramedullary nailing. Infection rates have been as low as 5% when the conversion occurred within the first month after injury (2). Abstracts 129-94-8–14 and 129-94-8–15 grapple with the dilemma of how to manage unhealed tibial shaft fractures after external fixation. In a retrospective review (Abstract 129-94-8–14), Siebenrock et al. identify lower deep infection rates with secondary intramedullary nailing (4.1%) as compared with secondary plate fixation (10.2%) and external fixation used as a definitive treatment (8.2%). The authors do not clearly stipulate whether their nails were inserted reamed or unreamed, or whether they were locked or unlocked. Their nonrandomized protocol introduces a significant bias and weakens their conclusion, and small numbers make the statistics less than robust. The reader should note the short time between injury and conversion to intramedullary nailing of approximately 6 weeks. Abstract 129-94-8–15, which contrasts reamed nailing with unreamed nailing as secondary treatment after external fixation of open tibial fractures, is also retrospective. The reamed group came from an earlier time in the evolution of their treatment protocols. The reader should note that in no patient was a locked nail used. They demonstrated a significant difference in deep infection rate; 7 of 16 treated with reamed nails and 1 of 14 treated with unreamed nails. Because of the historical progression of this treatment, the reader is wise to question whether superior débridement techniques before external fixation were used in the patients treated later in the study. However, this paper indicates that by avoiding reaming the surgeon can create fracture stability without providing the excess culture material for latent bacteria that may be present. The overwhelming themes of this growing body of literature would seem to favor early conversion to a secondary method of treatment and consideration for the concept of avoidance of reaming.—M.F. Swiontkowski, M.D.

References

1. McGraw JM, Lim EVA: *J Bone Joint Surg (Am)* 70-A:900, 1988.
2. Blachut A, et al: *J Bone Joint Surg (Am)* 72-A:729, 1990.

Nonunion of Tibial Shaft Fractures Treated With Locked Intramedullary Nailing Without Bone Grafting

Alho A, Ekeland A, Strømsøe K, Benterud JG (Univ of Oslo, Norway)
J Trauma 34:62–67, 1993   129-94-8–16

Background.—Intramedullary unlocked nailing is commonly used to treat nonunion of tibial fractures initially treated with external fixation. The outcome and advantages of locked intramedullary nailing for tibial nonunion were assessed.

Patients.—During a 7-year period, 25 patients with tibial nonunion 6–54 months after the fracture had occurred underwent intramedullary nailing. Grosse-Kempf slotted locked intramedullary nails were used. Eight patients had infected nonunions. Follow-up ranged from 12–99 months from the time of intramedullary nailing.

Results.—All nonunions healed. One patient required secondary nailing with cancellous bone grafting after the first nail fractured. Three patients (12%) had a recurrence of their infections, and in 1 patient deep venous thrombosis developed. All patients except 1 were able to return to their previous jobs. The overall results were rated excellent in 5 patients, good in 10, fair in 9, and poor in 1.

Conclusion.—Locked intramedullary nailing of tibial nonunion gives favorable results and appears almost to eliminate the need for cancellous bone grafting.

▶ This retrospective review of the use of reamed interlocked nailing without bone grafting for the treatment of established tibial nonunions suggests that even in the face of infection (8 of the 25 nonunions), union can be achieved predictably. Deep infection occurred in 3 patients. When established tibial nonunions are managed with reamed nailing, especially in the face of previous pin tract infection, patients should always be informed that deep infection may result. It is the editor's experience that once union is achieved (as it was in all but one patient in the index operation in this series), infection can be treated readily by removal of the implant and overreaming the canal with a brief period of parenteral antibiotics. Although this is a less than rigidly controlled scientific study, the authors' experience would seem to suggest that intramedullary locked nailing with reaming and without bone grafting will result in union in the vast majority of patients.—M.F. Swiontkowski, M.D.

Late Functional Outcome in Patients With Tibia Fractures Covered With Free Muscle Flaps

Laughlin RT, Smith KL, Russell RC, Hayes JM (Southern Illinois Univ, Springfield)

J Orthop Trauma 7:123–129, 1993

129-94-8–17

Objective.—Long-term functional outcome was examined in patients with grade III tibial fractures who were treated with free muscle flaps. Although such procedures are often used, limb salvage does not assure return to normal function.

Patients and Methods.—From July 1980 to September 1986, 70 patients received 78 microvascular flaps at one center. Fourteen patients had grade III tibial fractures covered with a free muscle flap within 3 months of the original injury. The group included 13 men and 1 woman; the average patient age was 32 years. Twelve patients were available for review, with follow-up averaging 7 years.

Results.—Eight of the fractures were classified as grade IIIB and 6 as grade IIIC. Amputation was subsequently performed in 4 patients, 2 who had microvascular free flaps performed within 14 days of the injury and 2 who had flaps performed 15–42 days after injury. There were no late amputations in the group of 5 patients who had flaps done 42–90 days after injury. In only 1 case was flap failure the reason for amputation. Flap survival was 86%. The 9 surviving patients with salvaged limbs had healed fractures in an average of 15 months. Infection was common, but all tibias that were initially infected were drainage-free for an average of 78 months. Eight of 9 patients whose limbs were salvaged and 3 of 4 who underwent amputation returned to work. One patient whose limb was salvaged was permanently disabled.

Conclusion.—Patients with severe tibial fractures should be made aware of the potential for long-term problems, the time required for reconstruction, and the expense of limb-salvage procedures. The cost of reconstruction and subsequent hospitalization is higher than that of late amputation, and late amputation has a higher cost than early amputation. However, long-term problems also exist for the amputee, with the added inconvenience of prosthesis maintenance.

▶ Bondurant et al. (1) did the orthopedic community a great service by alerting them to the medical and economic impact of attempted limb salvage in the face of futility. This paper, describing a series of 70 patients who received attempts at limb salvage, confirms the Houston group's warning. Although the flap survival rate was 86%, 6 of the limbs had established deep infection. With a total hospital cost of approximately $50,000 for patients with successful limb salvage and functional outcomes of the simplest type (return to work) showing equivalent results, we all must be alert to the fact that patients may benefit from wide consultation and early amputation with grade IIIC tibial injuries. The MESS score of Johansen et al. (2) is an attempt to guide clinicians. However, even this score contains a subjective assessment of the degree of soft tissue injury. We need much more scientific work in this area. Perhaps the multicenter, broad-based outcomes study on this topic recently commissioned by the National Institutes of Health will provide more definitive data.—M.F. Swiontkowski, M.D.

References

1. Bondurant R, et al: *J Trauma* 28:1270, 1988.
2. Johansen K, et al: *J Trauma* 30:568, 1990.

Treating Tibial Fractures With a Modified Sarmiento Method
Fritschy D, Peter R, Brigger A, Bonvin J-C, Rufenacht M (Univ Cantonal Hosp, Geneva)
Orthop Rev 22:217–222, 1993   129-94-8-18

Introduction.—Between 1976 and 1988, a modified version of the method developed by Augusto Sarmiento has been used for the closed treatment of tibial shaft fractures in 317 patients. The majority of injuries were caused by low-energy trauma. There were 230 spiroid comminuted fractures, 69 transverse fractures, and 18 oblique fractures. The average follow-up was 9 months.

Technique.—Traction is applied through a 3-kg transcalcaneal Steinmann pin and is maintained for 10–12 days. The fracture is then immobilized in a long leg cast, and the patient begins ambulating with crutches without weight-bearing for 3–4 weeks. The Sarmiento brace is applied with an additional piece of Orthoplast snugly fitting around the injured leg. Weight-bearing is allowed progressively and the Orthoplast brace is removed with complete roentgenographic healing.

Outcome.—The union rate was 98.7%. The average healing time was 12 weeks. The 4 failures had transverse or oblique comminuted fractures that required plate fixation or nailing. A total of 269 patients had no rotation abnormalities, 218 recovered complete range of motion in the knee, ankle, and foot, 222 had no muscle atrophy, and all but 2 had normal muscle strength. Average shortening was only 3 mm. Complications included fat embolism, external malrotation, fibular nonunion, and painful patellofemoral syndrome in 1 patient each.

Conclusion.—The modified Sarmiento method is ideal for the treatment of closed, spiroid, comminuted tibial fractures caused by low-energy trauma.

▶ Although there is increasing interest in operative management of closed tibial shaft fractures, no clear benefit to patient function has been demonstrated. The literature is lacking in this field, with very few comparative studies. In this retrospective review, the authors demonstrate the general effectiveness of the Sarmiento method of early weight-bearing in fracture braces. With an average shortening of 3 mm and a union rate of almost 99%, these results are hard to improve on. What we desperately need is a randomized trial comparing this method with closed interlocking nailing with patient-oriented functional assessment at 1 and 5 years. It is hoped that this information will be forthcoming.—M.F. Swiontkowski, M.D.

Tibial External Fixation, Weight Bearing, and Fracture Movement

Kershaw CJ, Cunningham JL, Kenwright J (Leicester Royal Infirmary, England; Nuffield Orthopaedic Centre, Oxford, England)
Clin Orthop 293:28–36, 1993   129-94-8–19

Objective.—Axial loading influences both the rate and pattern of fracture healing. Tibial fractures treated in plaster casts are subject to considerable movement during daily activities. The extent of movement at various sites with different external skeletal fixation systems is unknown. Axial fracture movement and loading during weight-bearing was examined in 45 patients treated with unilateral external skeletal fixation for tibial diaphyseal fractures.

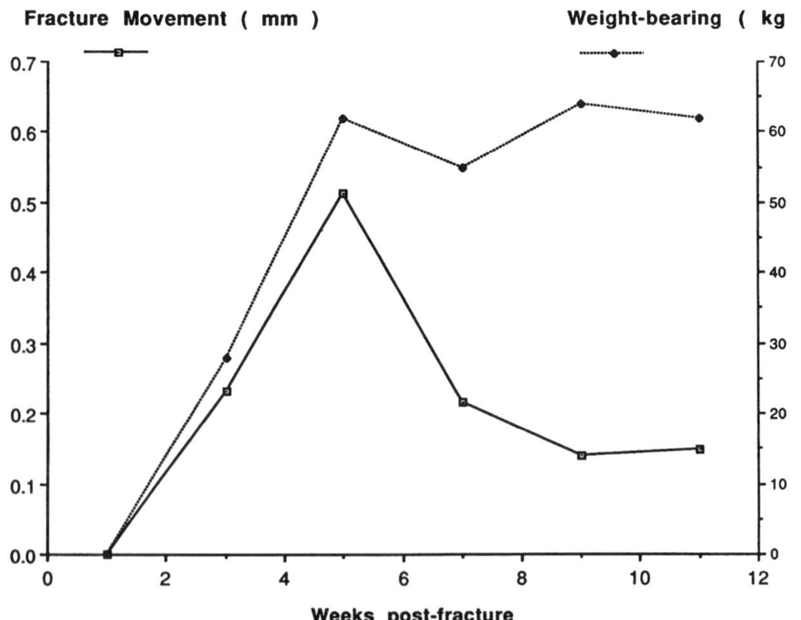

Fig 8–11.—Typical reading of an individual patient's fracture movement and weight-bearing ability recorded from the time of injury to fracture union and fixator removal. (Courtesy of Kershaw CJ, Cunningham JL, Kenwright J: *Clin Orthop* 293:28–36, 1993.)

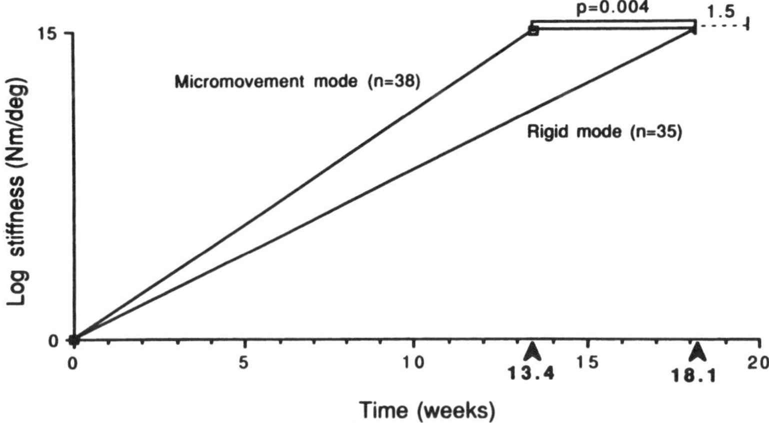

Fig 8–12.—The gradient of increase in bending stiffness for the 2 treatment groups is shown with the time in weeks taken to reach a bending stiffness of 15 N·m/degree. (Courtesy of Kershaw CJ, Cunningham JL, Kenwright J: *Clin Orthop* 293:28–36, 1993.)

Methods.—The patients all had serious tibial diaphyseal fractures treated with primary fracture stabilization by unilateral external fixation with the Dynabrace fixator. Weight-bearing was encouraged as soon as possible. Twenty-three patients had all clamps firmly attached to the fixator column, whereas 22 had a micromovement module attached to the fixator to enhance longitudinal axial fracture site motion. Fracture movement and loading were measured by a strain-gauged cantilever attached to the fixator column that allowed recording of screw displacement during weight-bearing. In addition, fracture movement was imposed in 22 patients in the first 2 weeks after frame application by a pneumatic activator attached to the micromovement module. This allowed measurement of the amount of force needed to produce movement.

Results.—From 7 to 12 weeks after the fracture, maximum axial fracture displacement was .6 mm; however, there was very little fracture movement in the first 5 weeks (Fig 8–11). Patients were bearing 75% of body weight by 10 weeks after the injury, and no mechanism of biofeedback was able to decrease weight-bearing. Activation of the micromovement module showed increased axial movement at the fracture site during weight-bearing by as much as 50%. Patients with imposed micromovement showed much greater displacement than patients with the frame in either fixed or micromovement mode. When 80 patients were randomized to receive external skeletal fixation of diaphyseal tibial fracture with or without micromovement, time to healing was significantly decreased in the micromovement group (Fig 8–12).

Conclusions.—Patients with tibial fractures may benefit from external fixation with micromovement. The difference in movement that occurs during weight-bearing is small, raising the possibility that the earlier healing observed in this study resulted from imposed micromovement in the early days after the fracture, when active loading by the patient is lowest.

Analysis of the External Fixator Pin-Bone Interface
Pettine K, Chao EYS, Kelly PJ (Mayo Clinic and Found, Rochester, Minn)
Clin Orthop 293:18–27, 1993   129-94-8-20

Background.—For patients with fractures treated by external fixation, pin loosening and infection represent serious complications. The stresses resulting in pin loosening probably have their effect at the interface between the pin and bone. However, there has been little research into the relationship between bone stress at the pin tract and the histologic response of bone.

Methods.—The mechanism of pin loosening was studied in dogs under 4 different in vivo loading conditions: no stress, constant static loading, constant static and dynamic loading, and repetitive dynamic loading. Tight and grossly loose pins were compared for their histologic, radiographic, and pin torque findings.

Findings.—There were more signs of gross loosening, including radiographic lucency of 1 mm or more in the cortical bone around the pin, in pins holding unstable fractures. Tight pins were associated with no histologic signs of bone remodeling in the pin tract, whereas loose pins were associated with extensive bone resorption and inflammatory infiltrates (Fig 8–13). When initial torque resistance was less than 68 newtons per cm, 69% of pins developed gross loosening, compared with only 9% of pins with a higher initial torque resistance. This was true regardless of

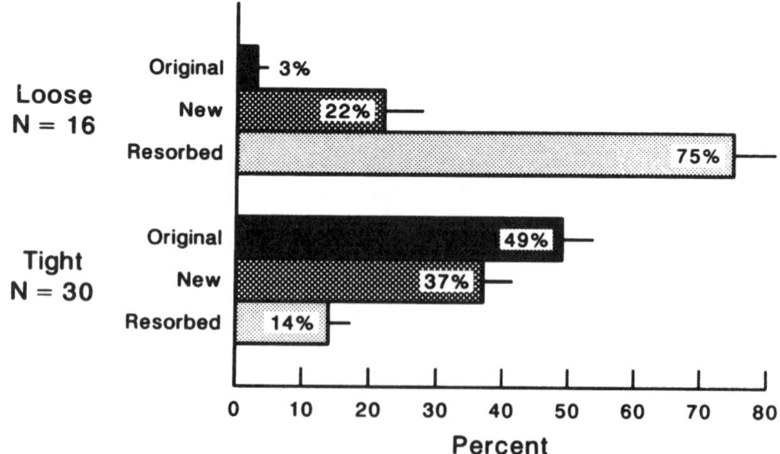

Fig 8–13.—Comparison of histologic results between tight pins (no. = 30) and loose pins (no. = 16), regardless of the experimental group or tibial side. (Courtesy of Pettine K, Chao EYS, Kelly PJ: *Clin Orthop* 293:18–27, 1993.)

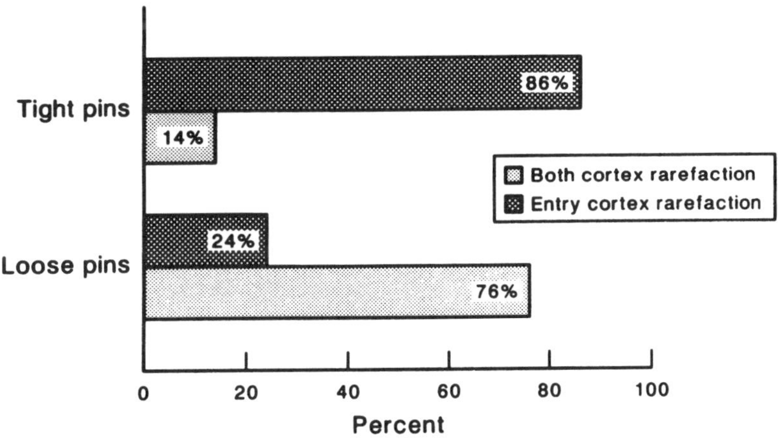

Fig 8–14.—Comparison of radiographic rarefaction results between the entry and exit cortices among the tight pins (no. = 40) and loose pins (no. = 24), regardless of the experimental group or tibial side. (Courtesy of Pettine K, Chao EYS, Kelly PJ: *Clin Orthop* 293:18–27, 1993.)

group assignment. Gross loosening was most likely in pins loaded under unstable fracture fixation conditions.

Conclusion.—In the external fixation of fractures, the 2 most important factors in preventing pin loosening may be final fixation rigidity and pin insertion technique. Static loading may result in pin loosening, which may be detected radiographically (Fig 8–14). The application of external fixation should include an assessment of fracture rigidity, with initial protected weight-bearing imposed if necessary. The minimal torque resistance value required to reduce pin loosening in human beings is being evaluated.

▶ Abstracts 129-94-8–19 and 129-94-8–20 significantly advance our knowledge of what goes right and what goes wrong with external fixation. Kenwright and Goodship long ago demonstrated the salutary effects of early imposed micromovement on the healing of experimental tibial fractures in a sheep model (1). They extended that work into the clinical situation and demonstrated a similar effect in patients with tibial fractures, even given the limitations of the difficulty of measuring fracture stiffness and healing in the clinical setting (2). Here they have further extended the work in a nonrandomized study comparing early weight-bearing with early weight-bearing plus imposed micromovement. The micromovement group showed significant reduction in time to healing, perhaps as a result of the fact that patients do not bear much weight early on (as is demonstrated by their data). Some weaknesses of this study are that it is not randomized and there is no information on the fracture patterns to which these frames were applied. Certainly, the advantage of micromovement deserves further investigation to determine how it can be applied to other clinical situations.

In assessing the clinical problem of pin loosening, the Mayo group (Abstract 129-94-8-20) has clearly spelled out the influence of the initial pin bone stability as reflected by high torque resistance. In essence, the more dense the bone, the less chance there is of the pin loosening. Initial fracture stability played a critical role in the rate of pin loosening; therefore, it would have been advantageous to have some information on fracture pattern in the first study. In the clinical setting it seems prudent to consider protective weight-bearing early on when the bone quality is poor or when the fracture pattern does not allow load bearing to occur through the tibia.—M.F. Swiontkowski, M.D.

References

1. Goodship AE, Kenwright J: *J Bone Joint Surg (Br)* 67-B:650, 1985.
2. Kenwright J, Goodship AE: *Clin Orthop* 241:36, 1989.

The Incidence of Osteitis in Open Fractures: An Analysis of 948 Open Fractures (A Review of the Hannover Experience)
Suedkamp NP, Barbey N, Veuskens A, Tempka A, Haas NP, Hoffmann R, Tscherne H (Freie Universität Berlin; Univ of Hannover, Germany)
J Orthop Trauma 7:473–482, 1993   129-94-8-21

Objective.—Because osteitis remains a major complication of open fracture, the factors responsible for post-traumatic osteitis were examined both retrospectively and prospectively in 948 patients having open fractures treated in 1981–1989. All the injuries resulted from high-energy blunt trauma incurred in a road traffic or industrial accident. Bone infection developed in 28 patients (3%).

Methods.—Injuries were classified using the Hannover Fracture Scale (table). Sterile dressings were applied at the scene of injury, and fractures were grossly reduced and splinted in the field. The wound was aggressively cleansed mechanically in the operating room and then disinfected with alcohol. All contaminated and nonviable soft tissue was débrided, and jet lavage irrigation was routinely carried out. Immediate bony stabilization is preferred. All primary open wounds were left open and covered with artificial skin. Once soft tissue control was achieved, either primary closure or split-thickness skin grafting was carried out.

Results.—Nineteen of 297 patients in a retrospective series who were treated in 1981–1983 had osteitis. Bone loss of more than 2 cm predisposed to infection, as did deep soft tissue injury involving more than half the circumference of the extremity. Osteitis was more frequent when more than 1 aerobic organism or both aerobic and anaerobic organisms were cultured. Vascular injury and compartment syndrome also increased the risk of osteitis developing. Of 651 patients monitored pro-

Hannover Fracture Scale	
Fracture type	
Type A	1
Type B	2
Type C	4
Bone loss	
<2 cm	1
>2 cm	2
Soft tissues	
Skin (wound, contusion)	
No	0
<¼ circumference	1
¼–½	2
½–¾	3
>¾	4
Skin defect	
No	0
<¼ circumference	1
¼–½	2
½–¾	3
>¾	4
Deep soft tissues (muscle, tendon, ligaments, joint capsule)	
No	0
<¼ circumference	1
¼–½	2
½–¾	3
>¾	6
Amputation	
No	0
Subtotal guillotine	20
Subtotal crush	30
Ischemia/compartment	
No	0
Incomplete	10
Complete	
<4 h	15
4–8 h	20
>8 h	25
Nerves	
Palmar–plantar sensations	
Yes	0
No	8
Finger–toe motion	
Yes	0
No	8
Contamination	
Foreign bodies	
None	0
Single	1
Multiple	2
Massive	10
Bacteriologic smear	
Aerobe, 1 germ	2
Aerobe, >1 germ	3

(continued)

Table *(continued)*

Anaerobe	2
Aerobe–anaerobe	4
Onset of treatment (only if soft tissue score >2)	
6–12 h	1
>12 h	3

Note: Fracture 0 I, 2-3 points; fracture 0 II, 4-19 points; fracture 0 III, 20-69 points; fracture 0 IV, >70 points.

(Courtesy of Suedkamp NP, Barbey N, Veuskens A, et al: *J Orthop Trauma* 7:473-482, 1993.)

spectively in 1984–1989, 9 contracted osteitis. Again, soft tissue damage was a significant factor (Fig 8–15). Annual rates of osteitis declined during the years of investigation (Fig 8–16).

Implications.—Antibiotic prophylaxis should be continued in patients with open fracture until definitive wound closure is possible. Antibiotics themselves will not reliably prevent bone infection if soft tissue coverage is difficult or if vascularity is impaired.

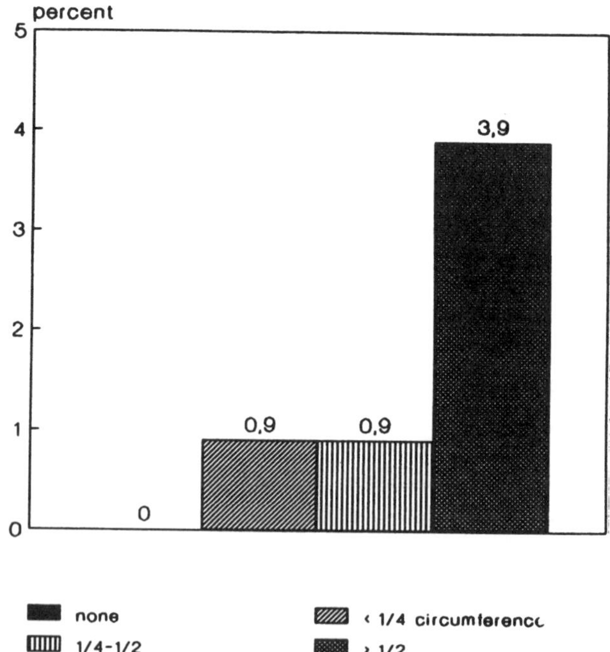

Fig 8–15.—Osteitis rates depending on deep soft tissue damage (P <.003) in open fractures, 1984–1989. (Courtesy of Suedkamp NP, Barbey N, Veuskens A, et al: *J Orthop Trauma* 7:473-482, 1993.)

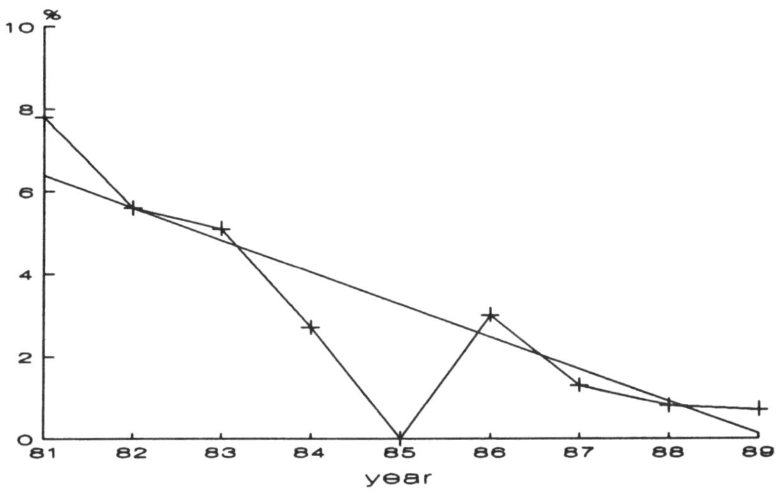

Fig 8–16.—Development of average osteitis rates, 1981–1989. (Courtesy of Suedkamp NP, Barbey N, Veuskens A, et al: *J Orthop Trauma* 7:473–482, 1993.)

▶ This most impressive series of almost 1,000 open fractures from the Hannover group provides a benchmark with which all centers can compare their experience. The authors demonstrate a declining rate of osteomyelitis during the years of investigation reflecting their experience with earlier soft tissue coverage for these open fractures. The most critical predictors of chronic osteitis included: bone loss, highly comminuted fracture types, type of bacteriologic contamination, soft tissue defects, compartmental syndromes, vascular injuries, and associative soft tissue infections. These are all related to the energy imparted to the limb at the time of injury. However, it seems from this retrospective experience that we can limit the rate of deep bone infection by aggressive débridement and early soft tissue coverage with muscle flaps.—M.F. Swiontkowski, M.D.

Fracture Classification System

Poor Reproducibility of Evans' Classification of the Trochanteric Fracture: Assessment of 4 Observers in 52 Cases

Gehrchen PM, Nielsen JØ, Olesen B (Aalborg Hosp, Denmark)
Acta Orthop Scand 64:71–72, 1993 129-94-8-22

Background.—The Evans' classification of trochanteric fractures is widely used for predicting the possibility of obtaining anatomical reduction and estimating the risk of secondary fracture dislocation. The system's reproducibility was evaluated through measurements of intraobserver and interobserver agreement.

Methods.—Preoperative radiographs obtained in 52 patients with trochanteric fractures were interpreted by 4 orthopedic observers familiar with the Evans' classification. The same observers were administered the same group of radiographs in a different order for interpretation 6 weeks later.

Results.—Interobserver agreement was poor; only 23 of the 52 radiographs were classified identically by all 4 observers. There was less intraobserver variation: the first and second classifications were identical for 35–44 of the 52 fractures.

Conclusion.—The reproducibility of the Evans' system for classifying trochanteric femoral fractures is poor. Review of the preoperative radiograph with an intensifier may be more helpful in selection of a course of treatment.

▶ Classification systems are under attack in the orthopedic literature today! Recent articles have shown the poor reproducibility of the Neer system for proximal humerus fractures. This article points out the same findings for Evans' classification for intertrochanteric fractures. Although one can simply conclude that these classification systems are poor, the editor believes that this is illustrative of the problem of beauty being "in the eye of the beholder."

Simply stated, the take-home message is that, when reporting clinical research using fracture classifications as an indicator of severity, one must use a consensus methodology to establish the classification or take mean values with three to four blinded observers. This will add some scientific rigor and increase the confidence in the classifications of fractures reported. For the time being, orthopedic surgeons need to continue to classify fractures for the published literature. The evolution may be toward even simpler classifications. This editor does not believe the systems are at fault but rather that authors must understand this phenomenon and avoid bias by increasing the number of observers used to determine classification.—M.F. Swiontkowski, M.D.

Interobserver Variation Using the AO/ASIF Classification of Long Bone Fractures
Johnstone DJ, Radford WJP, Parnell EJ (Charing Cross Hosp, London; Univ College Hosp, London)
Injury 24:163–165, 1993   129-94-8–23

Introduction.—A system for classifying long bone fractures was developed by the Swiss Association for the Study of the Problems of Internal Fixation (AO), refined with the cooperation of the International Society of Orthopedic Surgery, and published in 1990. A series of fractures was reviewed to evaluate the variability of the classification between observers.

Methods.—In the AO system, each long bone is coded with a number and subdivided into segments, usually 3, numbered accordingly. Fractures are classified according to severity as A, B, or C. Each fracture type

---

TABLE 1.—Description of Each Fracture With Commonly
Agreed AO Code and the Number of Correct Codings
in Parentheses

1. Comminuted intra-articular fracture distal radius (23–C1.2; 3 correct).
2. Simple transverse fracture through distal third radius and ulna at same level (22–A3.3; 17 correct).
3. Impacted four-part fracture through anatomical neck of humerus (11–C2.3; 6 correct).
4. Oblique juxta-articular fracture distal humerus (13–A3.1; 1 correct).
5. Displaced subcapital fracture hip – Garden grade III (31–B3.3; 7 correct).
6. Pertrochanteric fracture femur with avulsion of the lesser trochanter and spiral extension into subtrochanteric region (31–A2.3; 3 correct).
7. Simple spiral fracture middle diaphysis femur (32–A1.2; 10 correct).
8. Transverse fracture diaphysis femur with small butterfly fragment at junction of middle and distal thirds (32–B2.3; 3 correct).
9. Comminuted supracondylar femoral fracture with simple undisplaced intercondylar extension (33–C2.3; 4 correct).
10. Depressed medial tibial plateau fracture with vertical split (41–B3.2; 3 correct).

(Courtesy of Johnstone DJ, Radford WJP, Parnell EJ: *Injury* 24:163–165, 1993.)

---

is divided into 3 groups and further subdivided into subgroups based on severity, resulting in a 5-digit code. Eighteen orthopedic surgeons were invited to apply the system to 10 long bone fractures (Table 1), using an explanatory pamphlet provided by the AO Foundation. Only 3 of the surgeons had previous experience with the system. A consensus classification was derived from results of the individual classifications.

Results.—Only 57 of the 180 results obtained agreed with the final consensus. Surgeons with previous knowledge of the system had as many inaccurate codes (66%) as novice coders (69%) when compared with consensus codes. The highest correct score was for the second fracture presented, a simple transverse fracture of the radius and ulna. The greatest number of incorrect codes was for the oblique juxta-articular humeral fracture (Table 2).

Conclusion.—Coding of fractures by the AO system resulted in considerable interobserver variation. Most bone segment errors occurred when classifying the pertrochanteric fracture with the subtrochanteric extension. Miscoding of the fracture group was most common in the supracondylar elbow fracture and the medial tibial plateau fracture. Because of the large number of errors, a consensus of opinion should be sought if the AO system is used for research purposes or surgical audit.

TABLE 2.—List of Results for Each Fracture

Fracture	Correct	Incorrect	Segment	Type	Group	Subgroup
1.	3	15	0	7	5	3
2.	17	1	0	0	0	1
3.	6	12	0	3	4	5
4.	1	17	0	4	13	0
5.	7	11	0	1	4	6
6.	3	15	9	0	4	2
7.	10	8	1	0	2	5
8.	3	15	1	11	1	2
9.	4	14	1	4	5	4
10.	3	15	0	1	12	2
Total	57	123	12	31	50	30

Note: The number of correct results is shown in column 1 and incorrect results in column 2. The remaining columns show the number of incorrect codes and level of coding at which the initial error occurred.

(Courtesy of Johnstone DJ, Radford WJP, Parnell EJ: *Injury* 24:163–165, 1993.)

Clinical Dilemmas

Removal of Metal Implants After Fracture Surgery: Indications and Complications

Brown RM, Wheelwright EF, Chalmers J (Royal Infirmary, Edinburgh, Scotland; Princess Margaret Rose Orthopaedic Hosp, Edinburgh, Scotland)
J R Coll Surg Edinb 38:96–100, 1993   129-94-8-24

Objective.—There are concerns about the safety of the retention and of the removal of metallic implants after fracture surgery. A retrospective review was conducted of 297 internal fixation operations for fractures or joint injuries in 1982.

Findings.—Implants that were retained did not give rise to appreciable problems. A second operation for implant removal was undertaken in 42%, of which 19% had significant complications. When clear indications for implant removal existed, the results were usually favorable (table). Symptomatic relief was achieved in all but 1 patient who had implant removal for unexplained pain; pain was probably related to undiagnosed nonunion in the other patient. For the 29% of olecranon fractures with local complications, removal of the implant for clinical symptoms was not associated with any postoperative complications. Likewise, there were no significant complications among the 7 fractures of the radius or ulna, or both, with plates that were removed. For ankle injuries with diastasis screws removed after weight-bearing commenced, all 13 had full function and 2 had persistent wound infections. However, when implants were removed as a matter of routine, the infection rate

Indications for Removal of Implants and Resulting Complications

Reason for removal	No.	Complications	Type of injury
Routine	52	Implant not located	A/C dislocation
		Redislocation	A/C dislocation
		Redislocation	A/C dislocation
		Wound infection	Femur (K nail)
		Wound infection	Tibia (plate)
		Wound infection	Tibia (plate)
		Wound infection	Tibia (plate)
		Wound infection	Med. mall. (screw)
Patient's request	2	None	
Pain	9	Recurrent fracture	Patella
Neuritis	2	Continuing symptoms	M. epicondyle screw
Non-union (simple)	5	None	
Non-union (infected)	2	Pseudarthrosis	Humeral condyle
		Persistent infection	Humeral condyle
Skin reaction	1	None	
Wound infection (early)	6	Persistent infection	Bimalleolar + diastasis
Wound infection (late)	2	Persistent infection	Bimalleolar + diastasis
Skin necrosis	6	Refracture	Olecranon (TBW)
Prominence of implant	10	Delayed healing	Trimalleolar (screws)
Fixation failure	13	Continuing pain	Ulna Rush pin
		Continuing pain	Femur (K nail)
		Fascial hernia	Femur (K nail)
		Wound infection	Femur (K nail)
Fracture adjacent to fixation	1	None	

(Courtesy of Brown RM, Wheelwright EF, Chalmers J: *J R Coll Surg Edinb* 38:96–100, 1993.)

was 11%, and the overall complication rate was 15%. The incidence of complications related to fixation failures was 22%.

Conclusion.—Implants should be removed only when clear clinical indications exist. Routine implant removal after internal fixation of fractures is associated with an unacceptably high postoperative complication rate.

▶ All participants in trauma courses await with great anticipation the lecture on implant removal. However, nowhere in the body of musculoskeletal trauma literature does less information exist. These authors have done a real service to the orthopedic community by pointing out that in patients who are symptomatic (who have unexplained pain with an implant in place), one can achieve symptomatic relief with removal of the hardware. Routine implant removal was associated with a high rate of infection and a smaller risk of refracture. Because this review is retrospective and much of this surgery was no doubt carried out by junior registrars, the reader should consider with great caution recommending routine hardware removal in asymptomatic patients. Clearly, we need prospective studies using pain scales and general health status instruments to shed more light on this important clinical dilemma.—M.F. Swiontkowski, M.D.

The Use of One Compared With Two Distal Screws in the Treatment of Femoral Shaft Fractures With Interlocking Intramedullary Nailing: A Clinical and Biomechanical Analysis

Hajek PD, Bicknell HR Jr, Bronson WE, Albright JA, Saha S (Orthopaedic Associates, Albany, Ga; Louisiana State Univ, Shreveport; Specialty Orthopaedics, Spokane, Wash; et al)

J Bone Joint Surg (Am) 75-A:519–524, 1993   129-94-8-25

Background.—Most of the available nailing systems for interlocking intramedullary fixation of fractures of the femoral shaft involve the use of 2 transverse screws for distal fixation. It was hypothesized that 2 distal screws provide fixation that is more than adequate and that the elimination of 1 screw does not adversely affect the torsional rigidity, axial strength, or clinical results of interlocking nailing.

Study Design.—Sixteen femora obtained from 8 cadavers were examined to evaluate the torsional and compressive biomechanical characteristics of a system for intramedullary fixation with a slotted locking nail and either 1 or 2 distal locking screws. In addition, the use of 1 screw for distal interlocking fixation was evaluated in 27 patients with fractures of the femoral shaft. A Grosse-Kempf nail was inserted with a standard technique in all patients. Average duration of follow-up was 9 months.

Results.—In the cadaveric studies, there were no significant differences in the torsional rigidity and axial load to failure between specimens with 1 or 2 distal screws used for fixation. However, within the implant failure group, the mode of failure was uniformly different, with the screw failing in specimens with 1 screw and the nail failing in specimens with 2 screws, suggesting that 2 screws distally provide fixation that is more than adequate and that exceeds the strength of the nail, whereas 1 screw provides fixation similar in strength to that of the nail.

In the clinical study, all 27 fractures united. Average time to radiographic healing was 3 months. There were no nonunions or failures of the implant. Five patients had clinically unimportant migration of the distal screw.

Conclusion.—One distal screw provides adequate distal fixation in the treatment of fractures of the femoral shaft treated with interlocking intramedullary nailing.

▶ We have learned from excellent retrospective clinical work (1, 2) that static interlocking nailing is advisable for all femoral shaft fractures. Taking the easy way out and failing to interlock nails will lead to shortening of femoral shaft fractures of greater than 1 cm in 11% of patients. These authors address the remaining question of 1 vs. 2 screws, asking whether 1 screw is enough. In their biomechanical study, they demonstrated no difference in torsional rigidity or actual load to failure, and in a follow-up series of 27 patients there were no implant failures. The conclusion of only 1 screw being necessary seems appropriate. However, when the fracture is distal to the narrow part of the femoral shaft medullary cavity, 2 screws should be used to minimize the risk of nonunion.—M.F. Swiontkowski, M.D.

References

1. Brumback RJ, et al: *J Bone Joint Surg (Am)* 70-A:1441, 1988.
2. Brumback RJ, et al: *J Bone Joint Surg (Am)* 70-A:1453, 1988.

Preoperative Skin Traction for Fractures of the Proximal Femur: A Randomised Prospective Trial
Anderson GH, Harper WM, Connolly CD, Badham J, Goodrich N, Gregg PJ
(Leicester Royal Infirmary, England)
J Bone Joint Surg (Br) 75-B:794–796, 1993   129-94-8–26

Pros and Cons.—To control pain, many patients who are admitted with a proximal femoral fracture are managed by skin traction while awaiting surgery. In addition, some surgeons believe that traction helps maintain or improve the position of the fracture. However, there are risks, including skin damage, interference with lifting and turning the patient, and compromise of the vascular supply when circular bandages are applied.

Objective.—The effects of skin traction were examined in 252 patients awaiting surgery for a proximal femoral fracture. Patients were randomized to be nursed free in bed or to receive Hamilton-Russell skin traction with a 5-lb weight. Women outnumbered men by more than 3 to 1. The mean patient age was 81 years. Fractures were extracapsular in 137 patients and intracapsular in 115.

Findings.—Preoperative wait times were comparable in the 2 groups, as were daily pain scores (Fig 8-17) and analgesic requirements. Signifi-

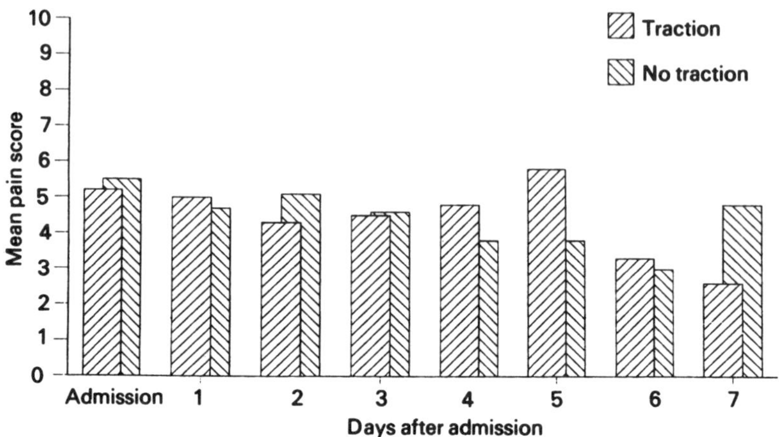

Fig 8–17.—Mean pain score at each day after admission. (Courtesy of Anderson GH, Harper WM, Connolly CD, et al: *J Bone Joint Surg (Br)* 75-B:794–796, 1993.)

cant pressure scores developed independently of whether skin traction was used. No patient had direct skin damage as a result of traction. Difficult reductions were no less frequent in patients having skin traction. The mean hospital stay was almost the same for the 2 groups.

Conclusion.—Skin traction is a time-consuming measure in patients with upper femoral fractures and does not confer significant benefit. Its routine use is not recommended.

▶ Many of us were trained to use preoperative skin traction for elderly patients with proximal femoral fractures. Traditional teaching tells us that this decreases muscle spasm and pain by immobilizing the limb. In this well-done, randomized, prospective trial the effect of skin traction on pain control was studied in 252 patients with proximal femoral fractures. Pressure sores developed in both groups and the mean hospital stay was almost identical in the two groups. Perhaps to some individuals' surprise, preoperative traction did not have any salutary effect on daily pain scores or analgesic requirements. When used with intracapsular fractures, this may be related to limiting hip capsular volume when the hip is in extension. The recommendation should be to have the patient supine with a pillow behind the knee, with frequent changes in position of the pelvis to avoid pressure sores while waiting for operative intervention.—M.F. Swiontkowski, M.D.

Fracture Blisters: Clinical and Pathological Aspects

Varela CD, Vaughan TK, Carr JB, Slemmons BK (United States Army Medial Activity, Wuerzburg, Germany; Med College of Virginia, Richmond; Univ of

Missouri, Kansas City)
J Orthop Trauma 7:417–427, 1993   129-94-8–27

Introduction.—Fracture blisters are tense vesicles or bullae arising on markedly swollen skin directly overlying a fracture. The frequency, histology, microbiology, treatment, and complications of fracture blisters in a trauma population were determined in a retrospective study.

Patients.—Fifty-one patients with 53 blisters were treated during a 3½-year period at 4 hospitals. The average follow-up was 9 months.

Location and Incidence.—All but 1 of the blister sites occurred at the skin overlying the tibia, ankle, and elbow, usually within 24–48 hours of acute injury. Of the 1,468 acute fractures that required hospitalization, 43 fracture blisters developed, for an incidence of 2.9%. The incidence of fracture blisters was significantly lower among patients with acute fractures who underwent open reduction internal fixation within 24 hours of injury (2%) compared with those in whom fixation was delayed for more than 24 hours (8%). The only open fractures that developed fracture blisters were open diaphyseal fractures of the tibia. Interstitial compartment pressures were markedly elevated in 2 patients studied.

Histology.—Histologic examination of 15 blisters showed subepidermal vesicles. All fluid cultures were sterile, whereas ruptured fracture blisters were colonized primarily with skin pathogens soon after blister rupture and continuing until reepithelialization. Blister fluid from a patient with AIDS was positive for the HIV antibody.

Treatment.—The treatment for fracture blisters consisted of application of dry dressing and casting, silver sulfadiazine dressing, or whirlpool débridement and silver sulfadiazine dressings. Blister healing was similar in these regimens. Patient management was affected in 13 (25%) of the 53 fracture blisters. Of these, patient care was affected in 10 patients (71%) with fracture blisters at the time of surgery. Two of these patients had postoperative wound infections; in these patients surgical incision was made through an intact blister or through the healing base of a ruptured blister. Other management problems included delayed surgery and changes in surgical plan. Fracture blisters that developed postoperatively did not affect patient care. The complication rate was significantly lower in fractures treated by closed means, although fracture blisters and swelling caused a delay in closed reduction and casting in 2 patients.

Conclusion.—Fracture blisters are relatively common and occur most frequently around areas of the musculoskeletal system with little soft tissue between bone and skin. Blisters are often sterile but become rapidly colonized when débrided. Nonsurgical treatment options have fewer risks attributed to fracture blisters. If indicated, surgery should be performed within 24 hours of injury and surgical incision through fracture blisters and the associated underlying damaged soft tissues should be avoided.

▶ We all face the clinical dilemma of what to do with fracture blisters when an open reduction is deemed appropriate. This important study has given us some very helpful information. Fracture blisters are relatively uncommon (2.9%). They occur in skin in which subcutaneous fat directly overlies bone. Blisters rarely occur postoperatively when surgery is done early. They are sterile, however, once a blister is open to the environment, skin pathogens rapidly colonize the epidermal lesion. Therefore, surgery directly through blisters is to be avoided until the blisters are completely healed and reepithelialized. The authors do not offer us detailed information as to how best to manage them after unroofing, and they seem to indicate that dry dressing with casts or splints or silver sulfadiazine dressing changes are equally effective. Conservative care should always be considered as an option when surgical incisions must be placed through blisters before reepithelialization.—M.F. Swiontkowski, M.D.

What to Do About a Dropped Bone Graft

Presnal BP, Kimbrough EE (Univ of South Carolina, Columbia)
Clin Orthop 296:310–311, 1993   129-94-8-28

Introduction.—The loss of harvested autogenous bone grafts to the operating room floor is a problem that is not widely discussed, although it is familiar to most orthopedic surgeons. Sterilization of essential autografts can damage the bone. To determine whether extensive sterilization procedures are required, bone specimens that had been deliberately dropped on the operating room floor were cultured.

Methods.—Bone samples that were to be discarded were collected for a 4-month period from 50 orthopedic and neurosurgical procedures. Two samples were obtained from each procedure. The first was placed on the operating room floor, left there for 1 minute, then placed in a culture tube; the second sample was taken from the operating field and placed into a culture tube under sterile conditions. The tubes were incubated in the microbiology department and monitored for culture growth. After the final cultures from the first half of the specimens were read, a single specimen was deliberately contaminated to test the laboratory's ability to obtain a positive result.

Results.—Most of the specimens were obtained from primary arthroplasties (60%) and lumbar laminectomies and iliac bone grafts (25%). Preoperative antibiotics had been used in the 39 orthopedic patients but not in the 11 neurosurgical patients. The only positive culture found was that of the purposefully contaminated sample.

Conclusion.—Sterilization procedures used for autogeneic bone reduce the desirable qualities of the graft for implantation. These findings indicate that a graft dropped on the operating room floor can be used, if necessary, without extensive and damaging efforts at sterilization.

▶ Everybody who actively practices orthopedic surgery has been present when there has been a bone graft dropped in the operating room. All have anecdotal experience regarding how to resolve this situation. These authors have provided us with some important information. One hundred samples were dropped on operating room floors that were not prepared in a special way. No positive cultures resulted. The limitation of this study is that placing a potentially contaminated bone graft into culture medium is different than placing a potentially contaminated bone graft into a well-vascularized bed with adjacent hematoma. However, it seems prudent not to carry out auto-claving or other damaging modes of sterilization. Perhaps a brief period of soaking in an antibiotic solution is a reasonable compromise, and, perhaps, one that would be more widely acceptable to all operating room personnel.—M.F. Swiontkowski, M.D.

Classification and Treatment of Volar Barton Fractures

Mehara AK, Rastogi S, Bhan S, Dave PK (All India Inst of Med Sciences, New Delhi)

Injury 24:55–59, 1993   129-94-8–29

Background.—Volar Barton's fractures with dislocation of the carpus have usually been treated initially with closed manipulation and immobilization in a plaster cast. Open reduction and internal fixation (ORIF) with miniplates is indicated when the fracture cannot be reduced adequately or in case there is redisplacement after closed reduction.

Patients.—During a 4-year period 82 patients were treated for volar Barton's fractures; follow-up of 78 patients was conducted for 2–3 years. Thirty-nine patients were treated satisfactorily with closed manipulation and immobilization; the other 39 required open reduction because check radiographs revealed inadequate reduction or subsequent displacement occurred.

TABLE 1.—Relation of Fracture Type to Treatment

	No.	Primary ORIF	Secondary ORIF	POP
Type I	48	5	13	30
Type II	24	0	15	9
Type III	6	6	—	—
Total	78	11	28	39

Abbreviation: POP, plaster of paris.
(Courtesy of Mehara AK, Rastogi S, Bhan S, et al: *Injury* 24:55–59, 1993.)

TABLE 2.—Analysis of End Results Related to Articular Step

				End result			
				Satisfactory		Unsatisfactory	
Type of fracture	Treatment modality	Residual articular step	Number of cases	Excellent	Good	Fair	Poor
Type I	CR & POP	<2 mm	18	6	7	3	2
(48 cases)	CR & POP	>2 mm	12	2	2	6	2
	ORIF	<2 mm	7	4	2	1	—
	ORIF	Nil	11	11	—	—	—
Type II	CR & POP	<2 mm	5	1	3	1	—
(24 cases)	CR & POP	>2 mm	4	—	—	3	1
	ORIF	<2 mm	11	6	3	2	—
	ORIF	Nil	4	2	1	1	—
Type III	ORIF	<2 mm	1	—	1	—	—
(16 cases)	ORIF	Nil	5	5	—	—	—

Abbreviation: CR & POP, closed reduction and plaster of paris.
(Courtesy of Mehara AK, Rastogi S, Bhan S, et al: Injury 24:55-59, 1993.)

Results.—Three distinct fracture types that correlated with the ease of reduction and later displacement were identified. Forty-eight patients had type I fractures, characterized by the displacement of a large single fragment. Five patients required primary ORIF, 13 patients underwent secondary ORIF when fragment displacement of more than 2 mm was seen on check radiographs, and 30 patients only had closed reduction and plaster cast immobilization. Twenty-four patients had a type II fracture, defined as a comminuted and displaced fracture with large or small fragments. Although closed reduction was achieved in all patients, 19 of them had redisplacement. Immobilization was continued in 4 patients who had just more than 2 mm of fragment displacement; the other 15 patients underwent secondary ORIF. Six patients had a type III fracture, defined as a large displaced fragment with an additional small cortical fragment lying beneath it. All 6 required primary ORIF. The relation of fracture type to treatment for all patients is shown in Table 1. The final outcome was good or excellent in 56 patients and fair or poor in 22. Among the nonsurgically treated patients, only 25% of those with more than 2 mm of postreduction displacement had a good or excellent outcome, compared with 74% of those in whom the fracture united with less than 2 mm of displacement. Good or excellent results were achieved in 35 surgically treated patients (89%). An analysis of the end results related to articular step is shown in Table 2. Surgically treated patients also had an easier course during rehabilitation. The extent of initial displacement was not related to the final outcome provided the fracture united with less than 2 mm of displacement.

Conclusion.—Open reduction and internal fixation is the optimal treatment for volar Barton's fractures because it produces the best outcome. Postreduction fragment displacement of more than 2 mm on check radiographs is prognostic of a poor outcome.

▶ This large retrospective clinical series documents the poor outcomes with conservative treatment of volar Barton's fracture. With only 25% of patients achieving a good or excellent outcome with conservative care, this option would seem to be eliminated given the availability of a skilled surgeon and an adequate operative facility. Although the study is limited by extreme bias, with no independent assessment of radiographs, measurement of displacement, adequacy of reduction, or nonblinded functional assessment, their conclusions are worthy of our attention. It seems that, whenever possible, these fractures should be treated with a volar approach and buttress plating.—M.F. Swiontkowski, M.D.

Compartmental Syndrome

Histologic Determination of the Ischemic Threshold of Muscle in the Canine Compartment Syndrome Model

Heckman MM, Whitesides TE Jr, Grewe SR, Judd RL, Miller M, Lawrence JH III (Emory Univ, Atlanta, Ga)
J Orthop Trauma 7:199–210, 1993   129-94-8-30

Background.—There are 2 hypotheses regarding the critical tissue pressure for fasciotomy in a compartment syndrome. The absolute pressure theory states that there is an absolute tissue pressure above which irreversible muscle damage occurs. The perfusion gradient theory states that tissue ischemia is a direct result of decreased tissue perfusion. Using a standard plasma infusion compartment syndrome model in a canine model, definition of the critical tissue pressure at which irreversible muscle damage occurs was attempted.

Methods.—The dogs were divided into 4 experimental groups with compartment pressures maintained as follows: at 30 mm Hg with support of the dog's diastolic blood pressures to a level > 50 mm Hg (i.e., > 20 mm Hg difference between diastolic and compartment pressure); at a pressure 20 mm Hg less than diastolic blood pressure; at a pressure 10 mm Hg less than diastolic blood pressure; and at a pressure equal to the diastolic blood pressure. The animals were watched closely for changes in hindlimb function and sacrificed 2 weeks later.

Outcome.—On light microscopy, none of the specimens subjected to 30 mm Hg showed evidence of tissue injury. Tissues subjected to pressures 20 mm Hg less than diastolic blood pressure demonstrated occasional cells undergoing regeneration but none had evidence of infraction or fibrosis. Specimens subjected to tissue pressures of 10 mm Hg less than diastolic showed scattered small areas of infarction and fibrosis with evidence of both regeneration and fibrosis, whereas more widespread infarction and scarring were evident in tissues subjected to 10 mm Hg of diastolic pressure. These findings were confirmed on ultrastructural studies.

Conclusion.—The ischemic threshold of muscle, beyond which irreversible tissue damage occurs, is associated more closely with the difference in compartment and perfusion pressure than with the absolute compartment pressure. This difference appears to be a tissue pressure less than 30 mm Hg of mean arterial pressure or about 10 mm Hg less than diastolic blood pressure. These data imply that fasciotomy should be performed when tissue pressure reaches within 10–20 mm Hg of diastolic blood pressure to abort an impending compartment syndrome and avoid irreversible tissue injury and its consequences.

▶ This well-controlled animal experiment confirmed recent clinical experience demonstrating the critical role of perfusion pressure in the development of compartmental syndrome. The authors identified the critical pressure of 10 mm of mercury less than the diastolic pressure, or within 30 mm of mean arterial pressure, as being productive of tissue necrosis in this compartmental syndrome model. With hypotension resulting from hemorrhage, the risks of compartmental syndrome increase even in limbs with minimal injury. Vigilance is the key, in this clinical setting, to avoid loss of limb function.—M.F. Swiontkowski, M.D.

Catastrophic Complication of Simple Cast Treatment: Case Report

Hawkins BJ, Bays PN (US Naval Hosp, Bremerton, Wash)
J Trauma 34:760–762, 1993   129-94-8-31

Objective.—Simple cast treatment of a relatively minor fracture that resulted in the death of a patient is described. This case illustrates the potential for life- and limb-threatening conditions after trauma and emphasizes the need for vigilance, even in seemingly minor musculoskeletal or vascular injuries.

Case Report.—Man, 36, sustained a closed, minimally displaced fracture of the left medial malleolus after falling 10 feet from a ladder. About 24 hours after treatment with a short leg cast at a provincial hospital in the Philippines, the patient returned to his physician with severe pain under the cast. The cast was extended and the pain continued. About 48 hours after injury the cast was removed, revealing severe blistering extending to the thigh. The patient was transferred to a United States Naval Hospital with a presumptive diagnosis of clostridial myonecrosis. His leg was discolored up to the medial groin and severely blistered below the knee (Fig 8–18). Blood pressure was 60/40 mm Hg, respirations were 28/min, and temperature was 104°F. The patient was anuric and remained so despite vigorous fluid resuscitation after emergency above-knee amputation. He was transferred to a United States Air Force Hospital for renal dialysis but died within 24 hours of cardiorespiratory arrest.

Discussion.—The history of this patient is consistent with acute compartment syndrome. Appropriate management would have been removal of the cast, but instead the rigid dressing was extended, the worst possible treatment. Failure to decompress the involved compartments led to development of crush syndrome after 48 hours. Clinical manifestations of the crush syndrome result from ischemic muscle cell death. Although treatment of renal failure usually prevents a fatal outcome, the morbidity from residual effects of crush syndrome remains very high.

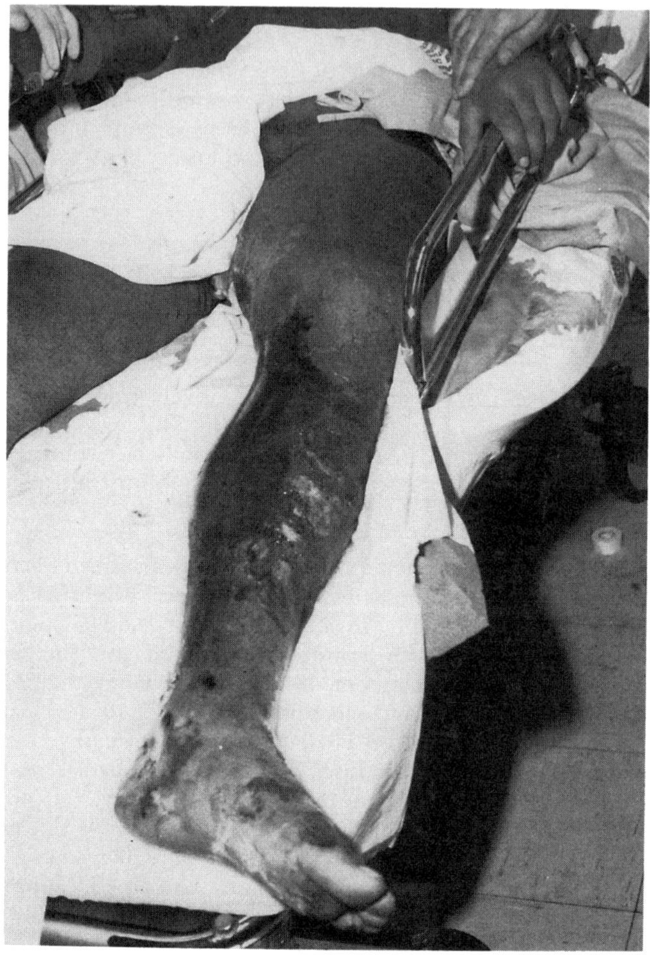

Fig 8–18.—The tensely swollen, blistered lower extremity. (Courtesy of Hawkins BJ, Bays PN: *J Trauma* 34:760–762, 1993.)

Skin Surface Pressures Under Short Leg Casts

Marson BM, Keenan MAE (Albert Einstein Med Ctr, Philadelphia)
J Orthop Trauma 7:275–278, 1993   129-94-8–32

Introduction.—Skin ulceration and compartment syndromes can result from excessive pressure when a cast is incorrectly applied. The surface pressures generated by 2 commonly used circumferential casting materials were compared.

Methods.—In the first part of the study, 15 plaster and 15 fiberglass short leg casts were applied to 17 normal volunteers. Electronic sensors were used to record skin surface pressures after application of the webril padding, application of the short leg cast, after univalving and bivalving, and after spreading of the casts. During the entire procedure the participants' legs were comfortably supported. In the second part of the study, 20 different orthopedic surgeons and technologists applied the same types of casts to a single participant. Sensors recorded pressures after webril application and casting.

Results.—No significant difference in webril pressures for the 2 materials was found in part I of the study. However, initial casting pressure was significantly higher than webril pressure for fiberglass and significantly lower for plaster (Fig 8–19). Bivalve pressures were significantly lower than casting pressures for both materials. In part II of the study, fiberglass pressures were again significantly greater than those caused by plaster. Mean pressures were 30.45 mm Hg for plaster and 61.1 mm Hg for fiberglass. Operator technique also affected pressure.

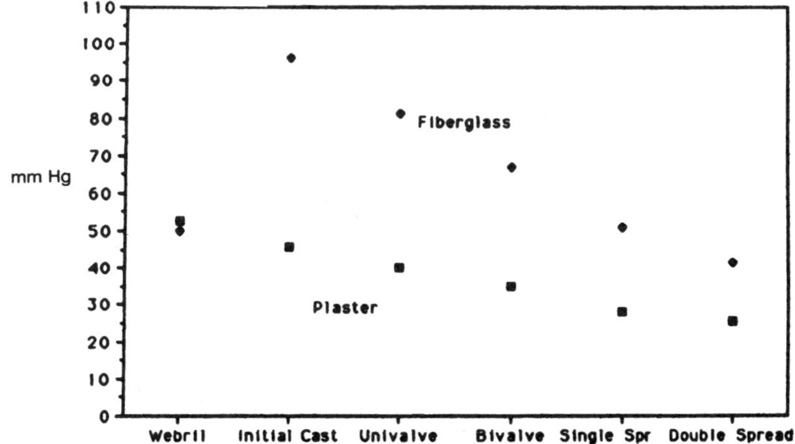

Fig 8–19.—Plot of mean pressures recorded for fiberglass and plaster after all stages of application, cutting, and spreading of casts. (Courtesy of Marson BM, Keenan MAE: *J Orthop Trauma* 7:275–278, 1993.)

Conclusion.—Plaster and fiberglass have different physical properties and are applied in casting with different techniques. The intrinsic recoil of fiberglass results in a greater potential for elevated skin surface pressures. Both bivalving and webril spreading are beneficial in decreasing pressure. Findings suggest that plaster casts are safer than fiberglass, particularly when swelling is likely or the patient's skin is vulnerable to breakdown. However, with any rigid dressing, extreme care must be used to prevent serious complications.

Pelvic Ring Injury

Posterior Pelvic Fixation Using a Transiliac 4.5-mm Reconstruction Plate: A Clinical and Biomechanical Study

Albert MJ, Miller ME, MacNaughton M, Hutton WC (Emory Univ, Atlanta, Ga)
J Orthop Trauma 7:226–232, 1993   129-94-8-33

Objective.—The goal of surgical management of unstable pelvic fractures is stabilization of the posterior sacroiliac ligamentous tension band. A technique of posterior fixation using a 4.5-mm reconstruction plate as a transiliac tension band was described.

Technique.—Three posterior incisions are made: one 6-cm midline incision and 2 lateral 8-cm incisions beginning at the posterior iliac spines and directed obliquely in an inferolateral direction (Fig 8–20). A 4.5-mm reconstruction plate is inserted through the posterior superior iliac spines and fixed to the ilium using cancellous screws.

Results.—Fourteen patients with acute unstable pelvic ring injuries with sacral fractures and 1 patient with a 14-year-old nonunion of the sacrum underwent posterior pelvic fixation using a transiliac 4.5-mm reconstruction plate. During an average follow-up of 15.2 months, all 14 evaluable patients achieved stable fixation with full ambulatory ability without external supports. There were no deep infections, no wound complications, and no failures of fixation. Comparative biomechanical testing using 4 fresh cadaveric and 15 artificial pelvises showed that the strength of the 4.5-mm reconstruction plate was equal to that of other alternatives of posterior pelvic fixation.

Conclusion.—A transiliac pelvic reconstruction plate provides sufficient posterior stability in unstable pelvic fractures and allows early patient mobilization to facilitate an aggressive rehabilitation program. Insertion of this low-profile plate requires only limited tissue dissection, and its length can be varied to fix associated iliac wing fractures. Screw placement for plate application is safely located within the ilium without risk of neurologic or vascular compromise.

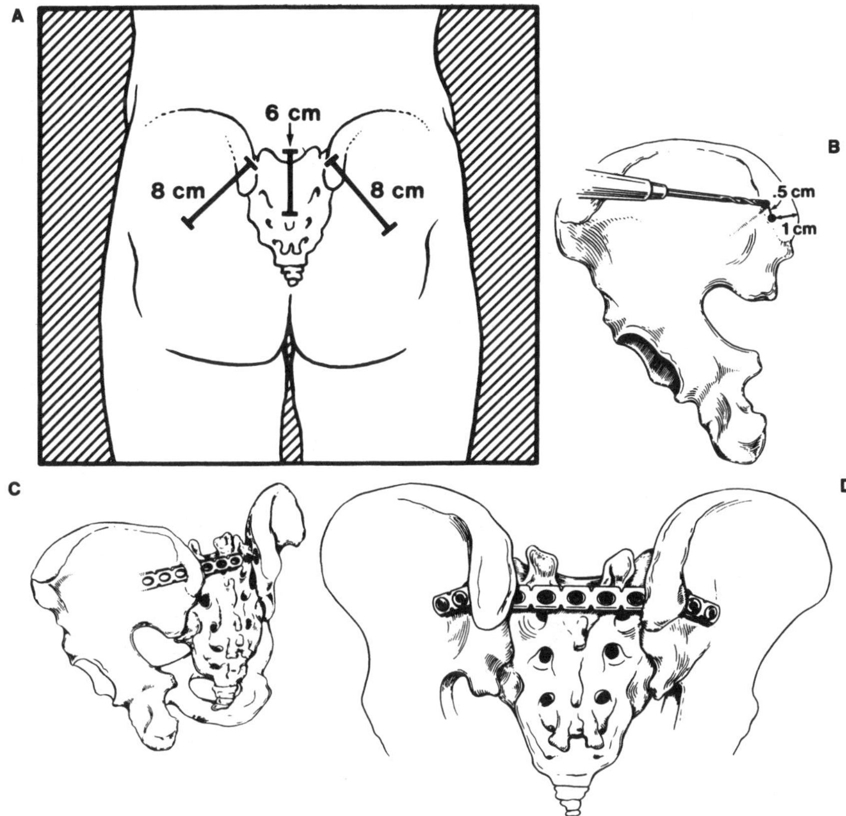

Fig 8–20.—A, incision placement for plate application. **B,** starting points to predrill the posterior superior iliac spine with a 4.5-mm-diameter drill. **C,** the plate is chiseled through the drill holes and directed toward the opposite posterior iliac spine. **D,** the plate is contoured in situ and fixed to the ileum using 6.5-mm cancellous screws. (Courtesy of Albert MJ, Miller ME, MacNaughton M, et al: *J Orthop Trauma* 7:226–232, 1993.)

Anterior Square-Plate Fixation of Sacroiliac Disruption: 2–8 Years Follow-Up of 23 Consecutive Cases

Ragnarsson B, Olerud C, Olerud S (Uppsala Univ, Sweden)
Acta Orthop Scand 64:138–142, 1993   129-94-8–34

Introduction.—Between 1983 and 1988, 21 consecutive patients with 23 sacroiliac (SI) joint disruptions were treated. All patients had rotationally and vertically unstable injuries.

Treatment.—All patients underwent open reduction and internal fixation with a square plate with 2 extended oval compression screw-holes, each allowing for 2 fully threaded, 6.5 mm AO/ASIF cancellous screws. The median follow-up was 5 years (range, 2–8 years).

Outcome.—Using the Harris hip scoring system, 12 patients had excellent and 6 had good results. The 3 patients with poor results had neurologic injury with radiating pain or palsy. Radiographically, the position of the SI joints remained unchanged in all patients.

Discussion.—For SI joint disruptions, the anterior approach to internal fixation provides good access to the anterior aspect of the sacroiliac joint with a small risk of wound complications. The 2-hole square plate offers the possibility for strong compression of the reduced joint to minimize the risk of redislocation.

▶ These two clinical papers attempt to address the problems associated with stabilization of posterior pelvic ring injury. Abstract 129-94-8–33 describes a method of using a 4.5-mm reconstruction plate as a posterior tension band. The authors were able to achieve stable fixation to allow mobilization of the patient and demonstrated in a cadaveric biomechanical model that this method of stabilization offers stability equal to that of sacral bars, single or double. Unfortunately, they do not compare their method with iliosacral screws, which is our current preferred method of stabilizing these injuries because it is minimally invasive and does not carry the risk of wound infection associated with these larger posterior incisions.

In Abstract 129-94-8–34, the anterior approach to sacroiliac disruption with the Olerud plate is evaluated retrospectively. This method is not applicable to sacral fractures as it is not possible to dissect medially enough to obtain fixation on both sides of the fracture without injuring the L5 nerve route. In 4 of 23 patients, residual displacements of 5–10 mm existed. Of critical importance is that the authors investigated the functional outcomes of patients with these injuries at a median follow-up of 5 years. Poor results were attributable to lumbosacral plexis injuries, resulting in radiating pain and weakness. In the future, clinical researchers need to pay more attention to investigating the relationship between the quality of the reduction and functional outcome.—M.F. Swiontkowski, M.D.

Acute Mortality Associated With Injuries to the Pelvic Ring: The Role of Early Patient Mobilization and External Fixation
Riemer BL, Butterfield SL, Diamond DL, Young JC, Raves JJ, Cottington E, Kislan K (Med College of Pennsylvania, Pittsburgh)
J Trauma 35:671–677, 1993   129-94-8–35

Background.—Early fixation for patients with pelvic ring injuries has gradually gained acceptance. Such injuries are frequently accompanied by significant bleeding. External fixation, while relieving pain, also allows for mobilization to an upright chest position, helping to control bleeding. The change in mortality after the introduction of a protocol for immediate mobilization of all patients, with the use of external fixation for control of pelvic bleeding and pain when necessary, was examined.

Statistical Analysis of Mortality Among Patients With Pelvic Ring Injuries and Hypotension

Variable	Year			Significance
	1981	1982	1983–1988	
Number of patients	61	68	476	
Number of patients with hypotension (SBP < 100)	16 (26%)	11 (16%)	83 (17%)	0.22
Number of external fixators for hypotension*	0	1 (9%)	43 (52%)	0.001
Number of deaths in hypotensive patients	7 (44%)	7 (64%)	17 (21%)	0.004

*Two fixators applied at days 2 and 4 as reconstructive procedures.
(Courtesy of Riemer BL, Butterfield SL, Diamond DL, et al: *J Trauma* 35:671–677, 1993.)

Method.—A total of 605 patients with pelvic ring fractures and dislocations were treated from 1981 through 1988. Mortality was retrospectively compared during 3 periods: 1981, preprotocol, when 2 fixators were applied on days 2 and 4 after injury; 1982, the transitional period, at the beginning of the orthopedic trauma service; and 1983 through 1988, when the protocol of early mobilization to an upright chest position with early external fixation, when necessary, for control of significant pelvic bleeding and pain was established.

Results.—During the preprotocol period 26% of patients died. In the transitional period mortality dropped slightly to 22%, and from 1983 through 1988 the number of deaths decreased significantly to 6%. During the study, the mean Injury Severity Score (ISS) of 23 patients did not change. Mortality in a group of consecutive patients with similar ISSs but without pelvic ring injuries did not change. The mortality rate in patients with systolic blood pressure of less than 100 mm Hg at admission decreased from 44% in 1981 to 21% in 1983 through 1988 (table). Deaths in patients with closed head injuries associated with pelvic ring injuries also decreased from 43% in 1981 to 7% in 1983–1988.

Conclusion.—An organized protocol of external fixation and early patient mobilization to upright chest position greatly decreases mortality related to pelvic ring injuries. When early fixation is indicated, particularly in the case of pelvic bleeding, it should be seen as a resuscitative procedure, and even in cases in which pelvic bleeding is suggested but not certain or in which control of pelvic pain is required, external fixation should be used.

▶ This group from Pittsburgh performed a retrospective analysis of the effect of internal fixation on mortality of patients with pelvic ring injury. They demonstrated a decline in mortality rates in patients who were not hypotensive as well as in those who were (from 41% to 21%). Although this retrospective review does not account for the effects of other improvements in treatment such as more aggressive management of an elevated intracranial pressure, the improvement in mortality figures remains impressive. Of note is the fact that the authors could not demonstrate a significant decrease in mortality rates in patients with pelvic ring injury and associated severe pulmonary injury or laparotomy. This type of review is certainly subject to bias and is flawed by the inability to control for the multiple factors that influence mortality. However, the negative aspects of using external fixators in patients with unstable pelvic fractures remain few. Our current restricted use of external fixators in patients with hypotension, in an attempt to avoid contamination of muscle and soft tissue for delayed open reconstruction, may be appropriate.—M.F. Swiontkowski, M.D.

The Computerized Tomography Subchondral Arc: A New Method of Assessing Acetabular Articular Continuity After Fracture (A Prelimi-

nary Report)

Olson SA, Matta JM (Hosp of the Good Samaritan, Los Angeles; Univ of Southern California, Los Angeles)

J Orthop Trauma 7:402–413, 1993   129-94-8-36

Background.—Displaced acetabular fracture is generally treated by open reduction and internal fixation. However, some of these fractures may be treated nonoperatively. Roof arc measurement was developed to diagnose the extent of intact superior acetabulum after a fracture, but the technique provides only an approximation of remaining superior acetabulum. A new method for evaluating superior acetabular involvement using CT has been developed.

Diagnostic Procedure.—Computerized tomography depicts the superior acetabulum as a series of subchondral bony rings or arcs. Scanning 10 mm below the vertex of the acetabulum evaluates an area equivalent to roof arc measurement criteria. If the CT scan does not reveal fracture lines involving the acetabular articular surface in this segment, nonopera-

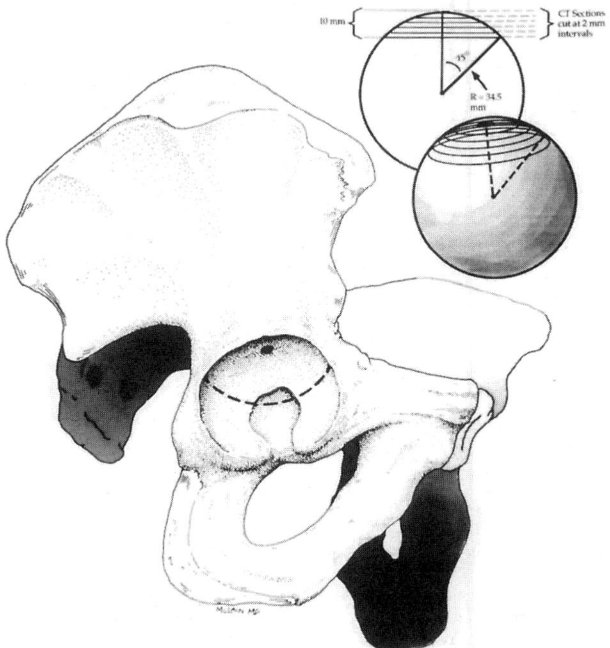

Fig 8–21.—The *line* shown in the acetabulum represents the level of the CT image at 10 mm inferior to the vertex of the acetabulum. The *circle* along the subchondral bone at 10 mm inferior to the vertex is equivalent to a fracture line for which all 3 roof arc measurements are 45 degrees. Evaluation of the superior 10 mm should be the equivalent of roof arc measurements of 45 degrees or more in almost all cases. The *inset* diagram illustrates evaluation of the superior acetabulum by CT to 10 mm inferior to the vertex in 2-mm intervals. (Courtesy of Olson SA, Matta JM: *J Orthop Trauma* 7:402–413, 1993.)

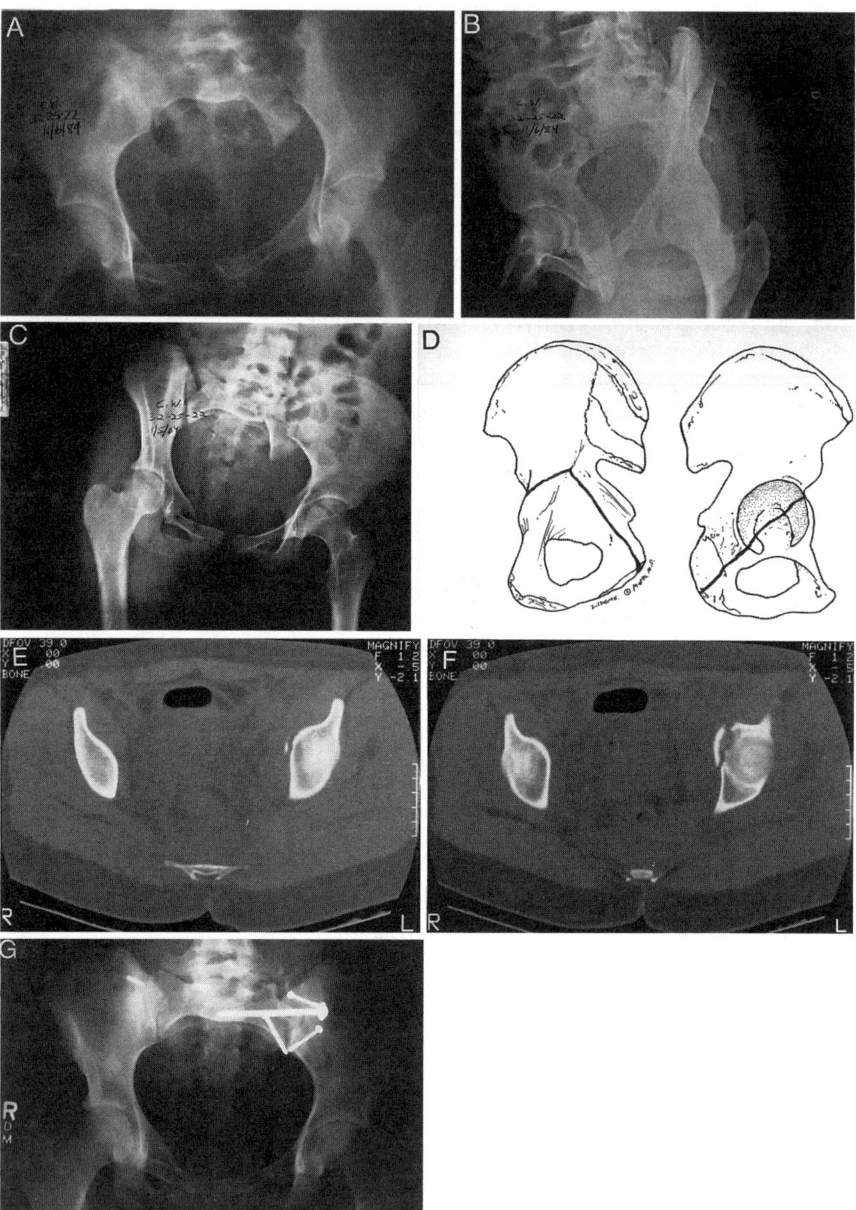

Fig 8–22.—The anteroposterior (**A**), obturator oblique (**B**), and iliac oblique radiographs (**C**) of a patient with a transverse acetabular fracture with an ipsilateral fracture dislocation of the sacroiliac joint as shown. The roof arc measurements for this patient are anterior (obturator oblique) 50 degrees, medial (anteroposterior) 45 degrees, and posterior (iliac oblique) 121 degrees. **D,** transverse fracture pattern. The CT images were taken at the vertex of the acetabulum (**E**) and at 10 mm below the vertex (**F**). The fracture begins at the pelvic brim (**E**) and the subchondral arc is intact. This fracture extends inferiorly to just begin to involve the subchondral arc at 10 mm below the vertex (**F**). This fracture pattern does not violate the articular surface in the superior portion of the acetabulum. A radiograph at 2-year follow-up shows healing of both injuries with nonoperative treatment of the acetabulum (**G**). The acetabulum has only slight narrowing of the articular space. (Courtesy of Olson SA, Matta JM: *J Orthop Trauma* 7:402–413, 1993.)

Patient Data

		Roof arc measurements				
Patient	Fracture type	Medial	Anterior	Posterior	F/U	Result
Patients fulfilling roof arc criteria, treated nonoperatively						
MC	T	65	60	75	2	G
GC	T	85	80	75	1	G
MG	AC	121	70	121	3	G
HH	TR	45	30	60	5	E *
FM	T	60	45	50	6	F
MM	AC	121	60	121	3	E
DR	T	55	85	45	1	G
JS	T	50	60	55	1	P
LS	TR-PW	55	60	80	3	G
TT	TR	65	55	80	2	G
CW	TR	45	50	121	2	E
Patients not fulfilling roof arc criteria, treated nonoperatively						
FB	AC	0	30	30	2	P
LB	TR-PW	121	15	21	3	G
CC	AC	15	50	21	1	F
MD	AC	0	0	0	1	E
WE	T	0	5	0	1	F
RF	AC	45	0	21	6	G
ML	T	0	75	0	3	P
JL	AC	25	20	20	1	P
RM	T	21	21	40	3	G
KP	TR	30	40	35	2	G
DS	T	21			2	P†
JS	AC	30	121	25	1	P

* Patient met roof arc criteria in the original series.
† Obturator oblique and iliac oblique views were not available for measurements.
(Courtesy of Olson SA, Matta JM: *J Orthop Trauma* 7:402–413, 1993.)

tive treatment of the fracture may be considered. The superior 10 mm may be evaluated with 3 images at 5-mm intervals including the vertex. However, CT images taken at 2- to 3-mm intervals (Fig 8–21) allow better evaluation of articular surface continuity in this area. This method requires only slight modification of CT evaluation (Fig 8–22).

Clinical Results.—Computerized tomography was used to evaluate 23 fractures in 22 patients with non–both-column injuries. Eleven fractures met the roof arc measurement criteria for nonoperative treatment; 82% of those fractures had a good or excellent result 1 year after treatment. Among the 12 fractures not satisfying the criteria for nonoperative treatment, 42% had a good or excellent result (table).

Discussion.—Computed tomography enhances the detail of superior acetabulum involvement in dislocated fractures. Criteria for selecting patients for nonoperative treatment include intact acetabular articular surface in the superior 10 mm of the joint on CT; femoral head congruence with out-of-traction superior acetabulum on the anteroposterior and 45-degree oblique radiographic pelvic views; and at least 50% of posterior wall articular surface intact at the most involved level in posterior wall fractures on CT.

▶ Through the seminal work of Letournel (1) and his disciples, it has become clear that surgeons who devote time and energy to developing the skills to fix acetabular fractures can do them safely and effectively. One question that remains: when is it in the patient's best long-term functional interest to fix an acetabular fracture? Dr. Matta has been on the cutting edge of trying to define these indications with his roof arc angles. He advances the concept in this study with CT scans that must be taken at 2- to 3-mm cut intervals. The critical area seems to be 10 mm below the vertex of the acetabulum. He demonstrated in a follow-up clinical series that 82% of patients who met the roof arc CT criteria had a good or excellent result one year after treatment, compared with 42% who did not meet the criteria.

Even with these limited data, there are factors besides fracture anatomy that affect functional outcomes. Much work is needed to clearly spell out the indications for an open reduction to optimize functional improvement. Factors other than the anatomical nature of the injury surely must play a role and are deserving of the same intensity of study.—M.F. Swiontkowski, M.D.

Reference

1. Letournel E, Judet R: *Fractures of the Acetabulum.* Berlin: Springer-Verlag, 1981.

Adult Respiratory Distress Syndrome, Blunt Trauma, and Reaming Effects

Primary Intramedullary Femur Fixation in Multiple Trauma Patients With Associated Lung Contusion: A Cause of Posttraumatic ARDS?
Pape H-C, Auf'm'Kolk M, Paffrath T, Regel G, Sturm JA, Tscherne H (Hannover Med School, Germany)
J Trauma 34:540–548, 1993   129-94-8–37

Background.—Primary stabilization of major fractures in patients with multiple trauma is thought to decrease complications, particularly in cases of pulmonary infection and adult respiratory distress syndrome (ARDS). Intramedullary nailing (IMN) is considered to be especially advantageous. However, a number of severely injured patients have experienced a deterioration in pulmonary function after intramedullary nailing, and ARDS, often with a lethal outcome, has developed. Whether there is an association between the increased incidence of ARDS and primary intramedullary stabilization of femoral shaft fractures in multiple trauma patients was investigated in a retrospective study.

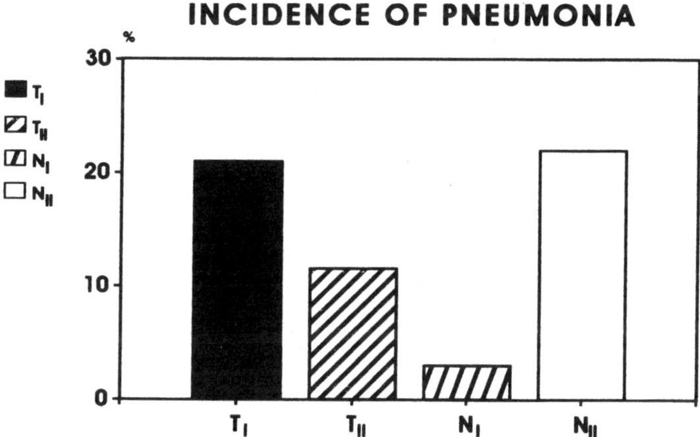

Fig 8–23.—Incidence of pneumonia in all subgroups. *Abbreviations:* T_I, thoracic trauma, primary IMN; T_{II}, thoracic trauma, secondary IMN: N_I, no thoracic trauma, primary IMN; N_{II}, no thoracic trauma, secondary IMN. (Courtesy of Pape H-C, Auf'm'Kolk M, Paffrath T, et al: *J Trauma* 34:540–548, 1993.)

Method.—The 106 patients admitted to the study had Injury Severity Scores of greater than 18, femoral midshaft fractures treated by IMN, and admission within 8 hours of injury. There was no death from head injury or hemorrhagic shock. The group was divided into those with severe chest trauma and those without and was further subdivided according to the time of femur stabilization: less than 24 hours after trauma (primary IMN) or more than 24 hours after trauma.

Results.—Patients without thoracic trauma who received early intramedullary nailing spent less time under intubation and in intensive care than the patients who underwent secondary stabilization. The patients

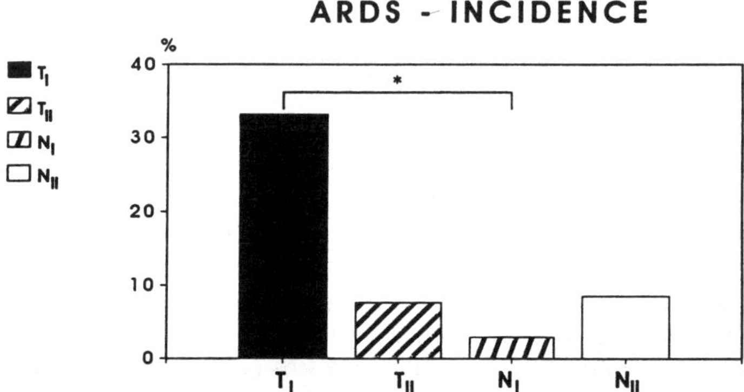

Fig 8–24.—Incidence of post-traumatic ARDS. *Abbreviations:* T_I, thoracic trauma, primary IMN: T_{II}, thoracic trauma, secondary IMN; N_I, no thoracic trauma, primary IMN; N_{II}, no thoracic trauma, secondary IMN. *Indicates significant difference between subgroups. (Courtesy of Pape H-C, Auf'm'Kolk M, Paffrath T, et al: *J Trauma* 34:540–548, 1993.)

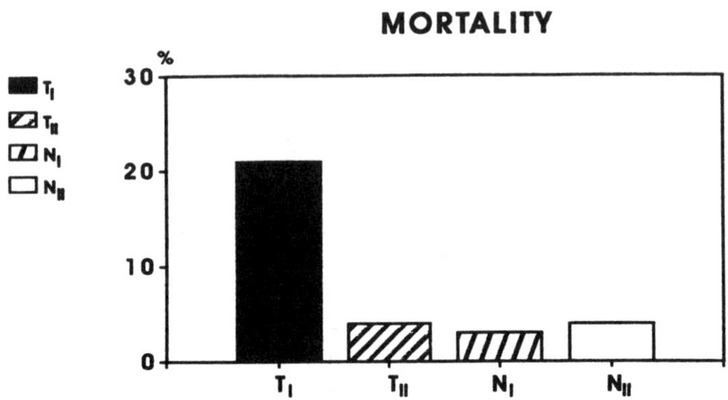

Fig 8–25.—Mortality in 106 multiple trauma patients. *Abbreviations:* T_I, thoracic trauma, primary IMN; T_{II}, thoracic trauma, secondary IMN; N_I, no thoracic trauma, primary IMN: N_{II}, no thoracic trauma, secondary IMN. (Courtesy of Pape H-C, Auf'm'Kolk M, Paffrath T, et al: *J Trauma* 34:540–548, 1993.)

without thoracic injuries who received delayed treatment had a higher incidence of pulmonary infections. The incidence of pneumonia in all subgroups is shown in Figure 8-23. However, when primary intramedullary fracture stabilization was carried out in patients with severe chest injuries, there was a high incidence of post-traumatic ARDS (Fig 8–24) and almost all patients with ARDS died (Fig 8-25).

Conclusion.—In the absence of severe chest trauma primary intramedullary femoral nailing appears to be beneficial. However, when multiple trauma is accompanied by thoracic damage, the early fixation of fractures by IMN carries the increased risk of ARDS. In these patients, definite fracture reduction should be delayed and alternative methods such as external fixation should be used.

Fat Emboli Syndrome in Isolated Fractures of the Tibia and Femur

Ganong RB (Truckee Tahoe Med Group, Olympic Valley, Calif)
Clin Orthop 291:208–214, 1993   129-94-8-38

Objective.—Most research on the fat emboli syndrome (FES) involves patients who have undergone multiple trauma. The incidence, morbidity, mortality rates, and treatment of FES in otherwise healthy young skiers with isolated fractures of the tibia and femur were defined.

Results.—Between November 1980 and May 1981, 56 skiing fractures of the tibia or femur were seen. Of these, 13 (23%) had FES, including 75% of femoral and 19% of tibial fractures and 33% of displaced, transverse tibial fractures. None of the 56 skiers required mechanical ventilation, and all survived with complete recovery from FES. Between 1980 and 1991, FES developed in 44 healthy young skiers with fractures of the tibia or femur and no other injuries. The mean patient age was 26 years.

• Findings in 44 Skiing Fractures of the Tibia and Femur With Resultant FES, 1980–1991

Sign	*Percentage of Cases With Sign*
Hypoxemia	93% mean p_{O_2} 45 mm Hg
Pyrexia	77% mean 38.5
Tachycardia	75%
Tachypnea	45%
Petechiae	41%
Abnormal chest reontgenogram	30%
Altered mental status	10%
Retinal changes	2%
Anemia	0%
Thrombocytopenia	0%
Day of onset of fat emboli syndrome	
Day 1	36%
Day 2	36%
Day 3	27%
> Day 3	0%
Duration of fat emboli syndrome	
One day	41%
Two days	23%
Three days	23%
> Three days	14%
Length of hospital stay	
Usual 19 patients	
> Usual 22 patients	
Number requiring mechanical ventilation	none
Number of deaths	none

(Courtesy of Ganong RB: *Clin Orthop* 291:208–214, 1993.)

Fat emboli syndrome developed by the third day of hospitalization. Most patients had hypoxemia, fever, and tachycardia, but none had thrombocytopenia, inappropriate anemia, or hypocalcemia (table). Most patients received supplemental oxygen, a few received steroids, and none required mechanical ventilation. The duration of FES was less than 4 days in 86% of the patients, and 50% required prolonged hospitalization. There were no complications, and all survived with no sequelae.

Conclusion.—Fat emboli syndrome occurs more frequently than previously recognized in healthy young skiers with isolated fractures of the tibia and femur. In this population, FES is not associated with mortality and causes little morbidity. Treatment consists of general supportive care, with specific care directed toward the underlying injury.

Clinically Inapparent Hypoxemia After Skeletal Injury: The Use of the Pulse Oximeter as a Screening Method

Moed BR, Boyd DW, Andring RE (Henry Ford Hosp, Detroit; Southeastern Orthopaedic Clinic, Wilmington, NC)

Clin Orthop 293:269–273, 1993   129-94-8–39

Background.—Early diagnosis of low arterial oxygenation and timely intervention may prevent progressive pulmonary dysfunction. Serial arterial blood gas (ABG) measurement, the recommended monitoring procedure, is invasive, expensive, and time-consuming. The use of the pulse oximeter in lieu of multiple ABG as a screening method for early diagnosis of clinically inapparent hypoxemia was evaluated.

Methods.—Forty-three patients with isolated fractures of the tibia, femur, pelvis, or acetabulum, or multiple long-bone fractures were hospitalized to undergo orthopedic surgery. With a portable pulse oximeter, standard transdigital pulse oximetry readings were obtained within the first 12 hours of admission and at 3 subsequent 24-hour intervals.

Results.—Fifteen patients had arterial hypoxemia, defined as oxygen-hemoglobin (O_2-Hb) saturation less than or equal to 94%; all were iden-

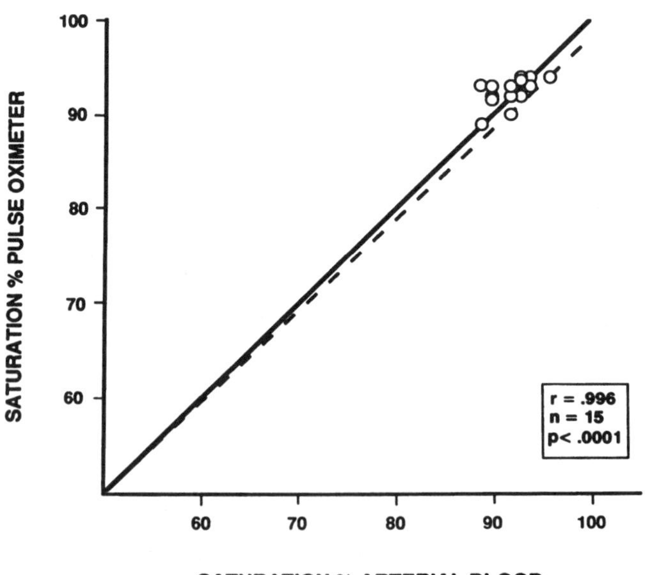

FIg 8–26.—The arterial oxygen-hemoglobin saturation values obtained with pulse oximetry readings as compared with ABG analysis using linear regression statistical analysis. The line of identity and the line of linear regression are solid and dashed, respectively. (Courtesy of Moed BR, Boyd DW, Andring RE: *Clin Orthop* 293:269–273, 1993.)

tified within the first 24 hours of admission. On linear regression analysis, pulse oximeter percent saturation correlated significantly with ABG percent saturation (Fig 8–26). Twelve of the 15 patients with percent saturation less than or equal to 94% on pulse oximetry had corresponding ABG partial pressure of oxygen values less than or equal to 80 mm Hg. In the remaining 3 patients, ABG O_2-Hb saturations were equivalent to pulse oximetry values.

Conclusion.—The pulse oximeter is an efficient, reliable screening device for clinically inapparent hypoxemia.

Influences of Different Methods of Intramedullary Femoral Nailing on Lung Function in Patients With Multiple Trauma

Pape H-C, Regel G, Dwenger A, Krumm K, Schweitzer G, Krettek C, Sturm JA, Tscherne H (Hannover Med School, Germany)
J Trauma 35:709–716, 1993   129-94-8-40

Introduction.—Early (within 24 hours) reamed intramedullary femoral nailing appears to be associated with the development of pulmonary complications and subsequent adult respiratory distress syndrome (ARDS) in patients with multiple trauma. An animal model showed that pulmonary dysfunction could be avoided if fracture fixation by a small-diameter nail was performed without previous reaming. Lung function in 2 groups of patients, one with primary femoral nailing with reaming

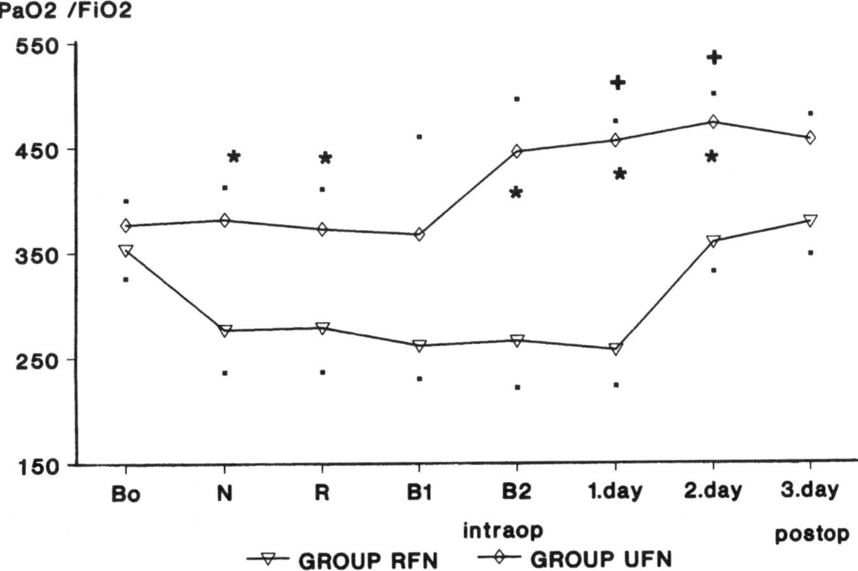

Fig 8–27.—Oxygenation ratio during and after surgery in both groups of patients. (Courtesy of Pape H-C, Regel G, Dwenger A, et al: *J Trauma* 35:709–716, 1993.)

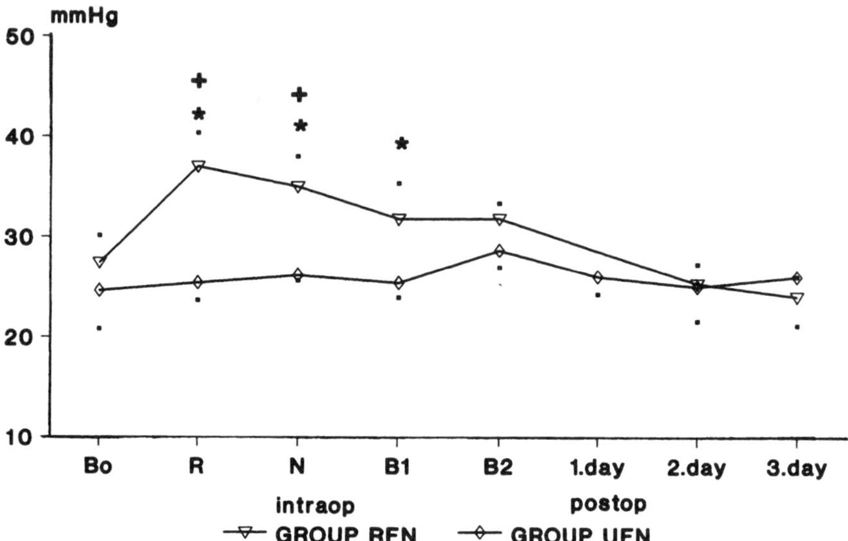

Fig 8–28.—Mean pulmonary artery pressure during and after intramedullary femoral nailing. Adjustment of correct position of the pulmonary artery catheter was determined before each measurement. (Courtesy of Pape H-C, Regel G, Dwenger A, et al: *J Trauma* 35:709–716, 1993.)

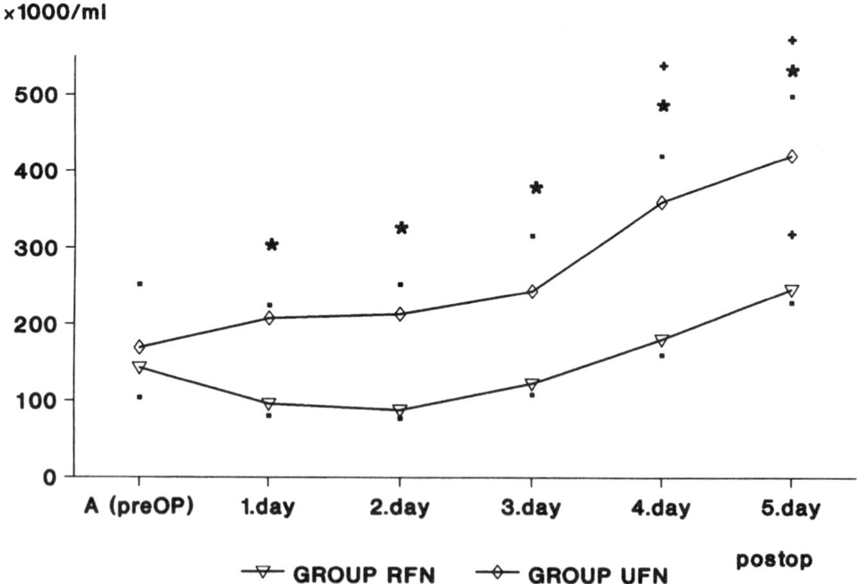

Fig 8–29.—Platelet count in the central venous blood. (Courtesy of Pape H-C, Regel G, Dwenger A, et al: *J Trauma* 35:709–716, 1993.)

(group RFN) and the other with unreamed femoral nailing (group UFN), was compared.

Patients and Methods.—Thirty-one patients were included, 17 in the RFN group and 14 in the UFN group. The groups were similar in demographic data and had comparable lung function at baseline. All had an Injury Severity Score > 20 but were without severe head or chest trauma. Lung function was assessed by oxygenation ratio and pulmonary hemodynamics by intraoperative pulmonary catheter measurements.

Results.—Lung function remained unchanged intraoperatively in patients undergoing UFN; a significant increase in oxygenation ratio was observed postoperatively. A decrease in the oxygenation ratio occurred in the RFN group on reaming of the medullary canal; the oxygenation ratio remained worse than that of the UFN group until day 2 after trauma (Fig 8-27). One patient in the RFN group had ARDS after day 4 and died. Neither group showed changes during or after nailing in positive end-expiratory pressure, respiratory minute volume, maximal inspiratory airway pressure, static compliance, or the ratio of inspiration to expiration. Although pulmonary artery pressure did not change during surgery in UFN patients, it increased significantly (from a mean of 27.2 mm Hg to 36.3 mm Hg) on reaming in RFN patients (Fig 8-28). Pulmonary artery pressure normalized in RFN patients 1 hour after nail insertion. In RFN patients, the platelet count decreased from a mean of 123 × 1000/mL on admission to 87.8 × 1,000/mL at day 2 after surgery. An increase occurred after postoperative day 3 (Fig 8-29).

Conclusion.—Patients with multiple trauma who underwent intramedullary nailing with reaming of the medullary canal showed a significant impairment of oxygenation. Unreamed intramedullary stabilization of the femur did not adversely affect the lung in patients with the same overall degree of injury. Although an increase in triglyceride levels in patients undergoing RFN was not detected, the reaming procedure appears to result in a higher amount of fat embolization.

The Detection of Fat Embolism by Transoesophageal Echocardiography During Reamed Intramedullary Nailing: A Study of 24 Patients With Femoral and Tibial Fractures

Pell ACH, Christie J, Keating JF, Sutherland GR (Edinburgh Royal Infirmary, Scotland)
J Bone Joint Surg (Br) 75-B:921–925, 1993   129-94-8–41

Introduction.—Several studies have linked intramedullary nailing and reaming for tibial and femoral fractures with the development of the fat embolism syndrome (FES), a complication associated with high morbidity and mortality. Transesophageal echocardiography was used to detect embolic material released from the fracture site into the systemic circulation.

Patients and Methods.—Twenty-four patients with a mean age of 38 years were included. Seven had femoral fractures and 17 had tibial fractures. Five patients had multiple injuries. All fractures were treated with a locking intramedullary GK nail, with nailing performed in all but 2 patients within 24 hours of injury. Transesophageal echocardiography was performed throughout the operation. Major criteria for the diagnosis of FES were petechial rash, hypoxemia, CNS depression, and pulmonary edema. A positive diagnosis required at least 1 major sign and 4 of 7 minor signs (tachycardia, pyrexia, retinal emboli on fundoscopy, lipuria, thrombocytopenia, decreased hematocrit, and fat globules in sputum).

Results.—Fourteen patients had only minimal evidence of emboli passing through the heart, but copious showers of small emboli were observed in 6 patients. In 3 of 4 patients with multiple large emboli (maximum dimension of more than 10 mm) FES occurred after operation. Two of the patients who had FES required ventilation; 1 of these patients died of fat embolism. In both of these patients nailing was delayed beyond 24 hours after injury.

Conclusion.—These preliminary findings suggest a role for transesophageal echocardiography in patients at risk for FES after nailing. The appearance of large emboli in association with reamed nailing has not previously been recognized. In all 3 patients with clinical FES, large volumes of embolic material had passed through the heart.

▶ The Hannover group is largely responsible for turning our attention toward the effect of reamed intramedullary nailing as associated with posttraumatic ARDS in patients with chest trauma. This has sparked a debate worldwide about the damaging effects of the act of reaming, reamer pressures, reamer design, and the critical role of a predisposing lung injury. In Abstract 129-94-8-37, the Hannover group defined "early" intramedullary stabilization as occurring within 24 hours of injury. A large group of patients seen in a 9-year period were investigated retrospectively. The incidence of ARDS was more than 4 times greater in patients with severe chest trauma, and the mortality rate was 5 times greater. Although this study certainly provokes questions, with unintentional patient selection bias and groups numbering in the 20s, the power of these statistics is weak. This phenomenon deserves further evaluation with well-controlled clinical studies.

Pape et al. (Abstract 129-94-8-40) used the same definition for ARDS and early primary intramedullary nailing and compared reamed vs. unreamed femoral nailing with small-diameter solid nails. They showed a significant deterioration in arterial oxygen pressure and increase in pulmonary artery pressure in patients with reamed femoral nailing. Based on the findings of their first paper, one wonders whether or not patient selection bias was the phenomenon active here. Certainly, the insult in passing a 10-mm reamer is the same in passing a 10-mm solid nail. The question is, then, do multiple passages of reamer with the "showering effect" lead to a cumulative damaging effect on the lung? Both papers seem to give a tentative "yes" to this question, but the topic is deserving of further study.

Pell et al. (Abstract 129-94-8-41) used transesophageal echocardiography to document the significance of reaming on pulmonary function. In six of the 24 patients small emboli (less than 1 cm in diameter) were observed, but, more significantly, in 4 patients emboli larger than this were observed. The fact that in the majority of these patients clinical ARDS developed and that 1 died brings an urgency to further scientific study of this phenomenon. Although it's clear that this study can be criticized for the fact that the observers of the ECGs were not blinded, were not multiple, and were probably subject to substantial bias, the findings of this study must be heeded. Further attention must be directed to limiting the showering effect by optimizing surgical instruments and techniques.

On a somewhat related topic, Ganong investigated the phenomenon of fat embolized syndrome in patients with ski fractures in Abstract 129-94-8-38. In this 11-year retrospective study, no patient required mechanical ventilation. However, fat embolization syndrome, as defined by fever, tachycardia, tachypnia, hypoxemia, and anemia developed in 23%. Although it is difficult to separate the effect of the injury from the treatment on these parameters, these signs (particularly hypoxemia) give rise to concern. The take-home message is to consider the diagnosis when these clinical symptoms arise and to follow-up quickly with pulse oximetry or arterial blood gas measurements, or both, when the suspicion is high.

In Abstract 129-94-8-39, the authors demonstrate the usefulness of pulse oximetry in monitoring patients after blunt musculoskeletal trauma. Fifteen of 43 patients had oxygen-hemoglobin saturation of less than or equal to 94% within 24 hours of admission. This method of monitoring is demonstrated to be effective and certainly is of little risk to the patient. The conclusion that this method is an efficient and reliable screening device is appropriate.—M.F. Swiontkowski, M.D.

Functional Outcomes Assessment

Physical Impairment and Functional Outcomes Six Months After Severe Lower Extremity Fractures
MacKenzie EJ, Cushing BM, Jurkovich GJ, Morris JA Jr, Burgess AR, deLateur BJ, McAndrew MP, Swiontkowski MF (Johns Hopkins School of Hygiene and Public Health, Baltimore, Md; Univ of Maryland, Baltimore; Univ of Washington, Seattle; et al)
J Trauma 34:528–539, 1993   129-94-8-42

Introduction.—Lower extremity injuries constitute the leading cause of all trauma hospitalizations in adults younger than age 65 years, and yet little is known about the long-term consequences of lower extremity fractures (LEFs). Patients with unilateral LEFs were studied prospectively to determine physical impairment and functional outcomes at 6 months and to examine the relationship between impairment and disability.

Patients.—Between May 1990 and December 1991, 444 patients aged 18–64 years were admitted for treatment of severe unilateral LEF after

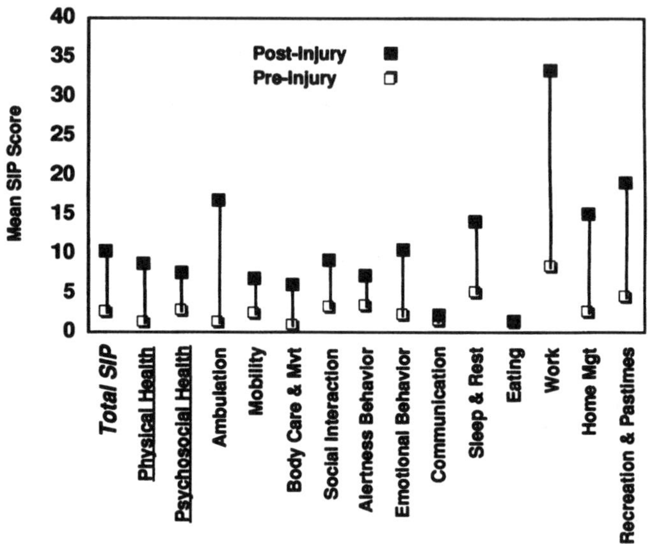

Fig 8–30.—Mean SIP scores: preinjury vs. 6 months postdischarge. (Courtesy of MacKenzie EJ, Cushing BM, Jurkovich GJ, et al: *J Trauma* 34:528–539, 1993.)

blunt trauma. Of these, 376 (85%) were successfully located and interviewed at 6 months after discharge, and 302 (68%) returned to the trauma center for clinical assessment. The patients were predominantly young (mean age, 32.4 years) white (72%) men who were working before the injury (77%). Impairment was measured in terms of range of motion, muscle strength, and pain. Disability was measured using the Sickness Impact Profile (SIP), a well-validated patient assessment of health status.

Outcome.—A significant proportion of patients remained physically impaired at 6 months after discharge. One half of the patients had range-of-motion scores above 15% based on guidelines developed by the American Medical Association. Most affected was the ankle joint, with 55% of patients having abnormal dorsiflexion or plantar flexion. More than one third of patients had abnormally weak extensors or flexors and ankle dorsiflexors compared with the unaffected leg. Only 10% of patients complained of substantial pain. The mean overall SIP score was 10.2, indicating a moderate level of dysfunction or disability. Analysis of the 12 categories that constitute the SIP showed that patients had difficulties sleeping, managing their home, getting back to work, and resuming their previous recreational activities (Fig 8–30). Only 48% had returned to work at 6 months. Both overall SIP scores and SIP subscores for ambulation strongly correlated with all measures of lower extremity impairment. However, the relationship between impairment and dysfunction in household management, work, and recreation were considerably weaker. The level of impairment, age, and gender explained 31% of the variance in ambulation scores and only 12% of the variance in SIP subscores for work, suggesting that factors other than the extent of physical impairment significantly influenced broader disability outcomes and ability to return to work.

Conclusions.—Significant impairment and disability persist at 6 months after treatment of severe unilateral LEF. Other factors over and above the extent of physical impairment may impede optimal recovery and return to preinjury levels of activity. Further research is necessary to define these factors and to identify and target appropriate rehabilitation services.

Open Tibial Fractures With Severe Soft-Tissue Loss: Limb Salvage Compared With Below-the-Knee Amputation

Georgiadis GM, Behrens FF, Joyce MJ, Earle AS, Simmons AL (Wayne State Univ, Detroit; New Jersey Med School, Newark; Case Western Reserve Univ, Cleveland, Ohio)

J Bone Joint Surg (Am) 75-A:1431–1441, 1993   129-94-8–43

Introduction.—Many patients with severe open fractures of the tibia ultimately require below- or above-the-knee amputation. The introduction 2 decades ago of microvascular transfer of free flaps was considered a major advance in the treatment of these injuries. Whether the use of free flaps has changed the long-term outcome of tibial fractures with severe soft tissue injury was assessed.

Patients and Methods.—The patients whose records were reviewed were managed at 1 center between 1982 and 1988. All had open tibial fractures associated with a large open wound and had been treated with a free-tissue transfer or an amputation. Sixteen patients with an average follow-up of 35 months had a successful limb-salvage procedure and could be personally examined (group 1). The average follow-up for the 18 patients who had below-the-knee amputation (group 2) was 44 months. Both groups were assessed for complications, operative procedures, hospital stay, hospital charges, and long-term functional results.

Results.—The limb salvage and early amputation groups were similar in mean age (33 and 32 years, respectively) and male/female ratio. Fifteen of 18 patients in the early amputation group but only 2 of 16 in the limb salvage group had a vascular injury (table). Patients who had limb salvage had a significantly longer hospital stay, more complications, and more operative procedures than those who underwent early amputation. Compared with group 2 patients, those in group 1 took significantly more time to achieve full weight-bearing, were less willing to work, and had higher hospital charges. Thirteen patients who had a successful

Patient Profile		
	Group 1 (Limb Salvage)	Group 2 (Early Amputation)
No. of patients	16	18
Duration of follow-up (mos.)*	35 (20-96)	44 (19-90)
Sex (M/F)	14/2	16/2
Age (yrs.)*	33 (19-51)	32 (16-56)
Mode of injury (no. of patients)		
Motorcycle accident	7	10
Automobile accident	1	0
Pedestrian hit by motor vehicle	7	4
Other	1	4
Vascular injury† (no. of patients)	2	15
Tibial fracture only injury (no. of patients)	5	6

*Mean value, with range in parentheses.
†The 2 groups differed significantly ($P < .001$) with respect to this characteristic, according to the chi-square goodness-of-fit statistic.
(Courtesy of Georgiadis GM, Behrens FF, Joyce MJ, et al: *J Bone Joint Surg (Am)* 75-A:1431–1441, 1993.)

limb-salvage procedure and 16 who underwent amputation completed a quality-of-life evaluation. Pain and sleep difficulties were common problems (Fig 8–31). Significantly more patients in group 1 considered themselves severely disabled. The limb-salvage patients also had more problems with recreational activities and job performance (Fig 8–32).

Conclusion.—Although modern microvascular free tissue techniques can successfully treat tibial fractures associated with large soft tissue defects, functional outcome is often less than adequate in these cases. Patients who underwent early below-the-knee amputation recovered faster, had fewer disabilities, and had a generally better quality of life. Costs were significantly higher for limb salvage than for amputation ($109,044 vs. $65,624).

▶ In Abstract 129-94-8–42, a multicenter prospective trial, the authors demonstrated the usefulness of the SIP, a widely used, highly validated general health status instrument, in patients with LEF. Patients with these fractures (acetabular fractures to hind-foot fractures with all variations of severity) demonstrate moderate disability 6 months after discharge. Usefulness of the SIP is confirmed by decreased range of motion and strength. The functional impact is highlighted by only 48% of the patients returning to work (patients who were employed in 77% of instances preinjury). This work confirms the complexity of functional issues, with impairment, age, and gender

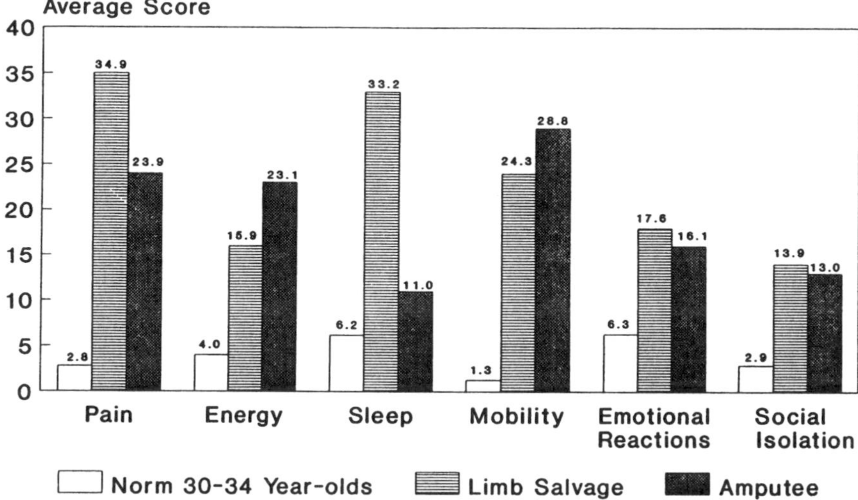

Fig 8–31.—Average scores on the Nottingham Health Profile (part I) for the patients who had had a limb salvage, those who had had an early amputation, and a healthy, age-matched reference group. The *numbers* indicate weighted responses in each category, with 0 representing no limitations and 100 representing maximum disability. (Courtesy of Georgiadis GM, Behrens FF, Joyce MJ, et al: *J Bone Joint Surg (Am)* 75-A:1431–1441, 1993.)

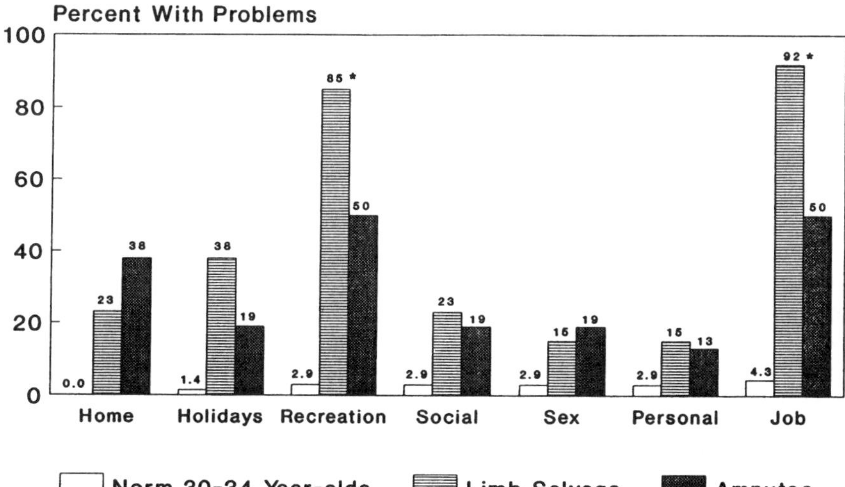

Fig 8–32.—Percentages of individuals who reported a health-related problem in the indicated areas of the Nottingham Health Profile (part II) in the group that had had a limb salvage, the group that had had an early amputation, and a healthy, age-matched reference group. The *asterisks* indicate a significant ($P < .05$) difference between the patients who had had a limb salvage and those who had had an early amputation (chi-square goodness-of-fit statistic). (Courtesy of Georgiadis GM, Behrens FF, Joyce MJ, et al: *J Bone Joint Surg (Am)* 75-A:1431–1441, 1993.)

accounting for only a limited amount of the variance in ambulation score. Quality-of-life instruments will clearly enhance the impact and quality of future clinical research and should be used widely.

The authors of Abstract 129-94-8–43 used the Nottingham Health Profile to assess quality-of-life impact on patients undergoing limb salvage, compared with those with below-the-knee amputation. Although this is a rather small group, the usefulness of the quality-of-life evaluation is again confirmed. All patients undergoing amputation had quicker times to full weight-bearing, higher ability to return to work, and lower hospital charges. More patients in this group, however, demonstrated moderate to severe life distress on the General Well-Being Schedule. The use of the quality-of-life instrument documented significant effects in both groups in all subscales in terms of functional domains. These scales add a complete picture of human function to studies addressing complex clinical decisions.—M.F. Swiontkowski, M.D.

Operative Techniques

Use of a Tourniquet in the Internal Fixation of Fractures of the Distal Part of the Fibula: A Prospective, Randomized Trial
Maffulli N, Testa V, Capasso G (Univ of Aberdeen, Scotland; Univ of Naples, Italy)
J Bone Joint Surg (Am) 75-A:700–703, 1993   129-94-8–44

Objective.—Operations involving the distal part of the limbs are often performed with the use of a pneumatic tourniquet to create a bloodless field. However, some adverse postoperative effects caused by the tourniquet have been reported. This prospective, randomized clinical trial was carried out to determine the complication rate associated with the use of a tourniquet during internal fixation of simple, closed fractures of the distal fibula.

Patients.—Of 80 patients aged 18–60 years with distal fibular fractions, 40 were randomly assigned to internal fixation with the use of a thigh tourniquet and 40 were operated on without a tourniquet. All fractures were operated on within 24 hours after the injury. Patients were examined daily during their hospitalization until a normal range of motion had been achieved, at which time a weight-bearing plaster cast was applied. The mean follow-up was 18 months; complete follow-up data were available for 72 patients.

Results.—The operation lasted a mean of 41 minutes in the tourniquet-treated group and 53 minutes in those treated without a tourniquet. The difference was statistically significant. In the tourniquet-treated group, deep vein thrombosis of the calf developed in 2 patients, 7 had possible wound infections, and 3 had frank infections. However, deep vein thrombosis did not develop in any of the patients treated without a tourniquet; none of these patients had frank wound infections, and only 4 had possible wound infections. Patients operated on without a tourni-

quet were able to return to work an average of 7 days earlier than tourniquet-treated patients.

Conclusion.—Routine use of a thigh tourniquet during internal fixation of a simple fracture of the distal part of the fibula is not recommended as its use increases the rate of postoperative complications and
prolongs the time to recovery.

▶ This editor's war cry has been "no tourniquets in trauma" for more than
10 years. This prospective, randomized series evaluating the effect of pneumatic tourniquets on the outcome of internally fixed lateral malleolus fracture
lends some scientific credence to this bias. The reader should note that all
fractures were operated on within 24 hours, as this makes good sense, and
the operative time was increased by a mean of 12 minutes when a tourniquet was not used. However, the lack of deep venous thrombosis and clinically proven wound infection in the patients treated without the tourniquet
speaks volumes against the use of these devices. Although this information
seems sound, a greater impression is made by the blinded functional assessment, which indicates the potential advantage of earlier functional return
when a tourniquet is not used. The authors do not offer a power analysis of
the statistics, which is unfortunate, but the group size seems adequate to
make their conclusions sound. This is one dogma that will continue, at least
for the present, in this editor's institution.—M.F. Swiontkowski, M.D.

Partial Patellectomy for Patellar Fracture: Tension Band Wiring and Early Mobilization

Hung LK, Lee SY, Leung KS, Chan KM, Nicholl LA (Chinese Univ, Hong Kong;
Margaret Trench Rehabilitation Centre, Kwun Tong, Hong Kong)
J Orthop Trauma 7:252–260, 1993   129-94-8–45

Introduction.—A partial patellectomy may require prolonged immobilization of the knee. The AO group has recommended placing a long
tension band wire loop to protect the tendon-to-bone repair and permit
early knee mobilization. Experience with 56 patients treated during a 10-
year period with tension band wiring and early mobilization was evaluated.

Patients and Methods.—Thirty-one of the patients were treated between 1977 and 1980 and retrospectively reviewed in 1981; 25 were
treated and monitored prospectively from 1984 to 1987, with the final
assessment completed in 1988. During these periods, partial patellecto-
mies accounted for 20% to 26% of all patella fractures treated. Thirty-
one of the 56 fractures were of the distal pole type. The patellar tendon-
to-bone repair was reinforced by a figure-of-eight tension-band wire
loop from the patella down to the tibial tubercle (Fig 8–33). Early mobilization and weight-bearing were started within the first postoperative
week.

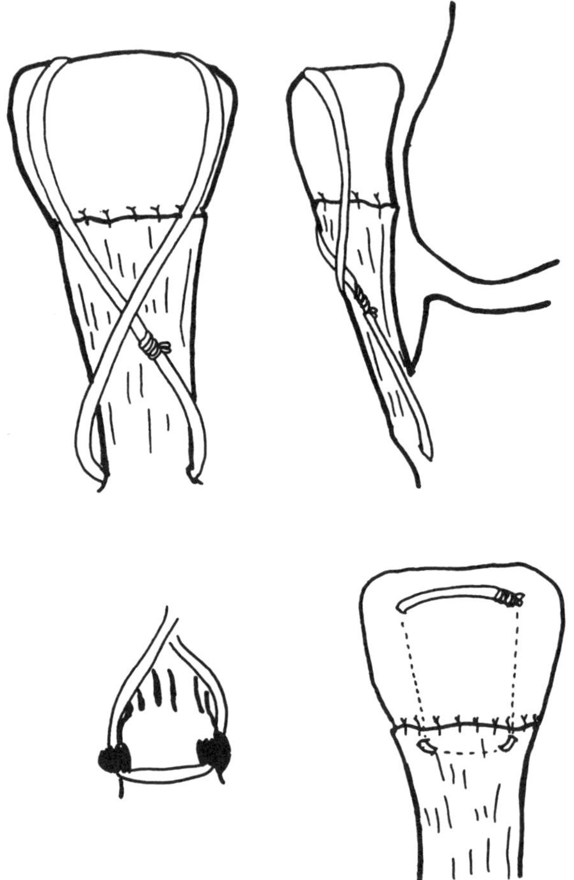

Fig 8–33.—Schematic drawing of the operative technique. The patellar tendon is approximated to bone with a Magnuson type of suture (nylon or wire), and the tension-band wire loop is applied on the outside. A screw across the tibial tubercle may be used for osteoporotic bone for distal anchorage of the wire. (Courtesy of Hung LK, Lee SY, Leung KS, et al: *J Orthop Trauma* 7:252–260, 1993.)

Results.—Patients were assessed for symptoms, functional activities, range of movement, and strength. Complications occurred in 52% of the first series of patients, but in only 12% of the second series (Table 1). Wire loops had to be removed from 5 patients in the first series and 2 patients in the second series because of symptoms. The 2 groups had a similar incidence of knee symptoms at follow-up (Table 2). Most patients had good recovery of knee function at 3-month evaluation (Table 3). There were no instances of disruption of knee extensor mechanism. Radiologic osteoarthritis after the fracture was common, perhaps because of alteration of the patellofemoral articulation after part of the patella was excised.

TABLE 1.—Complications

	Series I: 1977–1980	Series II: 1984–1987
Total no. of patients	31	25
Early		
Infection		
Superficial	2	1[a]
Deep	1	0
Septic arthritis	1	0
Wound gapping (not infected)	2	0
Faulty wire	2	0
Acute wire failure	2[b]	0
Late		
Wire knot and end symptoms	6	2
Total	16 (52%)	3 (12%)

*Revision for infected tension-band wiring.
†Both of these patients were treated by immobilization. There were no long-term sequelae in the knee extensor mechanism.
(Courtesy of Hung LK, Lee SY, Leung KS, et al: *J Orthop Trauma* 7:252–260, 1993.)

Conclusion.—Tension-band wiring allows early mobilization of the injured knee and good functional results in patients with comminuted patellar fractures requiring partial patellectomy. The procedure can be technically demanding and must be carried out meticulously. Patients should be monitored for the onset of radiologic arthritis.

TABLE 2.—Subjective Evaluation of Knee Functions

	Series I: 1977–1980		Series II: 1984–1987	
No.	31	25		
Follow-up (range)	22 mos (3–49)	5.5 wks (2.5–11)	3 mos	25 mos (8–48)
Pain (%)	16	50	20	14
Discomfort (kneeling and squatting) (%)	21	60	40	15
Weakness (%)	16	70	50	15
Stiffness (%)	21	50	45	18

(Courtesy of Hung LK, Lee SY, Leung KS, et al: *J Orthop Trauma* 7:252–260, 1993.)

TABLE 3.—Objective Assessment of Knee Function

	Series I: 1977–1980	Series II: 1984–1987		
No.	31	25		
Follow-up (range)	22 mos (3–49)	5.5 wks (2.5–11)	3 mos	25 mos (8–48)
Flexion >120° (%)	89	55	63	92
Extension lag <10° (%)	95	90	100	100
Power				
Extension				
MRC grade 4 (%)	—	70	47	5
MRC grade 5 (%)	100	30	53	95
Flexion				
MRC grade 4 (%)	—	78	43	5
MRC grade 5 (%)	100	22	57	95
Thigh girth	5	50	35	8

Abbreviation: MRC, Medical Research Council, United Kingdom.
Note: Difference between operated and normal control > 2.5 cm.
(Courtesy of Hung LK, Lee SY, Leung KS, et al: *J Orthop Trauma* 7:252-260, 1993.)

Factors Affecting Sliding of the Lag Screw in Intertrochanteric Fractures

Rha JD, Kim YH, Yoon SI, Park TS, Lee MH (Hanil Gen Hosp, Seoul, Korea)
Int Orthop 17:320–324, 1993   129-94-8-46

Introduction.—The sliding screw has been widely used for internal fixation of intertrochanteric fractures. This device allows compression and impaction of the proximal fragment, but failure can occur when there is excessive sliding of the proximal fragment. In a retrospective survey, the factors that cause excessive sliding of the lag screw were assessed.

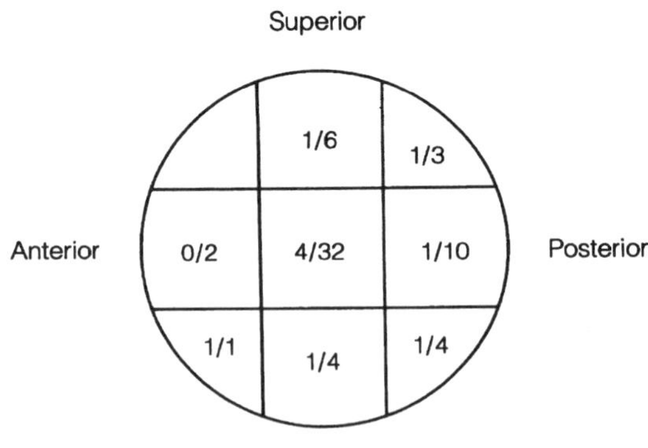

Fig 8–34.—Position of the lag screw in the femoral head. (Courtesy of Rha JD, Kim YH, Yoon SI, et al: *Int Orthop* 17:320-324, 1993.)

Displacement in Both Planes

In A-P view In lat. view	Ana. or lat. Ana. or post.	Medial Ana. or post.	Ana. or lat. anterior	Medial anterior
No. of patients	36	6	8	12
No. with exces- sive sliding	1 (2.8%)	1 (16.7%)	1 (12.5%)	7 (58.3%)

Abbreviations: Ana, anatomical; *lat,* lateral; *post,* posterior; A-P, anteroposterior.
(Courtesy of Rha JD, Kim YH, Yoon SI, et al: *Int Orthop* 17:320–324, 1993.)

Patients and Methods.—Sixty-two patients were available for follow-up at an average of 13.2 months after treatment for intertrochanteric fractures of the femur. The age range of the group was 40–89 years (mean age, 70.4 years). Anatomical reduction was attempted in every case, and 135-degree sliding compression screws and plates were used for fixation. Factors analyzed were patient age and sex, type of fracture, degree of osteoporosis, accuracy of reduction, and the position of the lag screw in the femoral head.

Results.—Excessive sliding occurred in 10 of 62 patients. The incidence of excessive sliding was significantly increased among patients older than 70 years. Excessive sliding occurred only in unstable fractures, and the incidence of these fractures was higher in patients older than 70 years (83.9%) than in those younger than 70 years (54.8%). Excessive sliding developed equally in each of the positions of the lag screw in the femoral head (Fig 8–34), but it was significantly increased when the distal fragment was displaced medially and anteriorly (table). Osteoporosis was not statistically correlated to excessive sliding.

Conclusion.—Excessive sliding is the major factor causing failure of fixation and unsatisfactory results in patients with intertrochanteric fractures. The incidence of this complication was increased in elderly patients (29%), in unstable fractures (23.3%), and when the distal fragment was displaced medially and anteriorly (58.3%).

Closed Intramedullary Femoral Osteotomy: Shortening and Derotation Procedures

Chapman ME, Duwelius PJ, Bray TJ, Gordon JE (Univ of California, Davis, Sacramento; Reno Orthopaedic Clinic, Nev; Oregon Health Sciences Univ, Portland)
Clin Orthop 287:245–251, 1993   129-94-8-47

Introduction.—Advancements in instrumentation and techniques have improved outcome in patients undergoing closed osteotomy of the femur for leg-length inequality or rotational deformities. A 10-year experience with closed femoral osteotomies was evaluated.

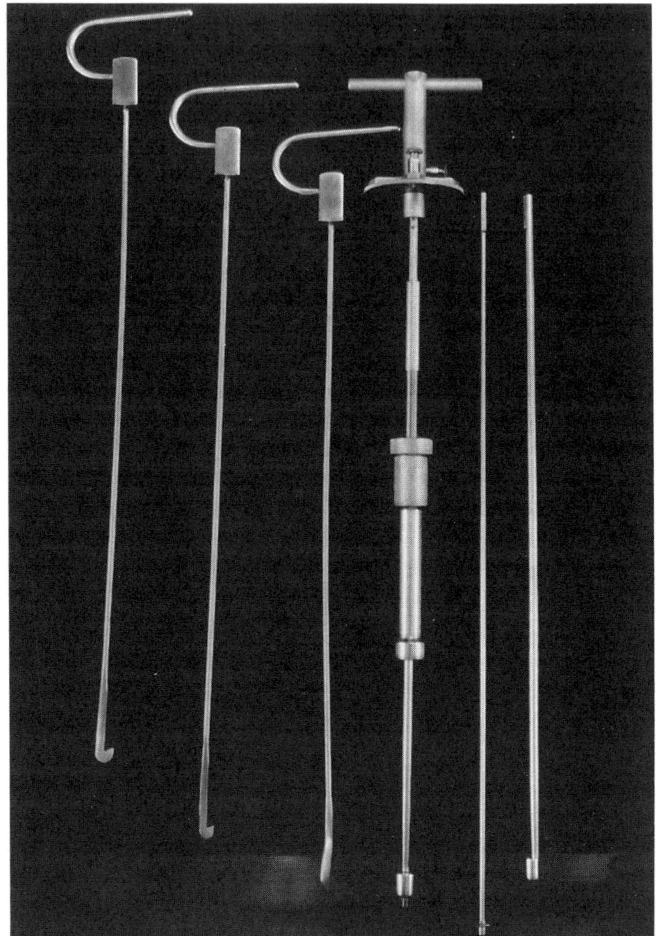

FIg 8–35.—Closed femoral osteotomy saw and back-cutting osteotomes. (Courtesy of Chapman ME, Duwelius PJ, Bray TJ, et al: *Clin Orthop* 287:245–251, 1993.)

Patients and Methods.—Included were 37 patients who were treated with closed femoral osteotomy from March 1978 until May 1987. Six had derotation osteotomies and 31 underwent femoral shortenings. The average age of the patients was 30 years. Most of the leg-length discrepancies were caused by a trauma or resulted from the complications of treatment. The range of discrepancies was 2–6.6 cm. Low back pain and limp were common problems in these patients. The technique of closed femoral shortening requires a fracture table, an image intensifier, flexible reamers, intramedullary nails capable of interlocking, Pearson's intramedullary saw, and a variety of intramedullary back-cutting osteotomes (Fig 8–35). Nails are removed only when symptomatic or if the patient engages in a high-risk vocation or avocation. Return to physically demanding activities should be delayed until full rehabilitation is achieved.

Results.—Patients were evaluated for an average of 3.3 years after the closed femoral osteotomy. The average duration of surgery was 3.4 hours and average hospital stay was 6 days. Twenty-four patients had equal measurements of leg length, 5 were corrected to within 5 mm, 1 to within 8 mm, and 1 to within 10 mm. Residual leg-length inequality was not functionally significant. All patients regained their full preoperative joint range of motion. Rotational deformities, which averaged 58 degrees preoperatively, were all corrected to within 5 degrees of normal. Two patients required reoperation because of severe bleeding into the thigh and 1 patient had a delayed union.

Conclusion.—Closed femoral osteotomy can successfully shorten, derotate, or correct mild angulation of the femur. The procedure is technically much simpler and more predictable than lengthening. Advantages include immediate weight-bearing, early union, and early return to function.

Multiple Relaxing Skin Incisions in Orthopaedic Lower Extremity Trauma

DiStasio AJ II, Dugdale TW, Deafenbaugh MK (Portsmouth Naval Hosp, Va; Hartford Hosp, Conn)
J Orthop Trauma 7:270–274, 1993   129-94-8–48

Introduction.—Lower extremity wounds caused by direct trauma or surgical intervention are often repaired by means of skin grafting, flap coverage, delayed primary closure, or closure by secondary intention. The use of multiple relaxing skin incisions (MRSIs) in patients with difficult lower extremity wounds was evaluated.

Methods.—Participants were 22 patients with musculoskeletal trauma to the lower extremities. The MRSIs were used when there was extreme tension (e.g., skin blanching, gapping) caused by swelling or soft tissue loss. The technique involves numerous small incisions (5–10 mm) full thickness through the dermis made with a no. 15 blade scalpel. The incisions are arranged in 1-cm–wide rows parallel to the primary wound or incision. Both the primary wound and MRSIs are covered with xeroform or other nonadherent gauze and then with a light compressive dressing (Fig 8–36). The wounds were evaluated in the early postoperative period for dehiscence, skin slough, superficial and deep infection, and neurovascular compromise.

Results.—The average patient age was 30 years. Vehicular trauma was the cause of 55% of the injuries. Fifteen injuries were to the tibia or fibula, or both, and 9 injuries were open. Associated injuries were seen in 10 patients. All 22 patients were available for follow-up after 1 year or

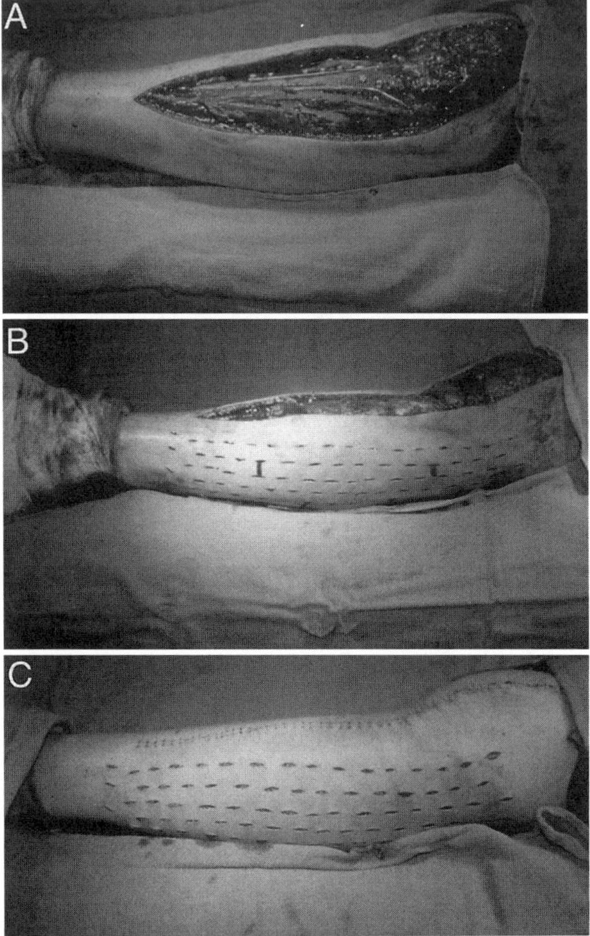

Fig 8–36.—**A,** wound status after open reduction internal fixation of bicondylar tibial plateau fracture; **B,** multiple relaxing skin incisions; **C,** staple closure with drains, no tension. (Courtesy of DiStasio AJ II, Dugdale TW, Deafenbaugh MK: *J Orthop Trauma* 7:270–274, 1993.)

longer. There were no cases of delayed wound healing or other complications. None of the patients had signs or symptoms of compartment syndrome or required further soft tissue coverage. Patients were satisfied with the cosmetic result of MRSIs.

Conclusion.—The technique of MRSI is easy, versatile, safe, and economical. In these patients with lower extremity trauma and without large, wide defects, MRSIs allowed closure of wounds without tension. No postoperative complications were related to wound closure. However, these incisions should be used with extreme caution in patients with compromised skin.

9 General Adult Reconstruction

General Knee Problems

Prediction of the Progression of Joint Space Narrowing in Osteoarthritis of the Knee by Bone Scintigraphy

Dieppe P, Cushnaghan J, Young P, Kirwan J (Univ of Bristol, England)
Ann Rheum Dis 52:557–563, 1993   129-94-9–1

Introduction.—Osteoarthritis of the knee joint is a principal cause of pain and disability in older individuals. Although symptoms improve with time in some patients, joint damage may progress in others. The hypothesis that subchondral bone activity, as detected by scintigraphy, will predict subsequent change in osteoarthritis of the knee was tested.

Patients and Methods.—Study subjects were 100 patients with a diagnosis of osteoarthritis of 1 or both knees. Radiographs and bone scans of the knees were obtained at study entry and at 5-year evaluation. Outcome data were available for 75 patients; 6 patients had no entry scans, 10 had died, and 9 were lost to follow-up. Entry and outcome radiographs were read in random order by a single observer unaware of pa-

TABLE 1.—Change in Radiographic Features of Osteoarthritis of the Knee in the 60 Patients Available for 5-Year Follow-Up and in Whom No Knee Operation Was Performed

Radiographic feature	Number (%) of knees showing change (n=120)
Osteophytosis	24(20)
Subchondral bone sclerosis	21(18)
Patellofemoral joint space	5(4)
Observer recording of a difference between paired films	57(48)
Loss of tibiofemoral joint space (mm)	
2	14(12)
1	33(28)
0	51(43)
−1	19(16)
−2	2(2)

(Courtesy of Dieppe P, Cushnaghan J, Young P, et al: *Ann Rheum Dis* 52:557–563, 1993.)

TABLE 2.—Predictive Value of Scintigraphic Findings at Entry in Relation to Subsequent Radiographic Change and Progression to an Operation on the Knee. Numbers of Patients Are Shown

Scan at entry	No radiographic change	Some radiographic change	Loss of ≥2 mm of joint space	Operation
No abnormality	40	15	0	0
Late phase/one compartment abnormality only	33	21	11	6
Late plus perfusion phase abnormality	4	12	3	16

(Courtesy of Dieppe P, Cushnaghan J, Young P, et al: *Ann Rheum Dis* 52:557–563, 1993.)

tient data. Scan findings and other entry variables were related to outcome. A change in osteoarthritis of the knee was defined as progression to an operation on the knee or a decrease in the tibiofemoral joint space of 2 mm or more.

Results.—The 94 patients for whom entry films were available had a mean age of 64.2 years. Fifty-two had bilateral osteoarthritis of the knee and 40 used walking aids. Most (76%) had pain at entry. Radiographic and scintigraphic abnormalities at entry included osteoarthritis of medial compartments (66%) and patellofemoral joints (71%). Forty-five knees had an abnormal perfusion phase scan and 121 had an abnormality on the bone phase. Fifteen patients (22 knees) were operated on during the study and 60 had no operation (Table 1). Fourteen additional knees met criteria for progression. Twenty-eight of 32 knees with severe scan abnormalities had progression; in contrast, none of the 55 knees with normal scans at entry progressed. Most of the knees without scan abnormalities at entry (73%) had no radiographic changes (Table 2). Pain severity—but not age, sex, symptom duration, or obesity—predicted a subsequent operation.

Conclusion.—Scan abnormalities predict subsequent outcome in osteoarthritis of the knee. For the 5-year study, a normal scan was a powerful negative predictor and a positive scan was a significant positive predictor of subsequent loss of joint space. Even with severe joint damage, however, some patients will do relatively well during a 5-year period.

▶ The lack of correlation between patients' symptoms and radiographic changes consistent with osteoarthritis of the knee is well known. The corollary is that you cannot predict whether a patient will progress, either radiographically or symptomatically, by judging the severity of changes on plain radiographs. This paper offers strong evidence that bone scintigraphy is predictive of the future course of osteoarthritis of the knee and that it can be used for both negative and positive predictive value. Perhaps a future study will address the usefulness of scintigraphy in predicting which patients will do well after tibial osteotomy or unicompartmental replacement of the knee.—C.B. Sledge, M.D.

Reliability of Grading Scales for Individual Radiographic Features of Osteoarthritis of the Knee: The Baltimore Longitudinal Study of Aging Atlas of Knee Osteoarthritis

Scott WW Jr, Lethbridge-Cejku M, Reichle R, Wigley FM, Tobin JD, Hochberg MC (Johns Hopkins Univ, Baltimore, Md; Univ of Maryland, Baltimore; Natl Inst on Aging, Baltimore, Md)
Invest Radiol 28:497–501, 1993   129-94-9-2

Introduction.—The appropriateness of the Kellgren-Lawrence grading system for longitudinal studies of radiographic progression of osteoarthritis of the hand, hip, and knee has been questioned by some researchers. The authors developed an original atlas of individual radiographic features of osteoarthritis of the knee and evaluated the inter-reader and intrareader reliability of trained readers using the atlas.

Subjects and Methods.—Good quality radiographs were selected from ones previously read using the Kellgren-Lawrence grades. The radiographs were from 25 male and 5 female patients who were participants in the Baltimore Longitudinal Study of Aging. The men had a mean age of 66.5 years, and the women had a mean age of 70.6 years. Four trained readers graded the standing anterior-posterior knee radiographs for 8 features of osteoarthritis: medial and lateral compartment osteophytes, joint space narrowing, and subchondral sclerosis; osteophytes of the tibial spine; and chondrocalcinosis. Radiographs were also graded using the Kellgren-Lawrence global scale.

Results.—Inter-reader reliability ranged from .63 to .83 and intrareader reliability ranged from .82 to .95 for all features of osteoarthritis except sclerosis and osteophytes of the tibial spines. The average interclass correlation coefficient indicated substantial agreement beyond chance. The average agreement between pairs of readers varied from 70.8% to 97.5% for the 8 individual features, but was only 51.4% for the global Kellgren-Lawrence scale.

Conclusion.—Trained readers using this atlas reliably measured the presence and severity of individual radiographic features of osteoarthritis of the knee. The individual features scale, in contrast to the Kellgren-Lawrence scale, is sensitive to change over time and can be used to study the symptoms and signs of knee osteoarthritis in relation to radiographic changes. Its excellent intrareader reliability should allow a single reader to be used in longitudinal cohort studies.

▶ It has been difficult to discuss either the natural history of osteoarthritis of the knee or its response to treatment because there has not been a satisfactory method of grading radiographic changes in any useful, quantitative fashion. The old Steinbrocker grading system had only 4 grades, covering the spectrum from normal to bony ankylosis; the Kellgren-Lawrence scale appears insensitive to change over time. The authors of this paper propose a cumulative score based on assessment of 8 characteristics of the knee with good inter-reader and intrareader reliability. Perhaps scintigraphy, as recommended in the previous paper (Abstract 129-94-9-1), added to the scale would improve its prognostic usefulness.—C.B. Sledge, M.D.

Patellar Tendon Rupture: Description of a Simplified Operative Method for a Current Therapeutic Problem
Persson K, Merkow RL, Templeman DC, Sieber J, Gustilo RB (Hennepin County Med Ctr, Minneapolis)
Arch Orthop Trauma Surg 112:47–49, 1992   129-94-9-3

Background.—A number of operative techniques have been proposed for the uncommon problem of acute patellar tendon rupture. A new technique that is simpler than the previously described techniques uses an implant with a very low-grade tissue reaction.

Technique.—Through a straight anterior incision, a 3-mm burr channel is drilled from medial to lateral, 1 cm dorsal to the tibial tubercle and at a right angle to the long axis of the tibia. The surgeon places a 5-mm Mersilene band with 2 needles through the burr channel, threading each strand proximally into the tendon in Bunnel fashion and out through the rupture site. Two additional 3-mm burr channels are placed through the long axis of the patella, from the deep to the proximal surface, converging at the proximal pole (Fig 9–1). The surgeon tags the deep synovial layer of the patellar tendon with interrupted sutures to provide a good gliding surface deep to the tendon. The Mersilene strands are passed through each burr channel and tied under tension, with the knots buried in the quadriceps tendon. The loop and deep synovial sutures are tied, with additional sutures in the superficial part of the patellar tendon and in the lateral and medial extensor retinaculum. Passive range of motion is checked on the operating table and should be 90–100 degrees.

Results.—The method has been used in 6 patients: 5 men and 1 woman, 32–69 years of age. One had bilateral injuries; that patient and 3 others had no other associated injuries. The rupture healed uneventfully after treatment in all patients. One patient had an infection and required removal of the Mersilene band.

Conclusion.—This Mersilene band technique represents a simple and effective technique for repair of patellar tendon rupture. It confers good stability with a minimum of foreign body implant. In most cases, the Mersilene band can simply be left in place.

▶ Ruptures of the patellar tendon are unusual but disabling and difficult to repair. The technique proposed by the authors appears to be simple and ef-

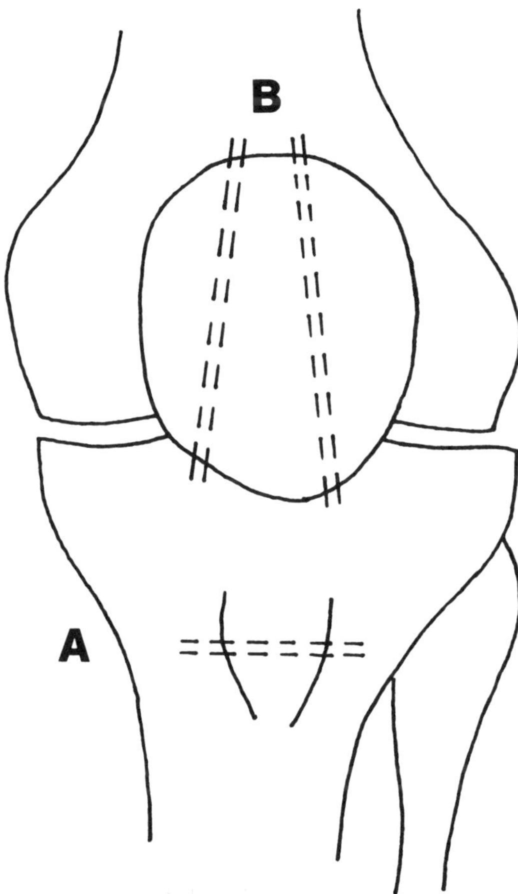

Fig 9–1.—Route of the burr channels (**A, B**) in the Mersilene loop tendon repair operation. (Courtesy of Persson K, Merkow RL, Templeman DC, et al: *Arch Orthop Trauma Surg* 112:47–49, 1992.)

fective. They report on 6 patients, with follow-up on 5; 4 of them had an excellent result and the fifth had a low-grade infection that responded to further surgical treatment. It appears that the use of a flexible Mersilene band is preferable to the use of wires, which would certainly break with activity.—C.B. Sledge, M.D.

Proximal Tibial Osteotomy: A Critical Long-Term Study of Eighty-Seven Cases

Coventry MB, Ilstrup DM, Wallrichs SL (Mayo Clinic and Found, Rochester, Minn)

J Bone Joint Surg (Am) 75-A:196–201, 1993   129-94-9-4

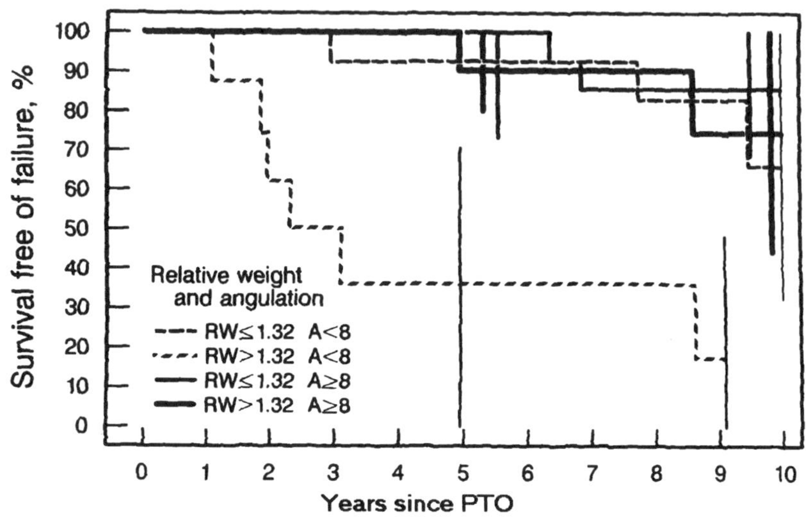

Fig 9–2.—Rate of survival free of failure, according to valgus angulation at 1 year after the operation (A) and the relative weight (RW) of the patient. Proximal tibial osteotomy, PTO. (Courtesy of Coventry MB, Ilstrup DM, Wallrichs SL: *J Bone Joint Surg (Am)* 75-A:196–201, 1993.)

Objective.—Experience from 1960 to 1976 with proximal tibial osteotomy in patients with unicompartmental degenerative osteoarthrosis of the knee has been described. Functional results correlated with pain relief; there was no loss of motion and there were few complications. There have since been a number of changes, including clearer surgical indications, standardized planning, and the use of direct measurements from weight-bearing radiographs. More recent experience with proximal tibial osteotomy was reported.

Methods.—The analysis included 87 valgus osteotomies in 73 patients performed from 1976 to 1981. All patients had osteoarthrosis of the medial compartment of the knee and were followed for a median of 10 years. Univariate and multivariate analyses and survivorship analysis of the clinical data were performed, using knee arthroplasty as the end point of failure. Further analyses used the end point of arthroplasty or the presence of moderate-to-severe pain in patients who declined arthroplasty.

Findings.—Two thirds of patients reported less pain at follow-up than before the operation, and more than half reported that they were able to walk farther. As pain decreased, walking ability increased. Maximum flexion and range of flexion decreased by a mean of 5 degrees. Seventy percent of knees were in less valgus angulation than at the 5-week postoperative examination, with a median loss of correction of 1 degree.

The only risk factors associated with duration of survival were relative weight and angular correction. Patients who had at least 8 degrees of valgus angulation, or who weighed 1.32 times their ideal weight or less at 1 year postoperatively, had a 90% probability of survival at 5 years and a 65% probability at 10 years. In contrast, patients with less valgus angulation and greater body weight had a 5-year probability of survival of 38% and a 10-year probability of 19% (Fig 9–2).

Conclusion.—In patients undergoing proximal tibial osteotomy, overcorrection of valgus alignment is a vital consideration. Failure is highly likely if alignment is not overcorrected to at least 8 degrees of valgus and if the patient is more than 30% overweight. Very little of the valgus angulation obtained at surgery is lost during long-term follow-up.

▶ Osteotomy of the proximal tibia was introduced to the American orthopedist by Mark Coventry in 1969. Since that time, the operation has waxed and waned in popularity and, in recent years, has definitely lost out to total knee arthroplasty. There are numerous reasons for that, but one of the most important ones is the lack of predictability and durability of the tibial osteotomy. This important long-term study should remove those uncertainties. Coventry and his co-authors demonstrate that proper surgical technique and proper patient selection can result in a 94% survivorship of a good result at 10 years. They emphasize the necessity to overcorrect into 8 degrees of valgus and select patients whose weight is no more than 17% above "ideal." Gender was not found to be associated with outcome, although previous studies had suggested that women do not do as well as men after this operation.

It is to be hoped that this paper will stimulate a renewed interest in this conservative operation, which can have excellent durability and avoid the complications of both unicompartmental and tricompartmental arthroplasties. It should be noted, however, that most surgeons have found that revision of a proximal tibial osteotomy to a total knee arthroplasty is technically more difficult and the results are slightly inferior to those achieved in patients who have not undergone the previous operation.—C.B. Sledge, M.D.

The Maquet Procedure in the Treatment of Patellofemoral Osteoarthrosis: Long-Term Results
Schmid F (Bezirksspital, Frutigen, Switzerland)
Clin Orthop 294:254–258, 1993   129-94-9–5

Introduction.—In 1963, Maquet suggested that painful patellofemoral osteoarthrosis resistant to conservative treatment should be treated with anterior displacement of the tibial tuberosity. This approach has remained controversial. Long-term results were examined in a series of patients treated with the Maquet procedure.

Subjects.—A series of 33 patients were treated for patellofemoral osteoarthrosis with the Maquet procedure. Three were lost to long-term follow-up, whereas the remaining 30 patients (35 knees) were followed for an average of 16 years. There were 19 men and 11 women in this series.

Results.—Before surgery, all knees were rated very poor. After surgery, 21 knees were rated very good, 7 were rated good, 4 were rated fair, and 3 knees were rated poor. Even in the knees rated poor, there was some improvement. In the 80% of knees rated good to very good, the diagnosis was correct and there were no postoperative complications. In the 20% of cases that did not yield good results, there were errors in diagnosis, resulting in additional problems being ignored, or the surgical technique was inadequate.

Conclusion.—The Maquet technique is an effective treatment for patellofemoral osteoarthrosis. However, a tibial tubercle elevation of at least 2 cm is necessary for success. Osteitis after skin slough must be prevented by relieving skin incisions.

▶ The Maquet operation has not been particularly popular in this country because of poor predictability, frequent complications, and the cosmetic aspects of tibial tubercle elevation of sufficient extent. This paper addresses the issue of predictability of results and reports 80% to be very good or good and only 20% to be fair or poor at a follow-up of from 10 to 20 years after surgery (mean, 16 years). The author stresses the fact that elevation of 2 cm is essential to provide a good result. Many would still believe that such an elevation produces an undesirable, if not unacceptable, cosmetic problem.—C.B. Sledge, M.D.

The Patello-Femoral Joint: A Critical Appraisal of Its Geometric Assessment Utilizing Conventional Axial Radiography and Computed Arthro-Tomography
Walker C, Cassar-Pullicino VN, Vaisha R, McCall IW (Robert Jones and Agnes Hunt Hosp, Oswestry, England)
Br J Radiol 66:755–761, 1993 129-94-9-6

Introduction.—Malalignment of the patellofemoral joint results in anterior knee pain and can lead to recurrent dislocation and degenerative change. Plain film skyline views of the joint are obtained to assess its functional relationships in patients with pain. The relationship of the geometric measurements obtained by skyline views and by CT was determined in 50 consecutive patients. The relative merits of the 2 techniques were assessed in a clinical setting.

Methods.—Fifty cases of anterior knee pain were assessed in skyline (Merchant's) views of the patellofemoral joint and by double contrast CT arthrography. Parameters examined were the congruence angle (CA), the lateral patellofemoral angle (PFA), and the trochlea depth (TD). The knees studied were from 40 patients ranging in age from 14 to 54 years. The shape of the patella was graded according to the system of Wiberg.

Results.—There was poor correlation between the 2 imaging methods. All of the 10 patients with PFA values less than zero on CT assessment

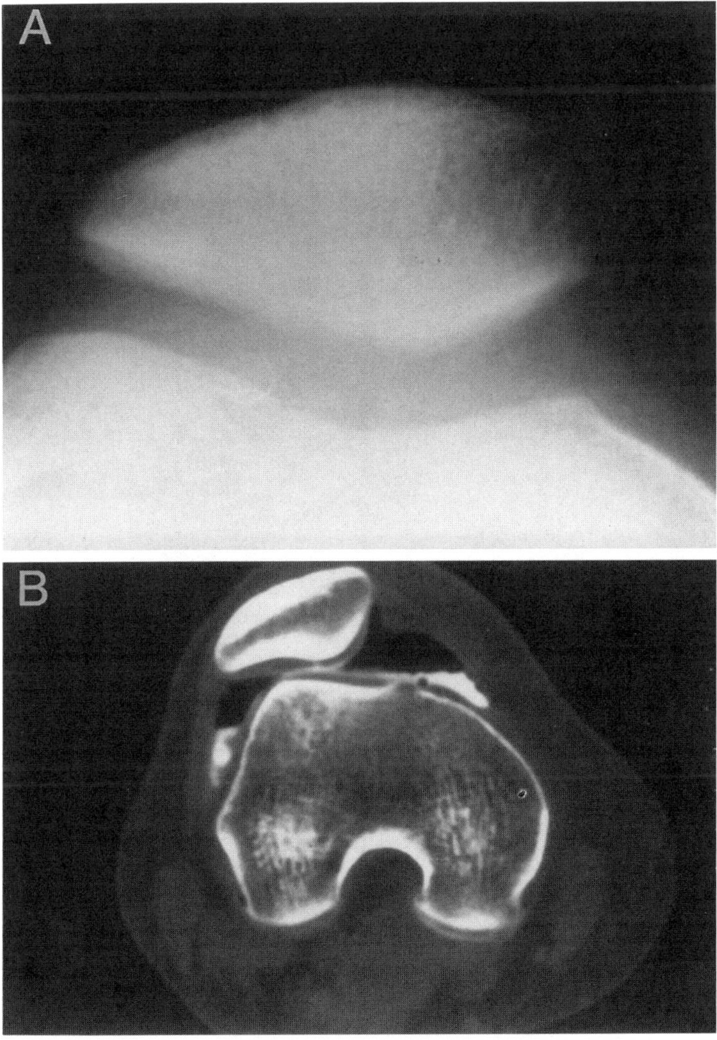

Fig 9–3.—Axial radiograph demonstrating normal patellofemoral indices (**A**), whereas the axial CT arthrogram (**B**) of the same knee shows a combination of lateralization and excessive patellar tilt. Morphological patellar features are different in both images. (Courtesy of Walker C, Cassar-Pullicino VN, Vaisha R, et al: *Br J Radiol* 66:755–761, 1993.)

had positive values on the skyline measurements, indicating a false negative rate of 20%. In 4 of those 10 patients, the measurements were greater than 15 degrees (Fig 9–3). The PFA was below 11 degrees in 35 of 40 cases with CT measurements above zero. Skyline measurement tended to overestimate TD, and there was a tendency toward a negative correlation in the plot of the CA measured on CT and skyline views. When Wiberg's system was used to classify the morphological type of

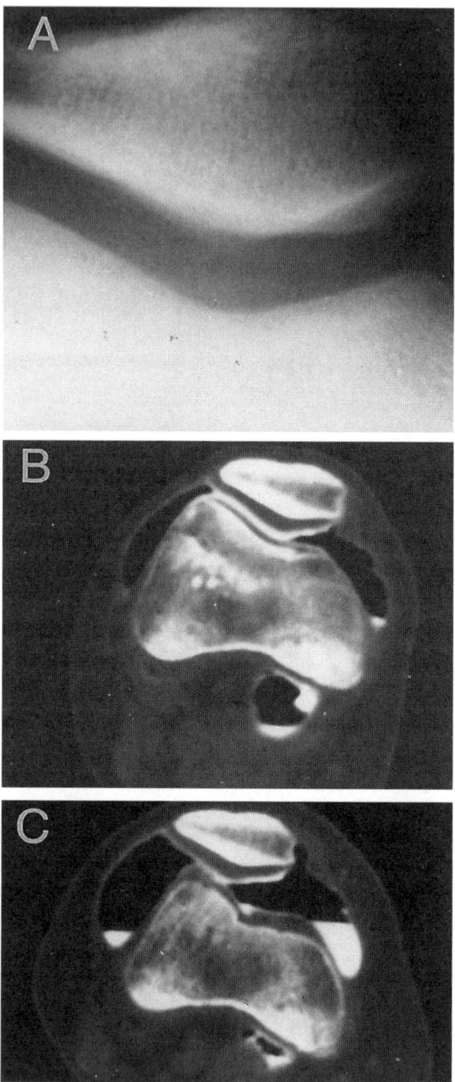

Fig 9–4.—Measurements of patellar position depend on the degree of knee flexion. Axial radiographs (**A**) and CT arthrogram in 30 degrees of flexion (**B**) show seemingly normal patellofemoral indices, which are clearly abnormal in CT arthrogram done in 10 degrees of knee flexion (**C**). (Courtesy of Walker C, Cassar-Pullicino VN, Vaisha R, et al: *Br J Radiol* 66:755–761, 1993.)

patellae, 70% were in group II on skyline views and 58% were in group II on CT. There was little correlation between morphological features of the patella and abnormal functional relationship of the joint.

Conclusion.—Skyline views are inaccurate, primarily because they cannot be obtained in less than 30 degrees of flexion. A large proportion of malaligned patellae appear to be corrected when viewed in 30 degrees of flexion (Fig 9-4). Surgery performed on the basis of skyline views would result in inappropriate operations. Although CT is preferable for the assessment of patellofemoral geometry, measurements must be made on a number of slices. Magnetic resonance imaging is expected to improve the diagnostic yield of CT in this setting.

▶ Anterior knee pain is common and is often ascribed to the patellofemoral articulation. In such instances, it is assumed that there is abnormal pressure on the cartilage of the patellofemoral joint resulting in pain, malacic changes, and cartilage degeneration. This very important paper examined 50 cases of anterior knee pain in which skyline views were obtained (30 degrees, 60 degrees, and 90 degrees of flexion) as well as axial CT imaging. The authors illustrate dramatic examples of maltracking of the patella with normal skyline views. They provide strong evidence to support their statement that surgery based on an abnormal skyline view is inappropriate.—C.B. Sledge, M.D.

The Relationship Between Quadriceps Angle and Anterior Knee Pain Syndrome

Caylor D, Fites R, Worrell TW (Univ of Indianapolis, Ind)
J Orthop Sports Phys Ther 17:11–16, 1993   129-94-9-7

Background.—Patellofemoral joint malalignment is an extrinsic factor in anterior knee pain syndrome (AKPS). This malalignment is commonly assessed by measuring the quadriceps angle (Q-angle)—the acute angle formed by the intersection of the line connecting the anterior superior

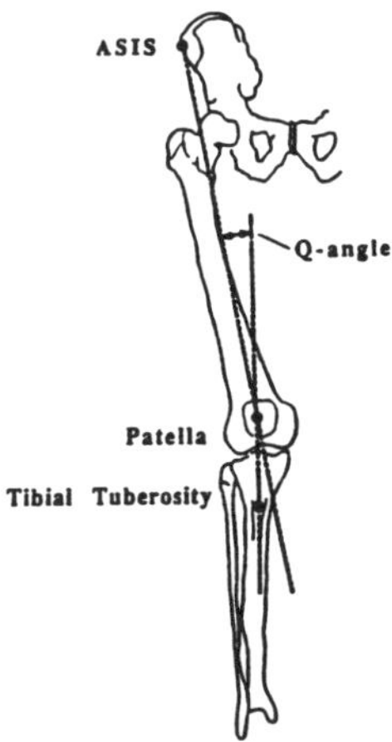

Fig 9–5.—Quadriceps angle (*Q-angle*) landmarks. (From Caylor D, Fites R, Worrell TW: *J Orthop Sports Phys Ther* 17:11–16, 1993. Courtesy of Moss RI, DeVita P, Dawson ML: *J Athl Train* 27:64–69, 1992.)

iliac spine with the midpoint of the patella and the line connecting the tibial tubercle with the midpoint of the patella (Fig 9–5). A study determined the reliability of the Q-angle measurement, quantified the Q-angle associated with knee flexion, and identified Q-angle differences between subjects with AKPS and asymptomatic subjects.

Methods.—The study included symptomatic knees of 50 patients with AKPS and both knees of 26 asymptomatic controls. The Q-angle was measured using a goniometer with subjects standing in 2 positions: with knees extended, and with the knee flexed and the heel on a 1.25-in. lift. The center of the patella and the tibial tubercle were located and marked. One end of a string was held at the anterior superior iliac spine (ASIS); the other end was taped below the midpoint of the patella. The goniometer was centered at the midpoint of the patella with 1 arm aligned with the string leading to the ASIS and the other arm aligned with the tibial tubercle. Each knee was measured twice in each position by 2 testers.

Results.—Intratester Q-angle values did not differ significantly in either position. The mean Q-angle was 12.4 degrees in symptomatic subjects and 11.1 degrees in controls; the between-group difference was not significant.

Conclusion.—The anterior knee pain syndrome appears to result from multiple factors. Therefore, patients with AKPS should be given a complete lower extremity evaluation: quadriceps strength, iliotibial band and hamstring flexibility, foot pronation, and patellar position (Q-angle tilt, glide, and rotation). Therapeutic intervention should also be multifaceted.

▶ Measurement of the Q-angle has been used as a predictor of abnormal tracking leading to anterior knee pain. This careful study looked at the difficulties of measuring the Q-angle, its change with degree of knee flexion, and its lack of relationship to the presence or absence of symptoms.—C.B. Sledge, M.D.

Knee Radiographs: A Substitute for Proper Clinical Examination Within the Accident and Emergency Department?

Pennycook AG, Rai A (Southampton Gen Hosp, England)
Injury 24:383–384, 1993   129-94-9-8

Background.—Most patients who are seen in accident and emergency departments with a knee injury undergo knee radiography. The clinical appropriateness and cost-effectiveness of this practice was evaluated.

Methods.—The records of 178 patients who had visited an accident and emergency department and undergone knee radiography were reviewed. The official radiologist's report, main clinical symptom or sign prompting radiography, and decision regarding the patient were noted.

Results.—There was no radiographic evidence of bony injury in 80.6% of 62 patients seen after a direct blow to the knee, in 90.4% of 104 seen with a twisting injury, or in any of 12 additional patients. The most frequent symptoms prompting a radiograph were bruising and decreased movement after a direct blow, and decreased movement and traumatic effusion after twisting injury. Overall, 49.4% of patients were discharged to their general practitioners, and 43.8% were referred to follow-up clinics. Only 12 patients were admitted to the hospital.

Conclusion.—Many patients who visit an accident and emergency department with a knee injury do not need an immediate radiograph. If symptoms and signs are minimal, particularly in twisting injuries, symptoms should be treated and the patient reassessed within 3 days. At that time, initial pain will have settled, permitting more careful examination of the knee and its ligamentous stability and, hence, determination of the need for a radiograph. This protocol would significantly reduce costs because fewer patients would require radiologic examination. Further, it would permit early detection of bony knee injury while minimizing patient exposure to unnecessary radiation.

▶ In a world without concerns regarding malpractice liability, clinical judgment based on careful history and clinical findings would obviate the need for many radiographs after minor trauma. The authors of this paper found that 90% of knee films in such a setting were entirely normal. They suggest reassessment 3 days after the injury and, if symptoms persist, x-ray studies at that time. The cost savings, if these rules were applied in this country, would be enormous, but some change in the legal climate would be necessary before this policy could be widely adopted.—C.B. Sledge, M.D.

Case Report 817
Kenan S, Abdelwahab IF, Klein MJ, Lewis MM (Mount Sinai Med School, New York)
Skeletal Radiol 22:623–626, 1993   129-94-9–9

Background.—Synovial chondromatosis, a condition of unknown etiology, is self-limiting. Primary chondrosarcoma arising from the synovium and chondrosarcoma secondary to synovial chondromatosis have been reported. In 1 patient, prolonged synovial chondromatosis of the knee joint transformed into a low-grade chondrosarcoma.

Case Report.—Man, 74, reported a long history of intermittent pain and swelling of the right knee and progressive loss of range of motion. He had undergone knee arthroscopy 5 years earlier. Radiographs of the knee revealed punctate calcification in the popliteal region with pressure erosion of the femoral intercondylar notch and lower patellar pole (Fig 9–6). On MR imaging, a large heterogeneous lobulated mass was seen occupying the entire knee joint and involving the popliteal fossa. The signal intensity of the mass was low on T1-weighted images

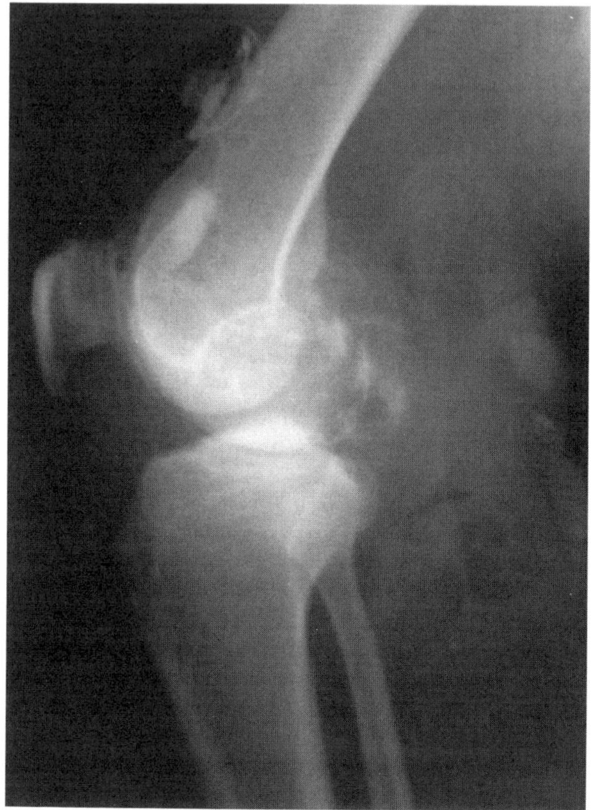

Fig 9–6.—Double-contrast arthrogram of the right knee revealing contrast and air at the periphery of an intra-articular mass that shows fine punctate calcifications. There is significant erosion of the lower pole of the patella. (Courtesy of Kenan S, Abdelwahab IF, Klein MJ, et al: *Skeletal Radiol* 22:623–626, 1993.)

and bright on T2-weighted images (Fig 9–7). On arteriography, the popliteal artery was found to be displaced and stretched over the mass. An open biopsy specimen revealed low-grade chondrosarcoma, with cartilage nodules containing atypical chondrocytes that lost their clustering arrangement in a myxoid background. A review of the histologic slides obtained from the arthroscopy showed synovial chondromatosis. During 2 subsequent surgical procedures, synovial chondromatosis and chondrosarcoma were found to be coexisting. Eighteen months after treatment, the patient was pain-free with improved range of motion.

Conclusion.—This patient had a long history of synovial chondromatosis of the knee joint, which transformed into low-grade chondrosarcoma. In a literature review, 19 cases of synovial chondrosarcoma secondary to synovial chondromatosis were identified (table).

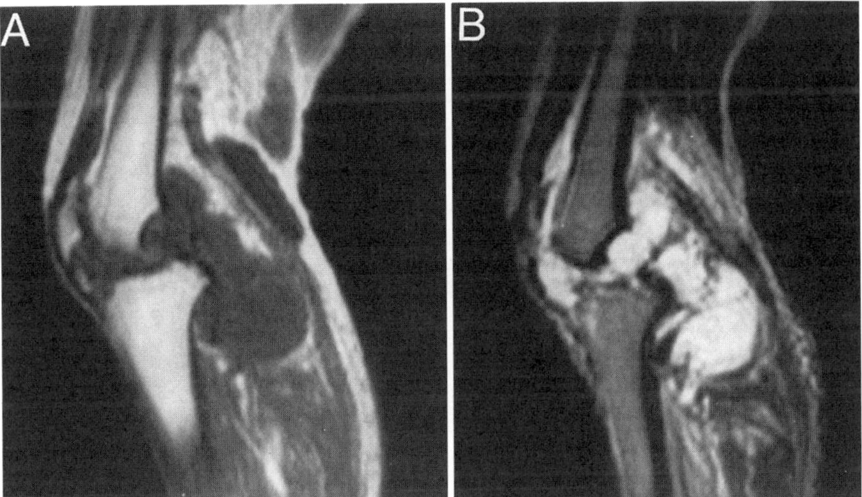

Fig 9–7.—Sagittal MRI of the right knee. **A,** T1-weighted image demonstrating an isointense intra-articular mass. **B,** T2-weighted image revealing a heterogeneous, high-signal-intensity lobular mass. The popliteal artery is displaced and stretched by mass. (Courtesy of Kenan S, Abdelwahab IF, Klein MJ, et al: *Skeletal Radiol* 22:623–626, 1993.)

▶ I usually do not include case reports in the YEAR BOOK OF ORTHOPEDICS, but this report of a case of chondrosarcoma secondary to synovial chondromatosis includes such a good review of the previous literature that it should be mentioned. The authors review the previous 19 cases in the literature, which include 6 patients with no evidence of disease at the time of report. This corrects my mistaken belief that these lesions were rapidly and uniformly fatal.—C.B. Sledge, M.D.

Literature Review on Synovial Chondrosarcoma Secondary to Synovial Chondromatosis

Authors	Age/sex	Duration of symptoms	Location	Treatment	Follow-up
Brannon et al. 1957 [2]	34/M	1 year	Hip	Synovectomy, hemipelvectomy	Lung metastases
Nixon et al. 1960 [16]	33/M	1 year	Knee	AKA	Lung metastases
[3]	72/M	3 years	Knee	Synovectomy, AKA	
Goldman & Lichtenstein 1964 [6]	58/M	10 years	Knee	Synovectomy, AKA	
	41/M	22 years	Knee	Synovectomy	
	37/M	3 years	Knee	Synovectomy	
Mullins et al. 1965 [14]	43/F	14 years	Knee	Synovectomy, hip disarticulation	Lung metastases
King et al. 1967 [10]	43/M	5 years	Knee	Synovectomy, AKA	NED
Dunn et al. 1974 [5]	67/M	25 years	Knee	Hip disarticulation	Lung metastases

Kaiser et al. 1980 [8]	47/F	15 years	Ankle	Synovectomies, BKA	NED
Hamilton et al. 1987 [7]	51/M	26 years	Knee	Hip disarticulation	NED
Perry et al. 1988 [17]	51/F	24 years	Knee	Synovectomy, AKA	Lung metastases
Manivel et al. 1988 [11]	50/M	15 years	Knee	Synovectomies	NED
Bertoni et al. 1991 [1]	47/F	3 years	Hip	Hemipelvectomy	NED
	57/F	10 years	Elbow	Shoulder disarticulation	Lung metastases
	64/F	4 years	Knee	AKA	Lung metastases
	66/F	–	Hip	–	–
	30/M	10 years	Knee	AKA	NED
	40/M	3 years	Knee	Synovectomy	NED

(Courtesy of Kenan S, Abdelwahab IF, Klein MJ, et al: *Skeletal Radiol* 22:623–626, 1993.)

Synovial Hemangioma: A Report of 20 Cases With Differential Diagnostic Considerations

Devaney K, Vinh TN, Sweet DE (Armed Forces Inst of Pathology, Washington, DC; Brown Univ, Providence, RI)
Hum Pathol 24:737–745, 1993 129-94-9–10

Background.—Because they are relatively uncommon, synovial hemangiomas may easily be omitted from the differential diagnosis of joint problems. This condition may mimic the more commonly seen pigmented villonodular synovitis (PVNS) or traumatic hemarthrosis; histologic criteria may be required for reliable identification. It has been suggested that a relationship between PVNS and synovial hemangioma exists, although the latter usually may be treated successfully with surgical excision. This retrospective study examined the clinicopathologic features of synovial hemangioma to determine whether PVNS is a related condition.

Materials and Methods.—Information for the study was obtained from the examination of Armed Forces Institute of Pathology consultation files for the 25 years beginning with 1960. A search for benign vascular lesions of the intra-articular synovium uncovered 26 cases. Twenty of those included hematoxylin-eosin–stained histologic specimens and were included in this study. The size, pattern, wall thickness and makeup, and cells of the sample blood vessels were examined.

Results.—Most patients had complained of pain and/or swelling, although 31% reported no pain. The knee was affected in 60% of patients and the elbow in 30%. Radiologic and arthroscopic studies revealed little about these conditions, aside from the presence of soft tissue masses within the joint that were visible in some cases. Specimens in 45% of the patients were pigmented and had a villus structure in 25%. These masses were pulled from synovial surfaces or from tendon sheaths and did not involve adjoining tissue. Histologic examination revealed examples of cavernous, lobular capillary, venous, and arteriovenous hemangiomas among these specimens.

Discussion.—These benign vascular lesions are difficult to diagnose without histologic confirmation. The essential features that differentiate the more dangerous and often recurrent condition, PVNS, are the presence of large numbers of proliferating histiocytes and multinucleated giant cells. When a similar condition affects the adjoining muscle and/or bone, it may be termed angiomatosis, which is associated with frequent recurrence after surgical removal. No association between synovial hemangioma and PVNS was found.

▶ Synovial hemangiomas are very uncommon lesions of the knee, but 20 cases were found in the files of the Armed Forces Institute of Pathology, leading to this review. Frequent incorrect diagnoses included PVNS and nonspecific synovitis. The authors point out the histologic characteristics of this lesion and clearly differentiate it from pigmented nodular synovitis and other lesions with which it is often confused.—C.B. Sledge, M.D.

Sports Injury

The Accuracy of the Clinical Knee Examination Documented by Arthroscopy: A Prospective Study

Oberlander MA, Shalvoy RM, Hughston JC (Hughston Orthopaedic Clinic, PC, Columbus, Ga; Tulane Univ, New Orleans, La)
Am J Sports Med 21:773–778, 1993   129-94-9–11

Objective.—A prospective study was designed to determine the accuracy of the clinical examination for diagnosing intra-articular injuries of the knee. Various diagnostic tests can document some intra-articular disorders with precision; these tests, however, involve invasive procedures, radiation, or considerable expense.

Patients and Methods.—During a 6-month period, 290 patients (296 knees) were evaluated by history, physical examination, and standard knee radiographs. Ninety-two of the knee injuries were acute and 204 were chronic. Forty-four patients had supplemental diagnostic studies including MRI (41), arthrograms (2), and previous arthroscopy (1). The preoperative diagnosis was compared with findings at arthroscopy. Each type of lesion was analyzed to determine the sensitivity, specificity, and accuracy of the diagnostic testing.

Results.—The clinical diagnosis was correct in 56% of the knees, incomplete in 31%, and incorrect in 13%. A total of 509 lesions were found at surgery. The preoperative diagnosis was correct in 72% of the cases with only 1 lesion identified at arthroscopy but in only 30% of the knees in which 3 or more pathologic entities were discovered. The sensitivity, specificity, and accuracy of the diagnostic testing varied for different types of lesions. Chondral fractures, fibrotic fat pads, tears in the anterior cruciate ligament, and loose bodies were the lesions most difficult to diagnose. Acute lesions and solitary lesions were significantly easier to diagnose.

Conclusion.—Multiple lesions are common in patients with knee injuries. The ability to diagnose all such lesions clinically is extremely low. Although the preoperative diagnosis was at least partially correct in 87% of the knees in this series, many lesions were missed. Chondral fractures, missed in 85% of the patients, were particularly difficult to identify. The use of MRI did not significantly improve intra-articular diagnoses.

▶ In this era of cost containment, it is important to document the accuracy of clinical examination so that unnecessary and expensive examinations, such as MRI and arthroscopy, can be avoided whenever possible. Unfortunately, this paper demonstrates that the clinical examination, even in the hands of experienced knee surgeons, is not very reliable. In this series of 296 knees, clinical examination was correct only 56% of the time. Injuries of the lateral meniscus were most difficult to detect on clinical examination as were lesions of the posterior horn of the medial meniscus. The reported accuracy of clinical diagnosis of severe anterior cruciate ligament injuries ranges from 38% to 95% correct. Chondral fractures were the most frequently missed lesions and were missed 85% of the time. It is significant that an anterior cruciate ligament tear was missed in 38% of the patients in the study, in contrast to previous studies. It is difficult, from this paper, to answer the more important question: How often are important lesions missed, especially lesions that might be picked up on MRI? To complete the diagnostic algorithm, that information would have to be obtained in addition to cost data so that a cost-effectiveness algorithm for diagnosis of the injured knee could be constructed.—C.B. Sledge, M.D.

Can MRI of the Knee Affect Arthroscopic Practice? A Prospective Study of 58 Patients

Spiers ASD, Meagher T, Ostlere SJ, Wilson DJ, Dodd CAF (Nuffield Orthopaedic Centre, Oxford, England)
J Bone Joint Surg (Br) 75-B:49–52, 1993   129-94-9–12

TABLE 1.—Accuracy and Predictive Value of the Surgeon's Clinical Decision to Perform Arthroscopy

True positive	23
True negative	12
False positive	16
False negative	7
Positive predictive value	*59%*
Negative predictive value	*63%*
Sensitivity	*77%*
Specificity	*43%*

Note: As related to those patients in whom there were lesions potentially treatable by arthroscopy or in whom biopsies were taken.

(Courtesy of Spiers ASD, Meagher T, Ostlere SJ, et al: *J Bone Joint Surg (Br)* 75-B:49–52, 1993.)

TABLE 2.—Accuracy and Predictive Value of MRI in Determining the Need for Arthroscopy

True positive	31
True negative	17
False positive	10
False negative	0
Positive predictive value	*74%*
Negative predictive value	*100%*
Sensitivity	*100%*
Specificity	*63%*

(Courtesy of Spiers ASD, Meagher T, Ostlere SJ, et al: *J Bone Joint Surg (Br)* 75-B:49–52, 1993.)

Introduction.—Compared with arthroscopy, MRI has proven to be accurate in the assessment of internal knee derangements. However, there are questions regarding the relative value of the 2 methods in the management of patients in whom internal derangements are suspected, with 1 report suggesting that MRI could avoid the need for diagnostic arthroscopy in one third to one half of the patients.

Methods.—The effectiveness of MRI in negating the need for arthroscopy was determined in a prospective study of 58 consecutive patients referred with suspected internal derangement of the knee. The 37 men and 21 women had an average age of 29 years. All had 3-dimensional gradient echo intermediate-weighted MRI studies of the symptomatic knee performed by a radiologist before arthroscopy was performed by the orthopedic surgeon; the latter had no knowledge of the MRI results.

Findings.—Arthroscopy detected 33 tears of the menisci; all but 1 was seen on MRI, and it was confirmed by a second look. There were 14 false positive tears. All complete cruciate ligament tears were seen, but MRI missed some partial tears and did not detect ligament laxity. The preoperative clinical examination had a sensitivity of 77% and a specificity of 43%, compared to 100% and 63%, respectively, for MRI. For articular cartilage lesions, MRI had a sensitivity of only 18% but a specificity of 100%. The relative abilities of MRI and clinical judgment to predict the presence of a lesion remediable by arthroscopic surgery, such as an unstable meniscal lesion, are shown in Tables 1 and 2. A 29% reduction in the number of arthroscopies could have been achieved if the decision had been based on the results of MRI.

Conclusion.—Magnetic resonance imaging is a reliable method for studying internal derangement of the knee. It detects complete tears of the cruciate ligaments sensitively and specifically, but it is less sensitive and specific for partial tears or ligamentous laxity. It is still sensitive, but less specific, for meniscal tears. Nevertheless, a substantial number of patients may be able to avoid arthroscopy, with the reduction in morbidity and time saved more than making up for the increased cost.

▶ A partial answer to the questions raised by the previous paper (Abstract 129-94-9–11) is provided in this paper in which the authors found out that MRI could have reduced the number of arthroscopies by 29% without missing any significant meniscal lesions. They point out the inaccuracy of MRI in diagnosing injuries to articular cartilage, but the development of intravenous contrast agents to enhance the intra-articular structures seen on MRI may improve that situation in the near future. Although the cost savings realized in this study were minimal, the authors correctly point out the value in avoiding arthroscopy (when not necessary) in terms of patient morbidity and overuse of facilities.—C.B. Sledge, M.D.

Knee Function After Anterior Cruciate Ligament Ruptures Treated Conservatively
Engström B, Gornitzka J, Johansson C, Wredmark T (Huddinge Univ, Sweden)
Int Orthop 17:208–213, 1993   129-94-9–13

Introduction.—Ruptures of the anterior cruciate ligament (ACL) are a common type of injury among athletes. Some studies have reported that rupture of the ACL need not prevent a return to strenuous sporting activity, but others contradict such findings. The natural course of conservatively treated ACL ruptures was examined in 39 patients who were excluded from ACL reconstruction because of primarily good functional stability.

Patients and Methods.—Thirty-nine patients with a mean age of 34 years took part in the study. All of their ACL ruptures had been treated conservatively. Twelve of the ruptures were chronic; 23 had occurred during athletic activity. Twenty-one patients had associated injuries at the time of the ACL rupture. Arthroscopy was used to confirm the diagnosis in 34 cases. Before and after rehabilitation, all patients performed a Cybex test and filled in the Lysholm score form. At a mean of 5.1 years after rehabilitation, patients were evaluated for subjective function, laxity, and muscle performance.

Results.—There was a significant increase in the knee extensor and flexor injured/uninjured torque ratio from the initial test to the test after rehabilitation and through follow-up. In all tests, extensor and flexor peak torque was significantly lower in the injured than the uninjured knee. There was a significant increase in the Lysholm score from the initial to the postrehabilitation test. Thirty patients reduced their activity level, 28 because of the knee injury. Instability and pain were common, and no patients were free of symptoms. The 1-leg-hop and instrumental knee joint laxity tests revealed significant impairment at follow-up.

Conclusion.—Most patients experience functional impairment after conservative treatment of ACL ruptures. Subjective scores were better indicators of functional stability than performance tests. Despite thorough initial rehabilitation, few patients were pleased with their knee function. The use of the pivot-shift test may help to predict which patients might benefit from conservative treatment.

▶ Patients with ACL ruptures are frequently advised to pursue a conservative course until it is obvious that important functions are adversely affected. This paper reports on a population of young patients treated conservatively and followed for an average of 5 years. Few patients were pleased with their function, and function was not found to be related to measures of knee joint laxity. The study confirms the current advice that patients electing conservative management for ACL rupture must anticipate decreased levels of functional activity and avoidance of strenuous athletics involving pivoting.—C.B. Sledge, M.D.

Proprioception After Rupture of the Anterior Cruciate Ligament: An Objective Indication of the Need for Surgery?
Beard DJ, Kyberd PJ, Fergusson CM, Dodd CAF (Nuffield Orthopaedic Centre, Oxford, England; Royal Berkshire Hosp, Reading, England)
J Bone Joint Surg (Br) 75-B:311–315, 1993   129-94-9–14

Background.—In deficiency of the anterior cruciate ligament (ACL), mechanical instability allows forward subluxation of the tibia on the femur and impairs knee function. Conservative management with physiotherapy is attempted before surgery. The success of conservative treatment and the need for surgery are usually assessed by the patient's evaluation. An objective measurement of the ability of the muscles to protect the subluxing joint by reflex contraction would facilitate the decision for or against surgery. In this study, the protective ability of the hamstrings, in terms of reflex contraction latency, was used as an indirect measure of the proprioceptive ability of the joint. Proprioception was defined as static awareness of the joint position, kinesthetic awareness, and closed-loop efferent activity required for the reflex response and the regulation of muscle stiffness.

Method.—Hamstring contraction latency, laxity, and functional results were measured in 30 patients with unilateral ACL deficiency and 20 controls.

Findings.—The mean latency of reflex hamstring contraction in the injured leg of patients with ACL deficiency was 99 ms compared with 53 ms in the unaffected limb. The differential latency and the frequency of reported episodes of giving way were significantly correlated, suggesting that functional instability may result, in part, from loss of proprioception.

Conclusion.—The latency of reflex hamstring contraction in 30 patients with ACL deficiency was significantly greater in ACL-deficient knees than in noninjured knees. Increased reflex hamstring contraction latency was directly related to the functional instability of the knee. This measure of proprioception can be used to provide objective data for the management of patients with chronic ACL deficiency.

▶ The previous paper (Abstract 129-94-9–13) pointed out the lack of correlation between patients' function and measures of knee laxity after ACL rupture. This paper offers what is perhaps an explanation for the lack of relationship between objective measures of knee stability and patient function. The authors found that faulty proprioception may increase functional instability, whereas patients with normal proprioceptive sensation may be able to compensate by reflex muscle contraction.—C.B. Sledge, M.D.

Anti-Inflammatory Drug Therapy After Arthroscopy of the Knee: A Prospective, Randomised, Controlled Trial of Diclofenac or Physiotherapy
Birch NC, Sly C, Brooks S, Powles DP (North Middlesex Hosp, London; Solihull Hosp, England; Lister Hosp, Stevenage, England)
J Bone Joint Surg (Br) 75-B:650–652, 1993   129-94-9–15

Background.—Arthroscopic meniscectomy is associated with considerable postoperative pain and swelling. The use of nonsteroidal anti-inflammatory drugs (NSAIDs) after such surgery has been advocated and tested, as has a regimen of physiotherapy. However, NSAIDs are expensive and have potentially deleterious side effects. The 2 methods were compared to determine which provides a better outcome.

Patients and Methods.—The study included 120 patients who had undergone meniscectomy at 2 hospitals. Patients were randomly assigned to the 2 treatment arms and a control group; the NSAID group received 75 mg of IM diclofenac sodium immediately after the surgery and 100 mg per day for the following 7 days. The physiotherapy group all received daily treatments from the same therapist. The operations revealed an assortment of conditions, including normal findings, torn menisci, degenerated cartilage, and loose bodies. Patients were assessed with the Noyes score before surgery and at 7, 14, and 42 days after surgery by a physician blinded to treatment method. Scores were analyzed with 2-way analysis of variance.

Results.—No significant difference in Noyes score was seen between the treatment and control groups at any of the postoperative follow-ups. Differences were within the limits of clinical variation. However, among the NSAID-treated group, 5 of 52 patients reported headache and gastrointestinal upset after the 7-day treatment. Those symptoms resolved at the 14-day follow-up.

Discussion.—Contrary to some previous studies, these results do not support the use of NSAIDs or physiotherapy after arthroscopy, particularly when the side effects are considered. Reasons for the different results obtained by other clinical studies may derive from the use of different assessment methods; the Noyes score used here is a relatively comprehensive assessment technique.

▶ It is common practice in many centers to give patients NSAIDs and physical therapy after arthroscopic procedures. This paper points out the lack of benefit from either treatment. The expense of physical therapy and the nearly 10% complication rate from NSAIDs leads these authors to recommend avoidance of both modalities.—C.B. Sledge, M.D.

Long-Distance Running Causes Site-Dependent Decrease of Cartilage Glycosaminoglycan Content in the Knee Joints of Beagle Dogs
Arokoski J, Kiviranta I, Jurvelin J, Tammi M, Helminen HJ (Univ of Kuopio, Finland)
Arthritis Rheum 36:1451–1459, 1993   129-94-9–16

Background.—Joint unloading by immobilization and diminished weight-bearing leads to transient or permanent atrophy of the articular cartilage. Although a certain amount of joint loading is probably needed to maintain normal cartilage properties, the role of increased joint loading on cartilage condition is not defined. The effects of running exercise on the thickness and glycosaminoglycan (GAG) content of articular cartilage was examined in young canine knee and humeral head cartilage.

Method.—After a 1-year program of running exercise up to 40 km/ day, samples were obtained from 12 different locations of the canine joints. A detailed, area-specific analysis measured the thickness of articular cartilage. The distribution of Safranin O stain that binds stoichiometrically to GAG was determined by quantitative microspectrophotometric analysis.

Results.—Depletion of GAG by running exercise was restricted to prominent weight-bearing areas of the joint. The GAG content was reduced in the lateral condyle of the femur, extending into the intermediate zone, and was significantly reduced in the superficial zone at the lateral condyle of the tibia and the head of the humerus. Running also decreased the GAG content of the uncalcified articular cartilage in the weight-bearing summits of the femoral condyles, but it had no significant effect on cartilage thickness at the summits or marginal areas of the femoral condyles. Similarly, the GAG concentration in the patellofemoral region was also unaltered by running.

Conclusion.—Depletion of GAG by long-distance running is site-dependent. It was restricted to prominent weight-bearing areas of the joint beginning from the superficial cartilage without signs of degeneration. The loss of GAG may be attributable to the breakdown of proteoglycans, which may affect the condition of articular cartilage, especially after long-term joint loading.

▶ Can the normal joint be overloaded to the point at which osteoarthritis develops? If so, shouldn't marathon runners and rowers all have arthritic joints? There has been no clear answer to that question, although Lane and co-workers (1) noted an absence of arthritic changes in long-distance runners. This study in dogs shows that the critically important cartilage component, proteoglycan, is depleted in response to vigorous levels of activity in the beagle. The authors attribute the lack of arthritic change to the fact that the proteoglycan can be replaced after depletion, whereas the underlying collagen structure, which cannot be replaced, was not injured. They point out, however, that the collagen network is more susceptible to injury when the proteoglycan is depleted and suggest that overload of the joint in that state could produce permanent damage.—C.B. Sledge, M.D.

Reference

1. Lane NE, et al: *JAMA* 255:1147, 1986.

Surgical Treatment of Acute Type-V Acromioclavicular Injuries in Athletes
Verhaven E, DeBoeck H, Haentjens P, Handelberg F, Casteleyn PP, Opdecam P (Free Univ of Brussels, Belgium)
Arch Orthop Trauma Surg 112:189–192, 1993   129-94-9–17

Background.—The optimal treatment for Allman's grade III acromioclavicular injuries is controversial because this grade has not been clearly defined. The Rockwood classification system corresponds with Allman grades I–III, except that grade III is further subdivided. A Rockwood type V injury is a very severe Allman grade III injury. Medium-term results of surgical treatment for acute type V acromioclavicular injuries in athletes were evaluated prospectively.

Methods.—Eighteen athletes with acute type V acromioclavicular joint injury underwent surgical implantation of a double velour Dacron coracoclavicular cerclage within 24 hours of injury. All patients were reassessed after a mean of 6 years. Follow-up entailed clinical functional evaluation using the Imatani system and comparison of presurgical and contemporary radiographs.

Results.—Satisfactory results were obtained in 66.7% of shoulders. All patients returned to preinjury levels of sports activity within a mean of 12 weeks; the sports involved were soccer, bicycle racing, motorcycle racing, and car racing. At follow-up, loss of reduction was apparent in 44.4% of shoulders. Additional complications included calcification or ossification of the coracoclavicular ligaments in 50% of patients, clavicular erosion at the graft site in 33.3%, and osteolytic changes of the distal clavicle in 33.3%.

Conclusion.—In this population of athletes, surgical treatment for acute type V acromioclavicular lesions provided fewer good results than similar treatment for type III lesions in a mixed population: Nearly half of the patients in this study experienced a loss of reduction. However, the degree of residual dislocation, the development of post-traumatic arthritis, or the presence of distal clavicular coracoclavicular ossification or osteolysis did not interfere with the clinical results or the level of postinjury sports activity.

▶ Will there ever be a consensus on how to treat acromioclavicular separations? Probably not. In this paper, the results of surgical treatment of severe, complete acromioclavicular separations were examined. There were frequent complications, including loss of reduction in 44% and a complete lack of correlation between the degree of residual dislocation, the development of post-traumatic arthritis, or other radiographic changes and the clinical result. One third of patients had a clinically unsatisfactory result. Perhaps the operative approach in this series, which involved the use of a Dacron loop without the repair of the ligaments and without excision of the distal clavicle, could not be expected to produce better results.—C.B. Sledge, M.D.

Blood Replacement After Hip and Knee Surgery

The Cost-Effectiveness of Preoperative Autologous Blood Donation for Total Hip and Knee Replacement
Birkmeyer JD, Goodnough LT, AuBuchon JP, Noordsij PG, Littenberg B (Dartmouth-Hitchcock Med Ctr, Lebanon, NH; Washington Univ, St Louis, Mo)
Transfusion 33:544–551, 1993   129-94-9–18

Background.—The frequency of preoperative autologous blood donation is rising dramatically. However, the cost-effectiveness of this procedure has not been fully explored. A decision analysis was done to determine the cost-effectiveness of autologous blood donation for hip and knee replacement.

Methods.—Data on red blood cell use in 629 patients having surgery at 2 tertiary care centers were used in the analysis. Cost-effectiveness was expressed as cost per quality-adjusted year of life saved.

Findings.—At centers 1 and 2, autologous blood donation for bilateral and revision joint replacement cost $40,000 and $241,000, respectively, per quality-adjusted year of life saved. For primary unilateral hip replacement, autologous blood donation cost $373,000 and $740,000 per quality-adjusted year of life saved at centers 1 and 2, respectively. The procedure was least cost-effective for primary unilateral knee replacement. Variations among procedures in the cost-effectiveness of autologous blood donation were explained by the differences between autologous blood collections and transfusion requirements. The poorer cost-effectiveness documented at center 2 was a result of higher transfusion rates in autologous blood donors than in nondonors.

Conclusion.—Autologous blood donation is not as cost-effective as most accepted medical procedures. Avoiding overcollection and overtransfusion of autologous blood may greatly improve its cost-effectiveness.

▶ Predonation of blood or subsequent autologous transfusion after hip or knee replacement surgery has become very common in this country with much of the stimulus coming from concern about the safety of allogeneic blood, especially regarding HIV transmission. The authors of this paper point out that, although autologous transfusion is safe and effective, it is not cost-effective, primarily because too many units are obtained before surgery and there is a strong tendency to give back the blood, even when clinical and laboratory parameters suggest that transfusion is not necessary. The costs associated with such overcollection and overtransfusion make the general practice of autologous blood collection expensive. Avoidance of those 2 errors, however, would improve the cost-effectiveness of the procedure. The finding that it costs from $1.147 to $1.467 million dollars for each quality-adjusted year of life saved in primary unilateral knee replacement suggests that for such a procedure, autologous predonation will never be cost-effective.—C.B. Sledge, M.D.

Effect of Postoperative Reinfusion Systems on Hemoglobin Levels in Primary Total Hip and Total Knee Arthroplasties: A Prospective Randomized Study

Mauerhan DR, Nussman D, Mokris JG, Beaver WB (Miller Orthopaedic Clinic, Charlotte, NC; Carolinas Med Ctr, Charlotte, NC)
J Arthroplasty 8:523–527, 1993   129-94-9–19

Introduction.—Blood transfusion is often required because of perioperative blood loss in patients undergoing total hip arthroplasty (THA) and total knee arthroplasty (TKA). Because of the risk of viral disease transmission, several studies have examined the feasibility of postoperative collection and reinfusion of shed blood in these procedures. This prospective, randomized study sought to quantify the effect of reinfusion of postoperative shed blood drainage on hemoglobin levels in patients undergoing elective primary THA and TKA.

Patients and Methods.—Patients were assigned to a standard postoperative collection-drainage system (ConstaVac) or a blood collection-reinfusion system (CBC ConstaVac). The systems differ in that the latter has an umbrella valve that ensures that the top 100 mL of fluid containing serum, fat, and bone debris does not leave the reservoir. All patients were encouraged to donate 2 units of autologous blood before surgery. Intraoperative blood transfusion was left to the discretion of the operating surgeon. Postoperative drainage volumes were recorded for both groups and the volume of reinfused blood was recorded for the study group.

Results.—Fifty-seven patients (35 TKAs and 22 THAs) received the CBC ConstaVac reinfusion system, and 54 (34 TKAs and 20 THAs) received a ConstaVac collection unit. Postoperative hemoglobin levels, recorded on postoperative days 1, 3, and 6, showed no statistically significant difference between the control and study groups. Hemoglobin levels and drainage volumes were similar in both THA and TKA study groups compared to their respective control groups. The mean volume of blood available for reinfusion in the first 6 hours was 360 mL in the study group. Only 2 of 57 patients would have had a significant enough volume in the second 6-hour period to allow additional reinfusion. Ninety-three percent of the units transfused were autologous units.

Conclusion.—Most transfusion requirements for elective primary THA and TKA can be met by a well-designed and administered autologous blood program. The risk of receiving homologous blood appeared to be a question of whether autologous blood was available, rather than whether a reinfusion unit was used. Thus, reinfusion units are not routinely needed in THAs and TKAs.

▶ An alternative to autologous predonation of blood is the use of recovery systems for blood shed during and immediately after arthroplasty. In this prospective, randomized study, no statistically significant difference in postoperative hemoglobin levels was found between the study group (in whom blood was reinfused after arthroplasty) and the control group (in whom postoperative drainage was discarded). The authors argue against the use of both reinfusion and autologous predonation blood together as being neither cost-efficient nor necessary.—C.B. Sledge, M.D.

Survival and Half-Life of Red Cells Salvaged After Hip and Knee Replacement Surgery

Umlas J, Jacobson MS, Kevy SV (Harvard Med School, Boston; Children's Hosp, Boston)
Transfusion 33:591–593, 1993 129-94-9–20

Background.—Studies of red blood cell survival after intraoperative salvage have not included hip and knee arthroplasty. Postoperative salvage and transfusion of unwashed hip and knee drainage may reduce the need for allogeneic blood. Only small volumes of red blood cells are lost after hip and knee replacement; thus, it would be important to know red blood cell viability. Survival and half-life of salvaged and peripheral red blood cells were compared in 6 patients undergoing hip or knee replacement.

Methods.—Fluid drainage from the joint was collected in an unanticoagulated bag for 3 hours after hip or knee arthroplasty; red blood cells were labeled with radioactive chromium and ascorbate. A sample of peripheral venous blood was drawn and labeled with nonradioactive chromium. Both labeled specimens were transfused and venous samples were drawn at 10, 15, and 20 minutes within the subsequent 18–24 hours, and after 2, 3, 5, 7, and 14 days.

Results.—The average survival and half-life of both sets of red blood cells were slightly less than normal. Nevertheless, survival and half-life were comparable in salvaged and venous red blood cells.

Comment.—The amount of red blood cells salvaged during the first 6 hours after hip and knee arthroplasty is generally small, representing only a small part of total perioperative red blood cell loss. Therefore, it may not be medically effective to collect red blood cells after these procedures even though their survival and durability are normal. The potentially life-threatening, profound hypotension and upper airway edema associated with the use of unwashed, postoperatively salvaged blood provides additional arguments against routine use of this material.

▶ Here is another convincing argument against reinfusion of drainage from hip and knee arthroplasties.—C.B. Sledge, M.D.

Infections

The Treatment of Infected Nonunions With Gentamicin-Polymethyl-methacrylate Antibiotic Beads

Calhoun JH, Henry SL, Anger DM, Cobos JA, Mader JT (Univ of Texas, Galveston; Univ of Louisville, Ky)
Clin Orthop 295:23–27, 1993   129-94-9–21

Background.—Amputation rates and failure of therapy for patients with chronic osteomyelitis are highest when an infected nonunion is present. Among the wide range of treatment techniques is polymethyl methacrylate (PMMA) antibiotic beads, which have recently been used to augment parenteral antibiotics for bone infection therapy. The local use of antibiotic beads was compared with the long-term use of systemic parenteral antibiotics in the treatment of the infected nonunion.

Method.—Fifty-two patients with infected nonunions were enrolled in the study. They were divided into group 1, which included 24 patients treated with débridement and intravenous antibiotics for 4 weeks, and group 2, which consisted of 28 patients treated with débridement, gentamicin–polymethyl methacrylate beads and perioperative broad-spectrum parenteral antibiotics. In both groups, nonunions were treated with the appropriate reconstruction. The treatment of infection was considered successful if no signs or symptoms of osteomyelitis were seen from the time of surgery through the end of the follow-up period. Nonunions were considered united if the patient was able to fully bear weight and had no pain or motion at the nonunion site, and if the union was confirmed by radiographs.

Results.—Infection was halted in 83.3% of patients in group 1, compared with 89.3% in group 2. Nonunions were successfully healed in 83.3% of group 1, compared with 85.7% of group 2. Four cases in group 1 and 3 in group 2 were considered failures and remained infected and unhealed. Cost analysis revealed that the only significant difference between the 2 groups was for outpatient home therapy for the parenteral antibiotic group.

Conclusion.—The use of PMMA antibiotic beads is a successful and cost-effective technique in the treatment of chronic osteomyelitis. This study showed no major complications from bead removal. The procedure does require a planned second surgery; however, the operation for placing an indwelling catheter is avoided, as is the need for 4–6 weeks of parenteral antibiotics.

▶ Gentamicin-impregnated polymethyl methacrylate beads were shown to be very effective in the eradication of infection in 2 groups of patients with nonunions. One group was treated with débridement and IV antibiotics for 4 weeks and the other group was treated with débridement and impregnated beads. The group treated with parenteral antibiotics had outpatient costs ranging from approximately $4,000–$48,000 for administration of the antibiotics. This produced an average additional charge of $14,000 in the group treated by IV antibiotics and, given the similar success rates in the 2 groups, argues for the use of implanted beads.—C.B. Sledge, M.D.

Treatment of Experimental Osteomyelitis With Antibiotic-Impregnated Bone Graft Substitute
Cornell CN, Tyndall D, Waller S, Lane JM, Brause BD (Hosp for Special Surgery/Cornell Univ, New York; Stanford Univ, Calif)
J Orthop Res 11:619–626, 1993   129-94-9–22

Introduction.—The current standard treatment of chronic osteomyelitis consists of complete surgical débridement of necrotic and infected tissues and prolonged parenteral antibiotic therapy. A possible alternative to parenteral therapy—depot administration of antibiotic agents—achieves high local levels of the drug with little risk of systemic toxicity. The use of gentamicin-loaded hydroxyapatite ceramic beads as a depot carrier in chronic osteomyelitis was examined.

Methods.—Osteomyelitis was induced in the left tibia of New Zealand White rabbits using a modification of the model of Norden. When radiographs confirmed development of osteomyelitis 21 days after inoculation, the animals were randomly assigned to 1 of 3 treatment protocols. The animals were anesthetized and the osteomyelitic cavity was débrided of all necrotic bone and grossly infected material. All cavities were irrigated with 100 mL of normal saline solution. Eight animals had no material packed into the bone defect (group I); 9 had the defect packed with 40 mg of plain hydroxyapatite beads (group II); and 13 had 40 mg of gentamicin-impregnated hydroxyapatite beads packed into the defect (group III). The animals were killed after 40 days of observation and secondary débridement. Nine more animals (group III+) were treated as in group III but were observed for an additional 59 days.

Results.—At the time of primary débridement, the infection was well localized to the proximal tibia in all animals. There was persistent infection at secondary débridement in all group I and group II animals but no evidence of purulence or infection in group III animals. Six of the group III+ animals had complete healing of the metaphyseal site 120 days after inoculation. The remaining 3 animals in this group had chronically unhealed sinus tracts over the site of infection. Intraoperative swab cultures showed no evidence of improvement or of increasing infection during the longer observation period of group III+.

Conclusion.—In this animal model, gentamicin-loaded hydroxyapatite beads effectively eradicated bacteria from the site of experimentally induced osteomyelitis. The success of the delivery system may be attributed to the use of gentamicin crobefat, a poorly soluble salt of gentamicin.

▶ The previous paper (Abstract 129-94-9–21) demonstrated that the major complication in the implantation of antibiotics impregnated with methacrylate beads was the need for a second operation to remove the beads. In this animal study, a bone graft substitute impregnated with antibiotics was shown to be effective in eradicating bacteria from a site of experimentally induced osteomyelitis and the necessity for a second operative procedure was avoided.—C.B. Sledge, M.D.

In Vitro Pharmacokinetics of Antibiotic Release From Locally Implantable Materials

Miclau T, Dahners LE, Lindsey RW (Univ of North Carolina, Chapel Hill; Baylor College of Medicine, Houston)
J Orthop Res 11:627–632, 1993   129-94-9–23

Introduction.—The IV administration of antibiotics to patients treated for open fractures or osteomyelitis has several drawbacks, including potential toxicity and a lack of adequate local tissue levels. An alternative method involves the local deposition of antibiotics using various substances as a delivery vehicle. This in vitro study compared 4 such substances for their antibiotic-releasing characteristics.

Methods.—The substances studied were cancellous bone graft (BG), demineralized bone matrix (DBM), plaster of paris (POP), and polymethyl methacrylate cement (PMMA). Tobramycin was mixed with each of the substances at a concentration of 25 mg/g of substance, and cylindrical pellets of uniform size (6 × 4 mm) were prepared. Six samples were tested for the BG and DBM groups, and 4 samples were tested for the POP and PMMA groups. The pellets were suspended in phosphate-buffered saline, and the antibiotic concentration in the buffer was determined by an immunoassay at 1, 2, 4, 7, 14, and 21 days.

Results.—By 24 hours, BG and DBM had eluted 70% and 45%, respectively, of their antibiotic load. Both substances released only negligible amounts of tobramycin after 1 week. Plaster of paris released 17% of its load and PMMA released only 6.7% on the first day. Trace amounts of the antibiotic could be detected with PMMA for as long as 2 weeks and with POP for up to 3 weeks. After the fourth day, PMMA and POP eluted significantly more antibiotic than either BG or DBM. The PMMA and POP pellets also maintained their integrity for significantly longer periods than did BG or DBM pellets. Some DBM pellets disintegrated as early as day 3.

Conclusion.—The 4 substances tested showed significant differences in their release of antibiotics and time to disintegration of the pellets. When long-term coverage is required, as for patients with established osteomyelitis, POP and PMMA may be advantageous. A brief period of coverage with high levels of the antibiotic, as for acute contaminated open fractures, might be achieved with BG or DBM.

▶ One of the critical factors when evaluating various implantable delivery systems for antibiotics is the rate of release of the antibiotic from the implantable material. This in vitro study demonstrated significant differences in the rate of release of antibiotics from the various materials and suggests that different carrier substances should be used depending on the clinical situation, how high a level of antibiotics is desired, and for how long.—C.B. Sledge, M.D.

Unicompartmental Knee Arthroplasty

Unicompartment Arthroplasty for Osteoarthrosis of the Knee
Sisto DJ, Blazina ME, Heskiaoff D, Hirsh LC (Blazina Orthopedic Clinic, Sherman Oaks, Calif)
Clin Orthop 286:149–153, 1993   129-94-9–24

Background.—How best to manage patients having single-compartment osteoarthrosis or osteonecrosis of the knee remains controversial. Unicompartmental knee arthroplasty (UKA) results in less loss of bone stock than total knee arthroplasty. In addition, it preserves both cruciate ligaments and the patellofemoral articulation, allows a greater range of motion, and probably carries a lower risk of infection.

Series.—The results of 61 medial compartment knee arthroplasties in 55 patients followed for 2–6 years after operation were reviewed. A Robert Brigham UKA was performed in all instances. The mean patient age at the time of surgery was 65 years. The knees were rated by the Knee Society Clinical Rating System.

Results.—The results were excellent in 70% of patients, good in 10%, fair in 10%, and poor in 10%. The preoperative scores for pain, range of motion, and stability averaged 54 out of a maximum 100 points, but after operation the scores averaged 87 points. At least 1 radiolucent line was associated with 16 femoral and 15 tibial components. Four of the 6 failures were in patients having lucent lines at both sites.

Recommendations.—Other investigators have concluded that, in properly selected patients, UKA provides a subjectively better knee than total knee arthroplasty, with a wider range of motion and little or no pain. High tibial osteotomy is indicated for active patients up to age 55 years. Sedentary patients aged 50 years and all those aged 55 years and older with single-compartment disease should undergo UKA. This procedure is also indicated for sedentary patients aged 70 years and older who have early to moderate changes in a second compartment. Suitable patients with advanced 3-compartment changes should have total knee arthroplasty.

The Natural History of Unicompartmental Arthroplasty: An Eight-Year Follow-Up Study With Survivorship Analysis
Swank M, Stulberg SD, Jiganti J, Machairas S (Northwestern Univ, Chicago; Tacoma Orthopaedic Surgeons, Wash)
Clin Orthop 286:130–142, 1993   129-94-9–25

Objective.—The results of unicondylar arthroplasty were reviewed in 82 consecutive knees operated on for primary unicompartmental osteoarthrosis from 1983 to 1987. The 72 patients were followed for an average of 5.5 years after surgery. Seventy-five knees had medial compartment arthroplasties, and 7 had lateral compartment arthroplasties.

Treatment.—Two similar component systems were used; both were designed to be inserted with or without bone cement. One system (Zimmer) uses fiber mesh as an ingrowth surface, whereas the other (Microloc) uses beads. Thirty-two knees received fiber mesh implants and 50 received Microloc implants.

Results.—After follow-up of 60 knees in 53 patients for a minimum of 4 years, 8 knees had been revised. One patient had died with a failed arthroplasty and 1 was awaiting revision. The total failure rate was 12%. Causes of failure included component loosening in 3 patients; progressive arthritis, polyethylene wear, and component failure in 2 patients each; and technical error in 1 instance. Six of 7 revisions have been converted to cemented total knee arthroplasties, which, so far, are functioning well. Impending failure was evident roentgenographically in 17% of patients, and another 15% had a gradual decline in knee function scores. No patient had progressive radiolucencies or lucencies exceeding 2 mm about the femoral or tibial component.

Discussion.—Extremities were reliably aligned in this series, but it proved difficult to achieve consistent positioning of the components, particularly the tibial implant. This and other studies have found increased rates of polyethylene wear and tibial subluxation when using implants that have flat femorotibial articular surfaces. In contrast to total knee arthroplasty, some factors influencing the outcome of unicompartmental arthroplasty are not predictably controllable by the surgeon.

Unicompartmental Arthroplasty for Osteonecrosis of the Knee Joint
Marmor L (Saint John's Hosp and Health Ctr, Santa Monica, Calif)
Clin Orthop 294:247–253, 1993   129-94-9-26

Introduction.—Osteonecrosis of the knee joint consists of avascular necrosis involving the medial femoral condyle of the knee and can be spontaneous or induced by steroids. Surgical treatment consists of arthroscopy, tibial osteotomy, total knee arthroplasty, or unicompartmental arthroplasty. A series of 32 patients with osteonecrosis of the knee joint who were treated with unicompartmental arthroplasty were studied.

Subjects.—Between 1975 and 1990, 10 men and 22 women with a diagnosis of osteonecrosis of the knee were treated. In 2 patients, both knees were affected. Only 2 of these patients had osteonecrosis induced by steroid treatment. The average follow-up was 5.5 years (range, 2–16 years).

Results.—In this series of 32 patients and 34 knees with osteonecrosis, good to excellent results were obtained in 89% of the patients. There were 4 treatment failures. Two of these failures were caused by the development of osteonecrosis in the lateral compartment, and 2 patients had persistent pain without a discernible cause.

Conclusion.—Unicompartmental arthroplasty is an effective treatment for osteonecrosis of the knee joint because of the low morbidity rate, rapid recovery, and the preservation of the cruciate ligaments, patella, and the opposite compartment, which results in better function and motion than tibial osteotomy or total knee arthroplasty. Total knee arthroplasty is preferable if there is evidence of advanced disease in the opposite compartment.

▶ Unicompartmental arthroplasty of the knee remains a controversial procedure; these 3 papers demonstrate why. The first paper by Sisto et al. (Abstract 129-94-9–24) reports 80% excellent and good results, with a 10% failure rate. The authors recommend the procedure for patients aged 55 and older with unicompartmental disease and for sedentary patients beyond 50 years of age. In contrast, Swank and associates (Abstract 129-94-9-25), although they had a similar failure rate of 12%, point to the many complications of unicompartmental arthroplasty and draw the conclusion that it is an unpredictable procedure in which, unlike total knee arthroplasty, the factors affecting its success or failure cannot be predictably controlled by the surgeon. The radiographs chosen for their illustrations, however, show consistent edge loading with the femoral component placed eccentrically on the tibial component leading to both edge loading and a tilting moment applied to the tibial implant. Those factors are within the control of the surgeon. Newer designs and techniques should reduce the number of complications related to improper relationship between the 2 components.

Marmor (Abstract 129-94-9-26) reports on the usefulness of unicompartmental replacement in patients with osteonecrosis of the medial femoral condyle. He obtained excellent or good results in 89% of the patients. The better results in his series may be related to the fact that in osteonecrosis the other compartment is usually entirely normal; therefore, one would not expect progressive arthritic changes in the contralateral compartment to be a reason for revision.—C.B. Sledge, M.D.

Total Knee Arthroplasty

RESULTS

Minimum Important Difference Between Patients With Rheumatoid Arthritis: The Patient's Perspective
Wells GA, Tugwell P, Kraag GR, Baker PRA, Groh J, Redelmeier DA (Univ of Ottawa, Ont, Canada; Ottawa Civic Hosp, Ont, Canada; Univ of Toronto)
J Rheumatol 20:557–560, 1993   129-94-9-27

Objective.—The relationship between a patient's personal assessment of his or her clinical condition and objective outcome measures obtained by a clinical evaluator was examined. A statistically significant difference between treated and control patients does not necessarily translate to a clinically significant difference, and it is important to identify the actual threshold for the clinically important difference.

Patients and Methods.—Forty adult patients with rheumatoid arthritis were recruited for the study. They participated in an evening of clinical assessment of tender and swollen joint count, pain, and physical ability conducted by a trained evaluator. Patients then had one-to-one conversations with other patients in which they discussed pain experienced the previous day, the effect of rheumatoid arthritis on activities of daily living, and feelings about their overall condition. Patients rated themselves relative to their conversational partner, and these subjective ratings were compared with the differences of the individual clinical assessments.

Results.—The mean age of participants was 58.5 years; 88% were women. The average duration of rheumatoid arthritis was 12.7 years. Tender joint count averaged 23 and swollen joint count averaged 8 in the clinical evaluator's assessments. On a scale from 1 (very good) to 5 (very poor), the average overall evaluator assessment of disease activity and the participants' personal assessment of their arthritic condition both averaged 2.6. Patients tended to judge themselves as less disabled than their conversational partners. They rated themselves as "somewhat better" when they had an average 7.2% better score on the Health Assessment Questionnaire, 6.2% less pain, and 9.1% better global assessment. They rated themselves "somewhat worse" when they had an average 16.2% worse score on the Health Assessment Questionnaire, 16.3% more pain, and 28.9% worse global assessment.

Conclusion.—Patients appear to perceive clinically important differences in an asymmetric manner. They perceived a smaller difference to be more meaningful when they felt better than their conversational partner than when they felt worse. In clinical studies, a separate reporting of patients who improve and those who deteriorate may provide a more meaningful summary of the expected outcome.

▶ The first 2 papers in this section (Abstracts 129-94-9–27 and 129-94-9–28) deal with some of the general aspects of evaluating the outcome of surgery in patients with lower extremity arthritis. This paper examines the general question of how to assess patients with rheumatoid arthritis. The authors begin the paper with a very important statement: "A statistically significant difference between treated and control patients does not necessarily mean a clinically significant difference. Clinical significance refers to the importance of a difference in terms of the magnitude of the outcome, whereas statistical significance indicates whether the hypothesis of no difference can be rejected."

If patients do not perceive that their condition is improved by a medical or surgical intervention, no amount of statistical manipulation can overcome that fact. The authors also point out that patients' functional losses are more important to them than corresponding gains; therefore, one should pay greater attention to complications than to the overall success rate.—C.B. Sledge, M.D.

Lumbar Spinal Stenosis and Lower Extremity Arthroplasty
McNamara MJ, Barrett KG, Christie MJ, Spengler DM (Vanderbilt Univ, Nashville, Tenn)
J Arthroplasty 8:273–277, 1993   129-94-9–28

Background.—Spinal stenosis causes back, hip, and leg pain in the elderly. Arthritis, a common source of pain in this age group, may be caused by avascular necrosis, spondyloarthropathy, or osteoarthropathy. A possible relationship between the development of spinal stenosis and arthritis of the hip or knee was investigated.

Methods.—Charts and radiographs of 2,515 patients with degenerative joint disease and 1,480 patients who underwent reconstructive arthroplasty at Vanderbilt University Medical Center between 1985 and 1990 were reviewed. Arthroplasties involved cemented and noncemented femoral implants, noncemented acetabular implants, or cemented knee components with patellar resurfacing; all were performed by 1 surgeon. Follow-up included radiographic evaluation and the Harris hip or Brigham knee score, and occurred at 6 weeks, 3 months, 6 months, and 12 months. The diagnosis of spinal stenosis was based on patient pain pattern and confirmed by MRI with or without myelogram and post-myelogram CT.

Results.—Fourteen patients (average age, 70.3 years) who had undergone hip or knee arthroplasty had symptoms of acquired lumbar spinal stenosis: 5 were seen with concomitant symptoms; in 9, spinal stenosis symptoms developed within an average of 9.3 months postarthroplasty. Surgical decompression was required to relieve stenotic symptoms in 2 patients of the concomitant symptom group and in 7 of the sequential symptom group.

Conclusion.—Patients with concomitant lower extremity joint degeneration and spinal stenosis may be successfully treated by arthroplasty. In other patients, severe lower extremity joint disease may mask the symptoms of spinal stenosis, and spinal stenosis may be anticipated during the first year after successful joint reconstruction surgery.

▶ In the age group of patients who are normally seen for arthroplasty of the lower extremity joints, lumbar spinal stenosis is a common finding. In this study, the authors examined the course of spinal stenosis in 14 patients who had the condition and underwent an arthroplasty of lower extremity joints. In the absence of disabling symptoms from spinal stenosis, the authors suggest that the arthroplasty be undertaken first, and then the severity of symptoms from stenosis can be more clearly evaluated. They also point out, however, that the symptoms of spinal stenosis are often unmasked by the increased functional capacity of the patients after arthroplasty.—C.B. Sledge, M.D.

Total Knee Arthroplasty Without Patellar Resurfacing: Clinical Outcomes and Long-Term Follow-Up Evaluation
Levitsky KA, Harris WJ, McManus J, Scott RD (Tufts Univ, Boston; New England Baptist Hosp, Boston; Harvard Med School, Boston)
Clin Orthop 286:116–121, 1993   129-94-9–29

Background.—There is ongoing debate regarding the need to perform patellar resurfacing in patients undergoing total knee arthroplasty (TKA). Whereas some reports advocate resurfacing in all patients with osteoarthritic knees, others recommend selective resurfacing only. The long-term outcome of TKA without patellar resurfacing in knees with osteoarthrosis was clarified.

Patients.—In 125 patients, TKA without patellar resurfacing was performed with at least 2 years of follow-up. The final analysis included 79 knees in 66 patients with osteoarthrosis (mean age, 77 years at follow-up). The surgeon made the decision to leave the patella unresurfaced based on the presence of satisfactory patellar articular cartilage, congruent patellofemoral tracking, anatomically normal patellar shape, and the absence of eburnated bone and signs of crystalline disease or inflammatory synovitis. Thirteen knees had lateral retinacular release to facilitate congruent patellar tracking.

Outcomes.—During an average follow-up of 7.5 years, no component revisions or reoperations were performed. The mean Knee Society score was improved from 23 to 90 after TKA and the mean function score from 58 to 92. Nineteen percent of patients had mild anterior knee pain. Nearly 90% of patients were satisfied with the result, and only 3% expressed mild dissatisfaction. Fourteen patients had mixed bilateral procedures, i.e., patellar resurfacing on 1 side but not the other. In this group, 46% of patients rated both sides equal, 46% favored the resurfaced side, and 8% preferred the unresurfaced side.

Conclusion.—In properly selected patients with osteoarthrosis, TKA without patellar resurfacing can give good long-term results. In this series, there were no mechanical complications and no patients needed reoperation. Selective patellar resurfacing might be appropriate in younger, more active patients on the basis of the criteria outlined.

Long-Term Complications After Total Knee Arthroplasty With or Without Resurfacing of the Patella

Boyd AD Jr, Ewald FC, Thomas WH, Poss R, Sledge CB (Univ of Rochester, NY; Brigham and Women's Hosp, Boston)
J Bone Joint Surg (Am) 75-A:674–681, 1993   129-94-9–30

Background.—The indications for patellar resurfacing are unclear. The prevalence, types, treatment, and consequences of long-term patellar complications after total knee arthroplasty (TKA) with an unconstrained prosthesis, with and without patellar resurfacing, were studied.

Methods.—Six hundred eighty-four patients with a total of 891 affected knees were studied. In 1 group, 303 patients had TKA on 396 knees with patellar resurfacing. In the other group, 381 patients with 495 treated knees underwent the same procedure without resurfacing. The mean follow-up was 6.5 years.

Findings.—The overall complication rate was 4% in the group with resurfacing and 12% in the group without resurfacing, a significant difference. The overall rate of patellar component loosening was 1%. In the group without resurfacing, chronic pain occurred in 13% of the 300 knees with inflammatory arthritis and in 6% of the 195 knees with degenerative osteoarthritis. This was also a significant difference. At a mean of 63 months after the index TKA, a revision to resurface the patella was done in all 51 knees that caused chronic pain and did not have patellar resurfacing.

Conclusion.—In patients with inflammatory arthritis or osteoarthritis, the patella should be resurfaced when this type of unconstrained prosthesis is used. Failure to resurface the patella in such cases may result in more revisions, including early revisions, for the treatment of chronic patellar pain.

▶ Levitsky and associates (Abstract 129-94-9–29) report on a large group of patients undergoing 79 knee arthroplasties without resurfacing of the patella with an average follow-up of 7.5 years. They report excellent clinical and functional evaluation of the patients at follow-up and suggest that younger, more active patients who meet their selection criteria may well have the patella unresurfaced at the time of arthroplasty. In a subset of patients, however, in whom 1 patella was not resurfaced and the contralateral patella was resurfaced at the time of arthroplasty, 46% rated both knees as equal, whereas 46% preferred the side with the resurfaced patella and only 8% preferred the side with the unresurfaced patella. The authors' findings confirm earlier reports that patients, in general, prefer a knee with a resurfaced patella in terms of pain relief.

The paper by Boyd et al. (Abstract 129-94-9–30) compared 396 knee arthroplasties with patella resurfacing to 495 arthroplasties without resurfacing. The rate of complications was significantly higher in those patients in whom the patella was not resurfaced. Thirteen percent of the patients in whom the patella was not resurfaced complained of pain at follow-up if their original diagnosis was rheumatoid arthritis and 6% if the diagnosis was osteoarthritis. The frequency of revision operation to resurface a previously unresurfaced patella was much higher than the frequency of revision operation for complications associated with a resurfaced patella. It is my current practice to resurface the patella routinely at arthroplasty.—C.B. Sledge, M.D.

The Effects of Axial Rotational Alignment of the Femoral Component on Knee Stability and Patellar Tracking in Total Knee Arthroplasty Demonstrated on Autopsy Specimens
Anouchi YS, Whiteside LA, Kaiser AD, Milliano MT (DePaul Biomechanical Research Lab, St Louis, Mo)
Clin Orthop 287:170–177, 1993   129-94-9–31

Objective.—Little is known about the effect of axial rotational alignment of the femoral component of total knee arthroplasty. A study was conducted on cadavers to determine the effects of rotational alignment on knee stability, patellar tracking, and patellofemoral contact points. The expectation was that the positions of the posterior femoral condyles would affect knee stability as the knee flexed.

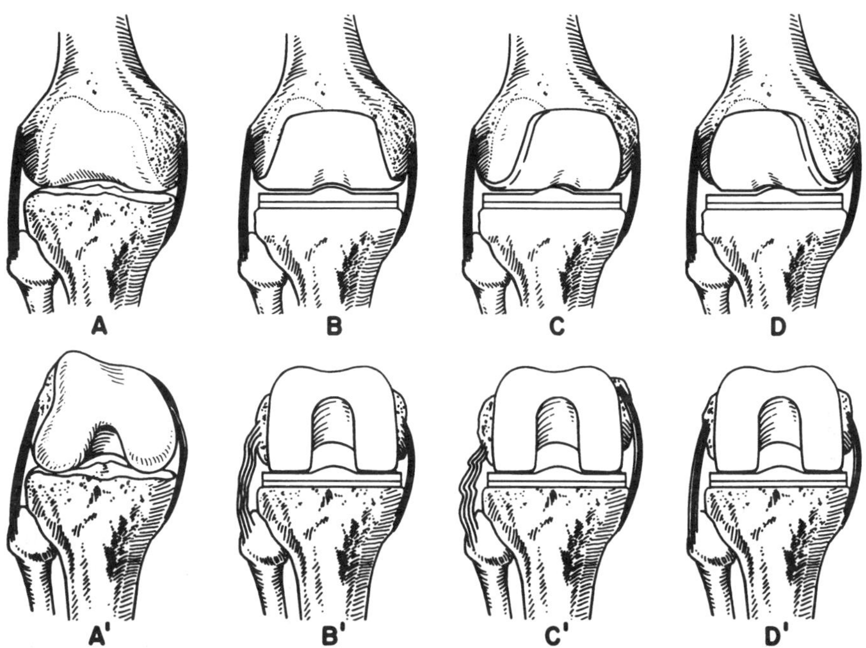

Fig 9–8.—**A** and **A'**, the normal ligament balance at 0 degrees and 90 degrees for weight-bearing flexion. **B** and **B'**, a neutrally aligned femoral component after total knee arthroplasty. **C** and **C'**, an internally rotated femoral component with resultant lateral ligament laxity. **D** and **D'**, an externally rotated femoral component. Rotation of the femoral component shifts the patellar groove either medially or laterally in extension without any effect on ligament stability. In weight-bearing flexion, the patellar groove is unchanged but the ligament balance is altered. (Courtesy of Anouchi YS, Whiteside LA, Kaiser AD, et al: *Clin Orthop* 287:170-177, 1993.)

Methods.—Four fresh-frozen anatomical knee specimens were mounted in a knee-testing device originally designed to test knee stability at various degrees of flexion. In this case, it was used to define the interaction between flexion, rotation, and varus-valgus deflections in regard to changes in the axial alignment of the femoral component. Stability, patellar tracking, and patellofemoral contact points were evaluated with the femoral component in 5 degrees of internal, 5 degrees of external, or neutral axial rotational alignment.

Results.—Varus-valgus stability of the knee was closest to control values in externally rotated specimens. A shift into valgus alignment was noted on flexion of internally rotated specimens. The externally rotated specimens were also most nearly normal in terms of patellar tracking and showed more even distribution of patellofemoral contact between the medial and lateral contact areas.

Conclusion.—Observations in cadaveric knees suggest that internal rotation of the femoral component of the knee with perpendicular resection of the tibia negatively affects knee stability, patellar tracking, and patellofemoral contact points. Similar effects of lesser magnitude are noted with neutral positioning. Patellar tracking and knee stability are both improved if the femoral component is placed in external rotation (Fig 9–8).

▶ Several maneuvers are useful in avoiding patellar maltracking after a total knee arthroplasty: lateral retinacular release, imbrication of the medial closure, and, as this paper confirms, slight external rotation of the femoral component of about 5 degrees.—C.B. Sledge, M.D.

Correction of Ligament and Bone Defects in Total Arthroplasty of the Severely Valgus Knee
Whiteside LA (DePaul Biomechanical Research Lab, St Louis, Mo)
Clin Orthop 288:234–245, 1993   129-94-9–32

Purpose.—Restoration of the normal angle and stability in the valgus knee requires correction of both bony and ligamentous abnormalities. Resection of the medial femoral condyle to a point that allows seating on the femoral component laterally results in severe overresection medially, damaging the femoral attachment of the medial collateral ligament. The use of a thick tibial component to correct the resulting ligamentous imbalance may make the knee excessively tight in flexion (Fig 9–9). An alternative method, in which the intact joint surfaces on the medial femoral condyle and medial tibial plateau are used as the reference level for resection of the distal femoral surfaces, has been introduced.

Technique.—The technique consists of a minimally constrained, cementless toal knee replacement using intramedullary alignment for the femur and tibia. The use of measured bone resection avoids raising the joint line and simplifies ligament balancing in flexion and extension. For patients with severe deficiency of the lateral femoral condyle, no bone is removed from the distal condylar surface; instead, bone grafting is performed to make up for the deficiency (Fig 9–10). In this way, ligamentous balance of the knee is maintained throughout the range of motion, based on the intact medial femoral condylar surface.

Experience.—This technique has been used in 135 knees with valgus deformity. The mean valgus angle improved from 16 degrees before knee replacement surgery to 7 degrees afterward. During 6 years of follow-up, there was no deterioration in either alignment or varus-valgus stability; however, posterior laxity tended to increase in knees with more than 25 degrees of deformity. Bone grafting of the medial femoral and tibial surfaces was required in knees with severe deformity. Less than 1% of patients had patellar subluxation or dislocation.

Conclusion.—In total knee replacement in joints with severe valgus deformity, resecting the femoral surface based on measurements from the intact joint surface is a simple and reliable way to ensure proper ligament tension in flexion and extension. The bony abnormality is precisely

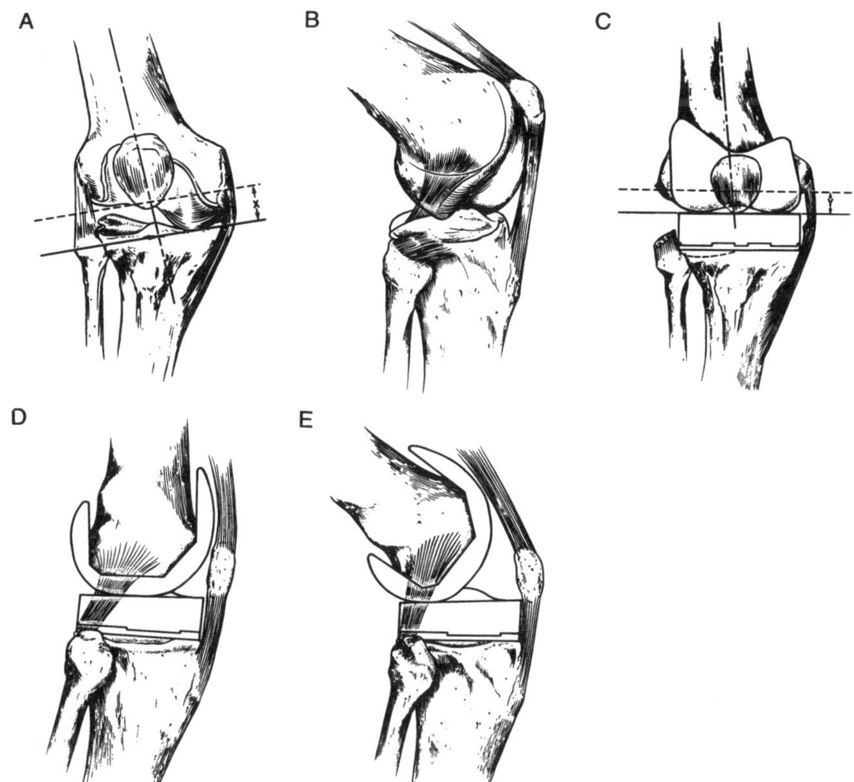

Fig 9–9.—A, anterior view of the knee with severe valgus deformity and deficient lateral femoral condyle. Resection to the level of the distal surface of the deficient lateral femoral condyle (x) overresects the medial femoral condyle and may damage the femoral attachment of the medial collateral ligament. **B,** lateral view depicts the usual conditions of the distal lateral and posterior femoral condyles. The distal surface is deficient, but the posterior lateral femoral condyle is relatively well preserved. **C,** replacement of the joint surfaces with a femoral surface (y) that is thinner than the distal femoral resection raises the joint line and requires a very thick tibial component to restore stability in flexion. The patella rides low relative to the new joint line. Lateral ligament release is necessary to achieve ligament balance. **D,** in full extension the femoral surface rides in the center of the tibial component, and the posterior cruciate ligament (PCL) is appropriately tensioned. The patella is low relative to the new joint line. **E,** when the knee is flexed, the PCL is excessively tensioned by the posterior femoral condyles, which have not been overresected as the distal condyles have been. The patella may impinge against the anterior surface of the tibial component. (Courtesy of Whiteside LA: *Clin Orthop* 288:234–245, 1993.)

corrected by the use of intramedullary alignment. Trial components to tension the ligaments provide a reliable means of balancing the ligaments that does not require any expertise or extensive experience.

▶ Severe valgus deformity is the most difficult situation faced in primary knee arthroplasty. This paper addresses the issues of ligamentous and bony defects in such knees and gives excellent advice on methods to correct those deficiencies.—C.B. Sledge, M.D.

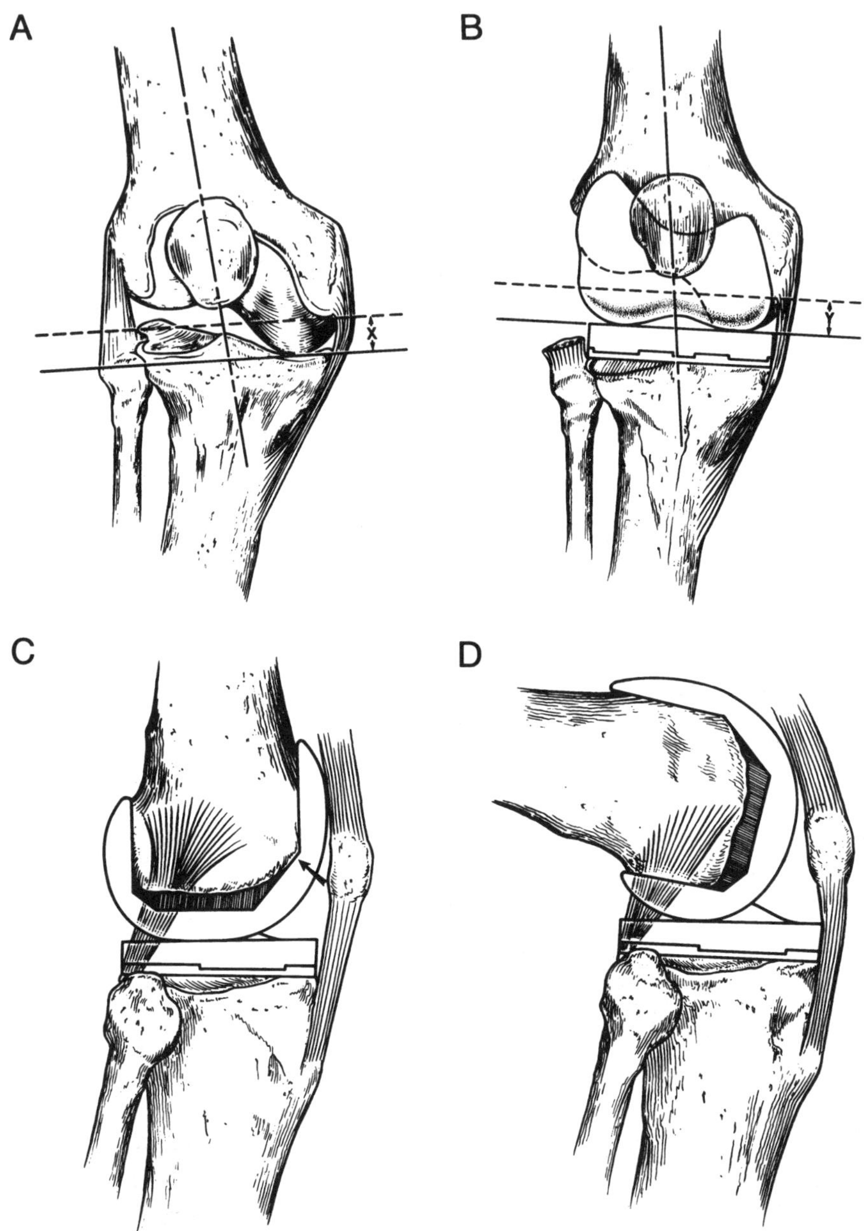

Fig 9–10.—A, anterior view of the knee with severe valgus deformity and defect of the lateral femoral condyle. The thickness of the distal portion of the femoral component (x) is measured for resection, but this leaves no resection of the distal lateral femoral condyle. **B,** replacement of the joint surfaces with a femoral surface of the same thickness as the portion resected (y) leaves the joint line in a normal position relative to the patella and to the intact medial half of the knee. The lateral bone surfaces are more widely separated by the space-occupying components. A thinner tibial component is used to ten-

(continued)

Proprioception After Knee Arthroplasty: The Influence of Prosthetic Design

Warren PJ, Olanlokun TK, Cobb AG, Bentley G (Royal Natl Orthopaedic Hosp Trust, Stanmore, England)
Clin Orthop 297:182–187, 1993   129-94-9–33

Background.—Proprioception has been shown to decline in the elderly, in patients with osteoarthritis, and in patients with anterior cruciate deficiency. The influence of prosthetic design on proprioception after knee arthroplasty was studied in osteoarthritic and prosthetic knees.

Methods.—Thirty-seven women and 13 men aged 56–85 years were tested for their awareness of knee joint position 1 year or more after total knee replacement. Nine volunteer control subjects were also tested. A special apparatus was used so that the leg being tested was completely relaxed.

Findings.—The special apparatus and more accurate measurements revealed a wider variability in joint position sense than had been found previously. Although the best performances in each group were comparable, osteoarthritic patients had the worst performances. A positive correlation was noted between joint position awareness in the osteoarthritic knee and in the opposite replaced knee. Knees with posterior cruciate ligament (PCL)-retaining Kinemax prostheses exhibited better joint position appreciation than PCL-sacrificing Insall-Burstein prostheses.

Conclusion.—These findings are consistent with those of previous observations that total prosthetic replacement confers some improvement in awareness of joint position. Increased awareness achieved by knee replacement with PCL retention may be consistent with the PCL making a significant contribution to joint position. This may be the direct result of retention of mechanoreceptors in the PCL.

▶ Proprioceptive function after knee arthroplasty has been a subject of discussion and investigation for several years. The absence of the cruciate ligaments and lack of proper tension in the collateral ligaments have been implicated as reasons why the prosthetic knee, after arthroplasty, might have diminished proprioceptive ability. In this study, it was found that retention of the PCL at the time of total knee arthroplasty led to improved proprioception when compared to implants that required posterior cruciate sacrifice. This is consistent with the findings of Andriacchi et al. (1) and Dorr et al. (2), who

---

Fig 9–10 (cont).

sion the ligaments of the medial side of the knee. **C,** lateral view of the knee in full extension. The femoral component rests on the anterior bevel surface (*arrow*), and the contained defect created by restoring the joint surface is filled with cancellous bone. A similar defect in the lateral tibial plateau is also grafted. The patella is in a normal position above the joint line. **D,** normal joint line position allows the knee to flex without overtensioning the posterior cruciate and medial capsular ligaments. Excessive rollback and patellar impingement are avoided. (Courtesy of Whiteside LA: *Clin Orthop* 288:234–245, 1993.)

reported improved function in patients with PCL retention when subjected to demanding functional challenges such as climbing stairs.—C.B. Sledge, M.D.

References

1. Andriacchi TP, et al: *J Bone Joint Surg (Am)* 64A:1328, 1982.
2. Dorr LD, et al: *Clin Orthop* 236:36, 1988.

Total Knee Arthroplasty in Active Golfers

Mallon WJ, Callaghan JJ (Duke Univ, Durham, NC; Univ of Iowa, Iowa City)
J Arthroplasty 8:299–306, 1993
129-94-9-34

Background.—Many elderly patients undergo total knee arthroplasty (TKA) to alleviate arthritis. Many patients who undergo TKA play golf for exercise. Because published data on activity and TKA loosening are not available, a study was conducted to assess total joint arthroplasties in active golfers.

Methods.—Eighty-three golfers who had a single TKA with at least 3 years of follow-up and who played golf at least 3 times per week were surveyed. Postoperative anteroposterior and lateral radiographs were requested from the patients' surgeons and evaluated for evidence of TKA loosening.

Results.—Although 84.3% of subjects reported no pain during play, 34.9% reported a mild ache after play. Radiographs were obtained for 54 golfers. Lucent lines were discernable in 53.7% of all prostheses, in 79.1% of cemented prostheses, and in 44.5% of uncemented prostheses. Radiographic loosening rates with hybrid TKAs were significantly lower than those of cemented or uncemented prostheses. Nevertheless, pain during and after play did not differ significantly among patients with the 3 types of prostheses. Radiographic loosening did not differ significantly between left and right TKA; however significantly more golfers with left TKAs experienced more pain during and after play.

Discussion.—The higher incidence of pain associated with a left TKA during and after golf may relate to the increased torque on the left knee in right-handed golfers. Playing golf with a TKA on the target side need not be discouraged; however, these patients should be cautioned about possible pain during and after playing.

▶ Patients seeking knee arthroplasty frequently mention their desire to continue with or return to the game of golf as a reason for seeking surgery. Traditionally, surgeons have counseled their patients not to return to such strenuous activities, but evidence one way or the other has been lacking. This remarkable study followed a group of extremely active amateur and professional golfers who had undergone arthroplasty and found that their game was improved and that they suffered no increase in complications related to their return to strenuous golf.—C.B. Sledge, M.D.

The Miller-Galante Knee Prosthesis for the Treatment of Osteoarthrosis: A Comparison of the Results of Partial Fixation With Cement and Fixation Without Any Cement
Rorabeck CH, Bourne RB, Lewis PL, Nott L (Univ Hosp, London, Ont, Canada)
J Bone Joint Surg (Am) 75-A:402–408, 1993   129-94-9–35

Introduction.—The Miller-Galante knee prosthesis has come into fairly widespread use since its introduction in 1984. Because its design promotes bone ingrowth in the femoral, tibial, and patellar components, it can be implanted with or without cement. However, there have been few clinical reports of the results with this prosthesis and few prospective comparisons of fixation techniques for total knee arthroplasty. The outcome of total knee replacement with the Miller-Galante I prosthesis and partial fixation with cement was compared with that of fixation without cement.

Methods.—From 1985 to 1988, 392 primary total knee replacements were performed using the Miller-Galante I prosthesis in 344 patients with osteoarthrosis. Of those, 183 knees in 163 patients had fixation without cement. The remaining 209 knees in 181 patients had partial fixation with cement; in this group, the tibial and patellar components were inserted with cement and the femoral component without cement. Patients were followed for an average of 3 years. Follow-up was complete except for 9 patients who died.

Results.—At follow-up, the 2 groups were no different in knee score, range of motion, radiographic findings, or complication rate. However, both had a high rate of complications caused by problems related to the extensor mechanism. Eight percent of the noncemented and 9% of the partially cemented group required reoperation. Thirteen patients required reoperation for recurrent patellar dislocation, 12 for abnormal wear of the polyethylene of the patellar component, 2 for avulsion of the patellar ligament, and 2 for unexplained knee pain. Eight patients had patellar fracture, which required surgery in 2 cases; 3 patients had deep infections, all requiring surgery.

Conclusion.—No difference was found in the results of Miller-Galante knee prosthesis fixation with and without cement. However, both forms of fixation are associated with a very high rate of complications related to the extensor mechanism. On the basis of this experience, the authors have ceased using the Miller-Galante prosthesis. They no longer use a metal-backed patellar component, although they continue to use tibial components without cement in young patients with apparent good bone quality.

▶ This paper reports on another excellent, randomized, prospective trial carried out by Rorabeck, Bourne, Lewis, and Nott. The authors took a single design (Miller-Galante knee prosthesis) and randomized the patients into a cementless group and a group with cementless femoral fixation but with cement for the tibia and patellar component fixation. The rate of complications in both groups was somewhat high and was primarily related to patellar problems. The authors conclude that this particular design has a flawed patellofemoral articulation (this design is now been superseded by the Miller-Galante II prosthesis).—C.B. Sledge, M.D.

Noncemented, Porous Ingrowth Knee Prosthesis: The 3- to 8-Year Results

Cameron HU, Jung YB (Univ of Toronto; Chung-Ang Univ, Seoul, Korea)
Can J Surg 36:560–564, 1993   129-94-9–36

Background.—The clinical outcomes of noncemented ingrowth-type total knee replacement prostheses have been fairly good in the short term. However, some concern has been expressed about fixation of the tibial component and wear of the patellar component. Sinkage and wear were assessed in patients with a noncemented total knee prosthesis.

Methods.—A total of 252 consecutive patients with total knee replacements were followed for 3–8 years. All had arthritis of the knee, primarily osteoarthritis, and were implanted with the Tricon M prosthesis, which has a metal-backed patella.

Findings.—Thirty-five prostheses needed revision. Eleven were done because of patellar wear only. In 13 prostheses, the tibial component and patella were revised because of wear. Six were revised for sepsis, 4 for reflex sympathetic dystrophy, and 1 for sinkage of the tibial component only. In the remaining 217 prostheses the results were good or excellent in 88%, fair in 6%, and poor in 6%.

Conclusion.—In this series, the single greatest cause of failure was polyethylene wear. This wear was associated with the metal backing of the patella and the use of thin polyethylene tibial components.

▶ In this group of 252 consecutive patients with uncemented total knee arthroplasties, 88% of results were good or excellent, and there was only 1 case of a tibial component revised for sinkage. Thirty-four other patients had revisions for a variety of problems but not for failure of fixation. The series suggests that it is possible to obtain satisfactory fixation, as judged at a 3- to 8-year follow-up, without the use of acrylic bone cement; however, given the absence of complications related to the use of cement, the goal still appears to be elusive. No advantage of cementless knee arthroplasty has yet been demonstrated.—C.B. Sledge, M.D.

Long-Term Results of the Total Condylar Knee Arthroplasty: A 15-Year Survivorship Study

Ranawat CS, Flynn WF Jr, Saddler S, Hansraj KK, Maynard MJ (Hosp for Spe-

cial Surgery, New York)
Clin Orthop 286:94–102, 1993   129-94-9–37

Series.—Survivorship was examined in a series of 112 consecutive Total Condylar knee arthroplasties followed since 1974. The 85 patients, 68 of whom were women, had an average age of 65 years at surgery. Fifty knees were operated on for osteoarthrosis and 62 for rheumatoid arthritis. The implants had an all-polyethylene tibial component and a femoral component measuring 59 × 62 mm.

Clinical Results.—Sixty-two knees evaluated for more than 11 years had an average range of motion of 99 degrees; 3 joints had less than 80 degrees of motion. Knee scores, according to the Hospital for Special Surgery grading system, were good to excellent in 92% of cases. Final follow-up of 45 knees after 14–16.5 years showed an average range of motion of 96 degrees and an average knee score of 85 points. Five revisions were carried out. Radiographs showed lucencies in 73% of the tibias, but only 2 components had loosened.

Survivorship.—Clinical survivorship was 94% at 15 years (Fig 9–11). When roentgenographic failures were taken into account, survival was 91% for patients with rheumatoid disease and 89% for those with osteoarthritis (Fig 9–12). The clinical-plus-roentgenographic survivorship was reduced to 71% in patients weighing more than 80 kg (Fig 9–13). This group included all patients with roentgenographic component loosening.

Conclusion.—The Total Condylar knee implant reliably relieves pain, provides 95 to 100 degrees or more of knee motion, and allows for good function. The implant appears to be very durable, with survivorship

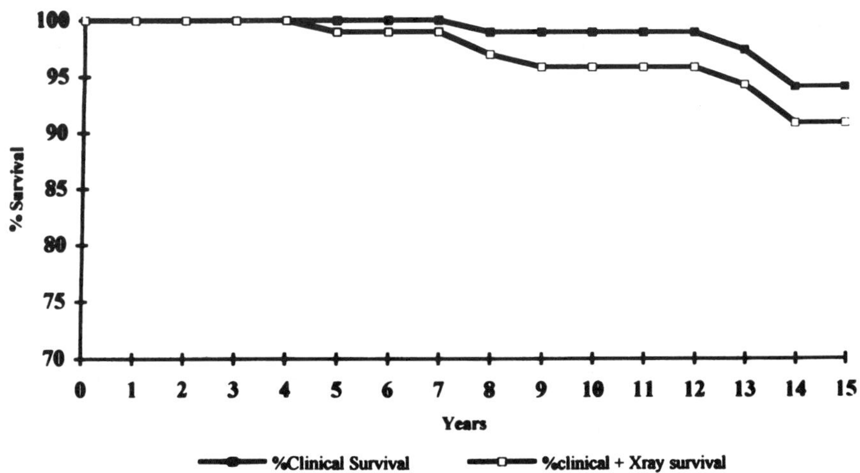

Fig 9–11.—Fifteen-year survival curve for Total Condylar prosthesis. (Courtesy of Ranawat CS, Flynn WF Jr, Saddler S, et al: *Clin Orthop* 286:94–102, 1993.)

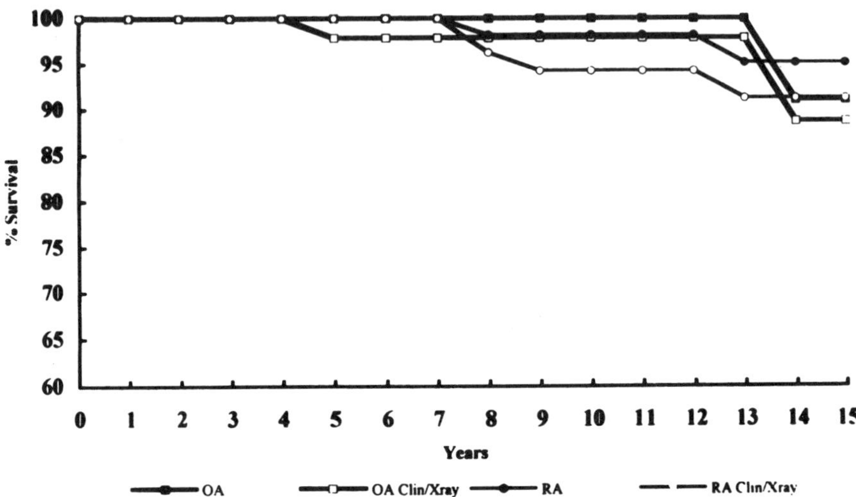

Fig 9–12.—Fifteen-year survival curve of rheumatoid arthritis vs. osteoarthrosis (Courtesy of Ranawat CS, Flynn WF Jr, Saddler S, et al: *Clin Orthop* 286:94–102, 1993.)

of 94% or better at 15 years. Tibial components made of polyethylene have worn minimally in well-fixed knees. Disadvantages include a lack of modularity and occasional problems in balancing the soft tissues in flexion.

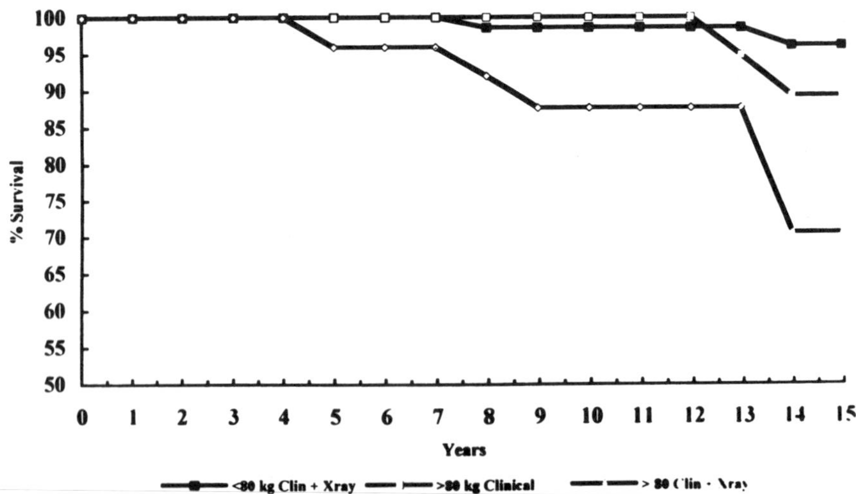

Fig 9–13.—Fifteen-year survival curve by body weight. (Courtesy of Ranawat CS, Flynn WF Jr, Saddler S, et al: *Clin Orthop* 286:94–102, 1993.)

▶ This paper presents an extremely long follow-up of 85 patients whose arthroplasty was carried out, on average, 15 years earlier. Survivorship was 94% on clinical criteria and 91% when radiographic failures were included. This is an outstanding result involving a cemented implant of a design that is no longer popular. It can only be hoped that further design refinements since the original Total Condylar have been improvements rather than mere changes and that follow-up studies in the future will reflect even better longevity. The authors conclude that "Total Condylar knee arthroplasty remains the 'gold standard' for longevity."—C.B. Sledge, M.D.

COMPLICATIONS

Operative Treatment of Distal Femoral Fractures Proximal to Total Knee Replacements

Healy WL, Siliski JM, Incavo SJ (Lahey Clinic Med Ctr, Burlington, Mass; Massachusetts Gen Hosp, Boston; Univ of Vermont, Burlington)
J Bone Joint Surg (Am) 75-A:27–34, 1993 129-94-9–38

Purpose.—Fracture of the distal femur proximal to a total knee replacement is an uncommon injury, with reported frequencies ranging from .3% to 2.5%. However, as the population ages and more total knee replacements are performed, these fractures may become more com-

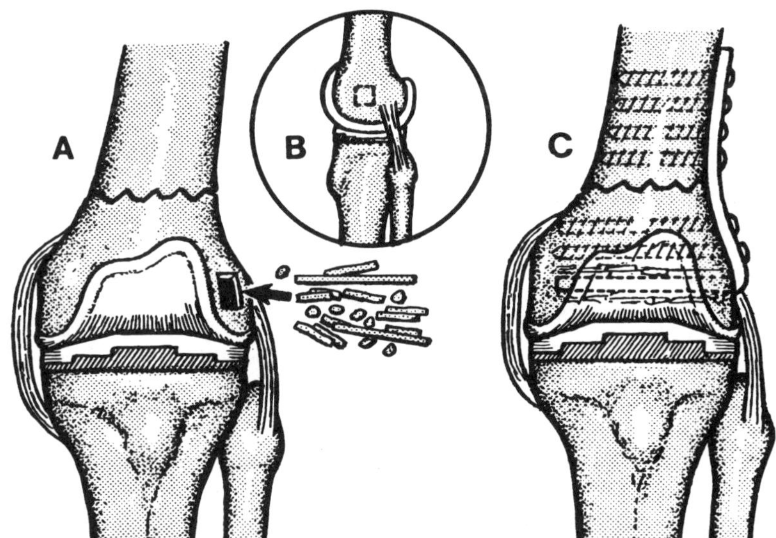

Fig 9–14.—Polymethyl methacrylate or bone graft may be used to augment the distal fixation of the implant used for treatment of the fracture in patients who have extreme osteopenia in the distal condylar fragment. **A,** a window is made in the lateral surface of the lateral condyle, and bone grafts are packed into the metaphysis. **B,** lateral view. **C,** fixation of the fracture with the implant in place and the distal fixation augmented with bone graft. (Courtesy of Healy WL, Siliski JM, Incavo SJ: *J Bone Joint Surg (Am)* 75-A:27–34, 1993.)

mon. There is debate as to whether notching of the distal femur as the result of knee replacement causes these fractures. Treatment recommendations have varied as well. The results of operative treatment in 20 patients with distal femoral fractures proximal to total knee replacements were reported.

Patients.—The patients were treated during a 5-year period. Most were women with osteoarthrosis and osteopenia; the mean patient age was 70 years. Twelve patients had serious medical illnesses that significantly affected treatment planning. The fractures occurred a mean of 36 months after total knee replacement; 19 were caused by low-velocity trauma. Twelve patients had comminuted fractures, 4 had short oblique fractures, 3 had transverse fractures, and 1 had a long spiral fracture. All patients were managed with open reduction and stable internal fixation, with bone grafting in 15 patients (Fig 9–14). The patients were followed for a mean of 27 months.

Results.—Only 2 of the fractures were associated with notching of the anterior aspect of the femoral cortex. None of the knee prostheses were loose. With open reduction and internal fixation, all of the fractures healed, 18 within a mean of 16 weeks. Union was delayed up to 40 weeks in the remaining 2 patients but was achieved with repeat open reduction and internal fixation plus autogenous bone grafting. All patients were able to return to their previous level of physical activity, with restoration of their preinjury tibiofemoral alignment and knee range of motion. The average Knee Society clinical and functional scores did not decrease after surgery.

Conclusion.—Open reduction and stable internal fixation is recommended for patients with distal femoral fractures proximal to total knee replacement. This approach, including bone grafting, can restore elderly patients to their preinjury level of function without pain or disability. Restoration and maintenance of normal tibiofemoral alignment of 5–7 degrees of varus angulation is a key consideration.

Internal Fixation of Supracondylar Fractures After Condylar Total Knee Arthroplasty

Zehntner MK, Ganz R (Univ of Bern, Switzerland)
Clin Orthop 293:219–224, 1993   129-94-9–39

Background.—Supracondylar femur fracture that follows total knee arthroplasty is difficult to treat. Choice of conservative vs. operative fracture management is controversial. Open reduction and internal fixation with the AO/ASIF condylar buttress plate was used to repair supracondylar femur fractures after condylar knee arthroplasty in 6 patients.

Technique.—With the patient in a supine position, a lateral incision is made shortly distal to the tibial tuberosity and extending proximally the length of the implant. The iliotibial band is divided, and the vastus lateralis is detached and

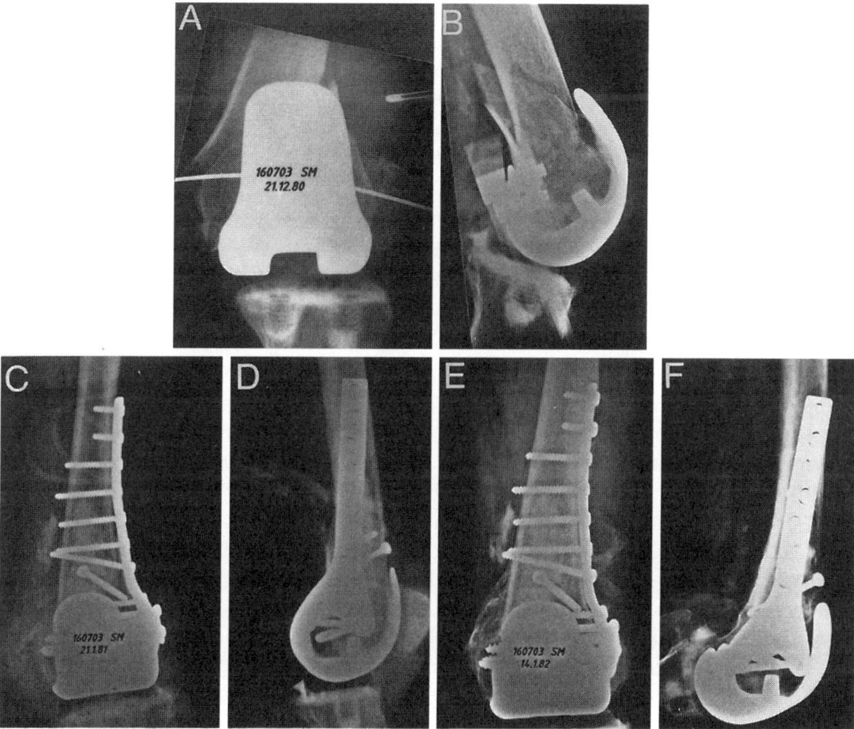

Fig 9–15.—A Neer grade II supracondylar fracture in a 78-year-old patient with rheumatoid arthritis and severe osteoporosis. **A,** preoperative anteroposterior view. **B,** preoperative lateral view. **C,** immediate postoperative radiograph: the additional use of bone cement is visible intramedullary and medially. The gap between cement and medial cortex shows that tightening of the screws was performed only after curing of the cement, thus displacing it. **D,** immediate postoperative lateral view. **E,** follow-up anteroposterior film at 1 year shows union with bridging callus formation and no loss of fixation. **F,** lateral view at 1 year. (Courtesy of Zehntner MK, Ganz R: *Clin Orthop* 293:219–224, 1993.)

lifted from the lateral intermuscular septum, leaving the periosteum attached to the bone. The knee joint is opened in the same direction as the deep dissection, and the condyle-proximal main fragment alignment is checked. A corresponding condylar buttress plate is provisionally fixed to the condylar fragment. The proximal fragment is reduced and rotated to align with the plate. The plate tensioning device is placed and the fracture site is compressed by careful application of tension. After 2-plane radiography verifies correct implant alignment and position, additional screws are inserted into the condylar fragment. Low-viscosity cement is injected into the screw holes in patients with severely osteoporotic bone. Two-millimeter overlength screws are inserted into the distal cortex and tightened fully after the cement has hardened (Fig 9–15). The wound is closed over 2 aspirative drains and a conventional dressing is applied. After 48 hours, the suction drains are removed, and knee mobilization and touch-down weight-bearing are begun.

Results.—All fractures healed uneventfully within 14 weeks. Loss of fixation with secondary displacement, infections, and component loosening did not occur. Follow-up radiographs revealed restoration of alignment to an average 5 degrees of valgus. Four patients were pain-free; 2 had minimal pain that did not interfere with daily function. All patients regained prefracture ambulatory status, although 5 needed 2 crutches outdoors.

Conclusion.—Open reduction and internal fixation using the condylar buttress plate may prevent malalignment and allow early ambulation and knee motion. In patients with severe osteoporosis, bone cement may be used to strengthen screw fixation without compromising fracture healing.

▶ Healy and associates (Abstract 129-94-9–38) report on the operative treatment of distal femoral fractures proximal to total knee arthroplasty and report excellent results, with all fractures healed and returned to the level of activity enjoyed before the fracture. Zehntner and Ganz (Abstract 129-94-9–39) report similar results in a group of 6 patients in whom open reduction and internal fixation was carried out. It seems reasonable to conclude from these 2 papers that, whenever feasible, surgical treatment is the treatment of choice for these fractures unless they are undisplaced, the patient is too ill to undergo surgery, or the quality of bone and comminution of the fracture preclude satisfactory internal fixation.—C.B. Sledge, M.D.

Surgical Decompression for Peroneal Nerve Palsy After Total Knee Arthroplasty
Krackow KA, Maar DC, Mont MA, Carroll C IV (Johns Hopkins Univ, Baltimore, Md; Northwestern Univ, Chicago)
Clin Orthop 292:223–228, 1993   129-94-9–40

Background.—The risk factors for development of peroneal nerve palsy subsequent to total knee arthroplasty (TKA) have been identified; however, treatment of the palsy has not been defined. Spontaneous improvement may occur over several months to several years; but incomplete resolution of pain, loss of pedal dorsiflexion, and diminished distribution of peroneal nerve sensation may impede rehabilitation. Surgical peroneal nerve decompression has been used as a treatment for peroneal nerve palsy subsequent to TKA in 5 patients.

Technique.—With the patient in the lateral decubitus position, a longitudinal posterolateral incision is made. The incision is centered at the level of the fibular head and parallel to the biceps tendon and fibula to allow proximal identification and distal tracing of the nerve. The nerve is released proximally from its fibrous enclosure at the fibular neck and distally to where it dives deep to the peroneus longus. The proximal fibular neck attachment of the peroneus longus is released to allow full decompression (Fig 9–16).

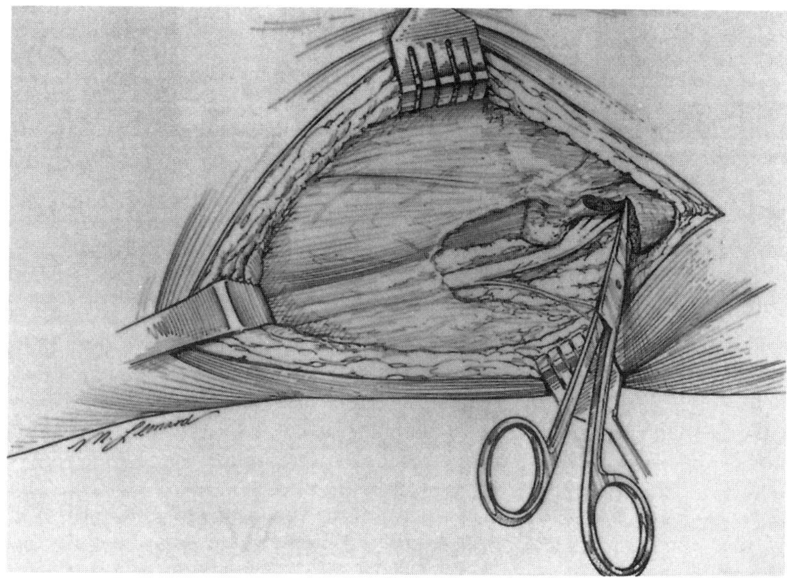

Fig 9–16.—The proximal fibular neck attachment of the peroneus longus is released to free the peroneal nerve completely. (Courtesy of Krackow KA, Maar DC, Mont MA, et al: *Clin Orthop* 292:223–228, 1993.)

Results.—All patients reported subjective symptomatic improvement within 3 months. Four patients had full peroneal nerve recovery; all were able to discontinue ankle-foot orthoses.

Discussion.—Some peroneal nerve palsies observed immediately after TKA respond to simply removing constricting dressings and allowing 30 to 40 degrees of flexion. Palsies that do not respond within the first several hours require further consideration. Intrinsic factors, such as a large expanding hematoma, indicate surgical exploration to relieve the pressure on the nerve. It is difficult to define the optimal timing of exploration of post-TKA peroneal nerve palsy on the basis of only 5 cases. Nevertheless, any patient who does not show clinical resolution or electromyographic improvement over the subsequent 3 or more months should undergo surgical exploration.

▶ Peroneal palsy after TKA is an uncommon complication. Five patients were identified in this study and were explored from 5 to 45 months after arthroplasty. Four of the 5 patients had complete recovery, leading the authors to conclude that decompression, even when carried out late, is worthwhile for patients with this injury who are not improving on a conservative course.—C.B. Sledge, M.D.

Extensive Osteolysis Around an Aseptic, Stable, Uncemented Total Knee Replacement

Berry DJ, Wold LE, Rand JA (Mayo Clinic and Found, Rochester, Minn)
Clin Orthop 293:204–207, 1993   129-94-9–41

Background.—Risk factors for osteolysis in aseptic cemented hip joint prostheses include prosthesis-bone micromotion, stress shielding or concentration, foreign body reactions, and hypersensitivity to metal ions. Whether these mechanisms may lead to osteolysis around knee prostheses is uncertain. Significant osteolysis occurred around an aseptic, well-fixed, stable, uncemented total knee prosthesis in 1 patient.

Case Report.—Man, 63, was seen with pain and swelling in the right knee 5 years after tricompartmental total knee arthroplasty (TKA) using uncemented cobalt-chromium tibial and femoral prostheses with a porous coating. Physical examination suggested metal-on-metal crepitus on knee motion. Radiographs revealed probable loosening of the tibial component, thinning of the medial tibial polyethylene, and osteolysis of the anterior femoral cortex (Fig 9–17). Revision of the TKA revealed micromotion between the tibia and the tibial component with only fibrous tissue holding the tibial component to the bone. The medial tibial polyethylene surface was completely worn through. Extensive lytic lesions were present in the medial and lateral condyles beneath the femoral component and in the anterior femoral cortex adjacent to the femoral prosthesis. A .5-cm trough of bone loss surrounded the periphery of the tibial component. In all areas of bone loss, hypertrophic synovium abutted bone. Pathologic examination of deep femoral synovial tissue obtained in areas of bone deficiency suggested marked chronic inflammation with histiocytic response and focal giant-cell reaction, as well as polyethylene, chromium, cobalt, and titanium wear debris.

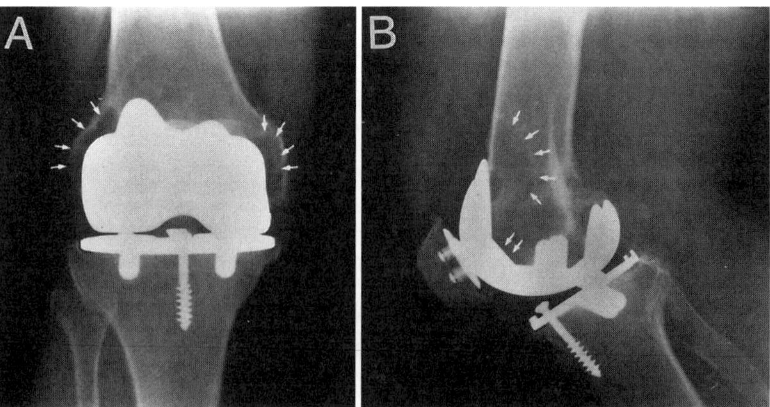

Fig 9–17.—Extensive osteolysis (*arrows*) of the distal femur. **A,** anteroposterior view; **B,** lateral view. (Courtesy of Berry DJ, Wold LE, Rand JA: *Clin Orthop* 293:204–207, 1993.)

Conclusion.—The development of focal osteolysis around well-fixed, uncemented TKA components may be analogous to that in uncemented total hip prostheses. The process may relate to polyethylene and metal wear debris; thus, knee prosthetic designs and materials should minimize production of these particles. If radiographic and clinical evidence reveals significant polyethylene wear or metal-on-metal contact, osteolysis around the arthroplasty components should be considered.

▶ Osteolysis is being increasingly recognized as a complication of total hip arthroplasty and has been related to fine-particulate polyethylene wear particles intruding into the interface between the femoral component and the surrounding bone, especially in uncemented devices. This report from the Mayo Clinic reports extensive osteolysis in both the femur and the tibia in a patient who had undergone an uncemented TKA 5 years previously and in whom there was extensive wear of the tibial polyethylene component. The frequency of this complication remains to be determined, and whether it is more frequent around uncemented devices is also not clear.—C.B. Sledge, M.D.

Heterotopic Ossification Following Primary Total Knee Arthroplasty
Harwin SF, Stein AJ, Stern RE, Kulick RG (Albert Einstein College of Medicine, New York; Montefiore Med Ctr, New York)
J Arthroplasty 8:113–116, 1993   129-94-9-42

Introduction.—Heterotopic ossification (HO) after total knee arthroplasty (TKA) is a rare complication that is frequently asymptomatic. It was hypothesized that the location of HO and its severity depend on the specific cause of the HO and the individual patient's predisposition to this complication. This hypothesis was retrospectively evaluated in 158 primary TKAs.

Patients and Methods.—The TKAs were performed in 144 patients from 1985 to 1989. The group of 144 patients was predominantly female (100 patients) and had a median age of 68.2 years. Osteoarthritis was the diagnosis in 103 patients, rheumatoid arthritis in 51, and avascular necrosis in 4. The patients were graded before and after surgery using the Hospital for Special Surgery TKA score. Records were examined for the presence of recognized risk factors for HO and to determine whether a manipulation under anesthesia was performed. All patients were radiographed at 3, 6, 9, 12, 18, and 24 months, and annually thereafter.

Results.—The incidence of HO in this series of patients was 3.8%. All 6 cases occurred in women, 5 of whom had osteoarthritis. None had evidence of gout or a history of previous knee surgeries. Two of 3 patients who underwent manipulation had HO. The mean preoperative and postoperative Hospital for Special Surgery TKA scores for patients with HO were 45 and 91, respectively. Heterotopic ossification was defined as grade I in 1 patient, grade II in 2 patients, grade IIIa in 2 patients, and grade IIIb in 1 patient.

Conclusion.—Female sex and osteoarthritis predominated in the patients with HO, and manipulation was a significant variable. Patients with grades I, II, or IIIa HO had no pain or functional limitation secondary to HO. Disability associated with this complication appears to occur only in cases of massive HO. Because symptoms can resolve spontaneously, mass excision of HO is not usually required. Female patients with recognized risk factors for HO, especially hypertrophic osteoarthritis and/or previous HO, should undergo prophylactic irradiation and/or indomethacin treatment if they are likely to have extensive dissection of the anterior femur and/or manipulation in the early postoperative period.

▶ Another uncommon complication of TKA is HO, usually seen on the anterior surface of the femur immediately proximal to the femoral component. The authors identified female sex, extensive dissection, and postoperative manipulation as risk factors. This complication has been so infrequent in my own experience (which includes many female patients and, in earlier series, frequent manipulation) that I must assume that it is the result of differences in technique involving more extensive dissection of the soft tissues over the distal anterior femur. It is quite standard to clear enough of the anterior femur to determine the proper level of condylar resection to avoid notching the femur, but any more dissection is unnecessary and perhaps contributes to this problem.—C.B. Sledge, M.D.

Dislocation Following Primary Posterior-Stabilized Total Knee Arthroplasty
Lombardi AV Jr, Mallory TH, Vaughn BK, Krugel R, Honkala TK, Sorscher M, Kolczun M (Ohio State Univ, Columbus; Raleigh Orthopedic Clinic, NC; Grace Hosp, Detroit; et al)
J Arthroplasty 8:633–639, 1993   129-94-9–43

Background.—Among the several posterior-stabilized total knee arthroplasty (TKA) systems currently available, the Insall-Burstein Posterior Stabilized Condylar Prosthesis I (IB-I) has been used most widely. In 1988, the IB-II system was introduced to address modularity. A further alteration in 1990 resulted in the IB-II modified system. Many reports of the system's success and complications have appeared in the literature since its introduction. The current study documents dislocations occurring after primary posterior-stabilized TKA.

Methods and Findings.—From 1981 through 1991, a total of 3,032 primary TKAs were done with the IB-I, IB-II, or IB-II modified systems. Fifteen posterior dislocations occurred, 4 with the IB-I system 2 or more years after surgery, 10 with the IB-II system less than 6 months and up to 33 months after surgery, and 1 with the IB-II modified system 9 months

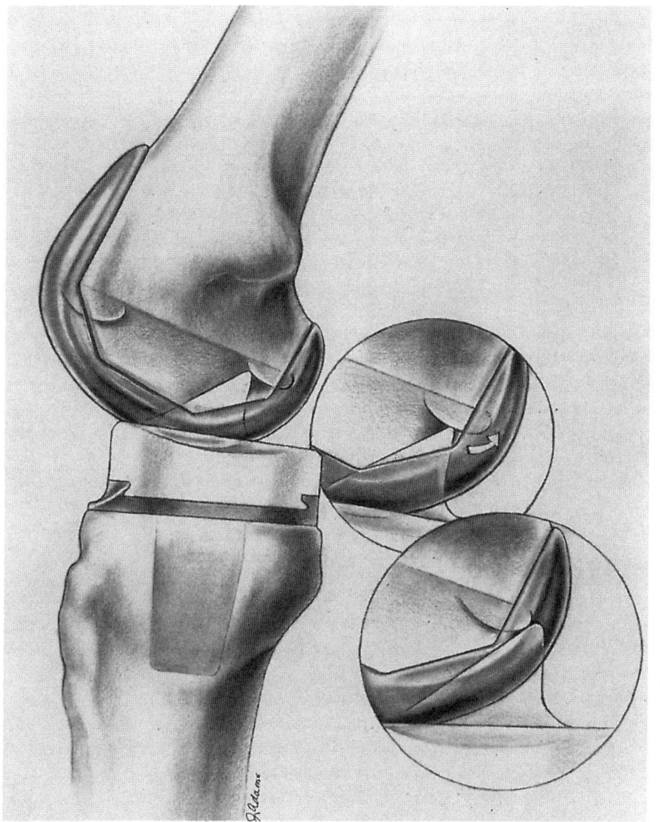

Fig 9–18.—Slight flexion mechanism. With knee in slightly flexed posture, either hamstring contracture or posteriorly placed force causes posterior subluxation; the spine impinges, further flexion occurs, and inability to extend the knee fully results. (Courtesy of Lombardi AV Jr, Mallory TH, Vaughn BK, et al: *J Arthroplasty* 8:633–639, 1993.)

after surgery. Dislocation rates between the IB-I and IB-II modified arthroplasties and the IB-II arthroplasties differed significantly. The 15 cases of dislocation were analyzed retrospectively to search for causes. Postoperative flexion was the only variable studied that distinguished patients with dislocations from those without dislocations (Figs 9–18 and 9–19). In 11 patients, conservative treatment was successful.

Conclusion.—Dislocation can complicate primary Insall-Burstein Posterior Stabilized Condylar TKAs. Adequate soft tissue balance must be achieved to insure stability. Surgeons should be alerted to patients in whom ligamentous stability is in question or flexion-extension gap mismatch is possible. When the range of motion exceeds 95–100 degrees during hospitalization, flexion restriction with an adjustable brace should be considered, with emphasis on quadriceps rehabilitation. In most patients, conservative treatment of dislocation is effective. For cases of re-

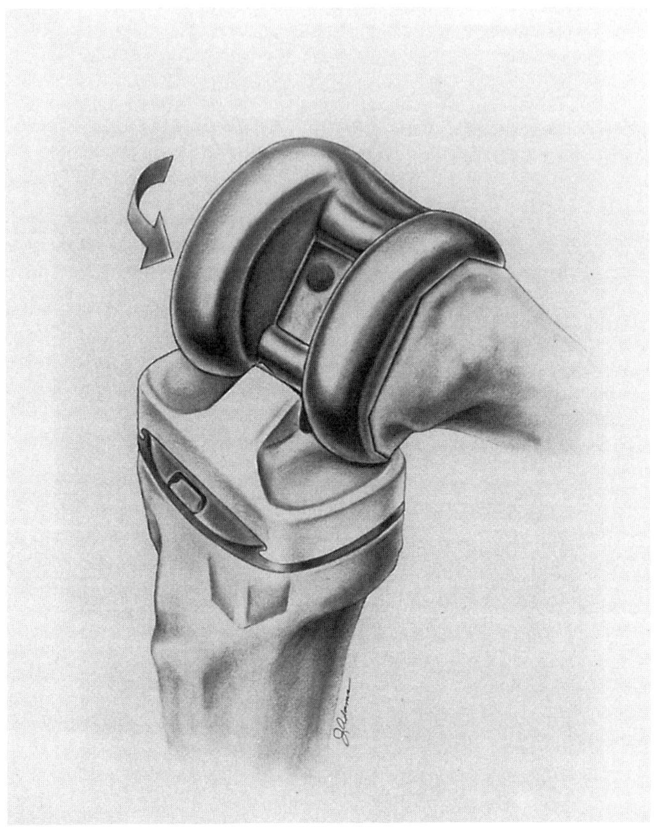

Fig 9–19.—Maximal flexion mechanism. With knee in maximal flexion, rotation, dislocation, and spine impingement occur with resultant inability to extend the knee fully. (Courtesy of Lombardi AV Jr, Mallory TH, Vaughn BK, et al: *J Arthroplasty* 8:633–639, 1993.)

current dislocation with the IB-II arthroplasty, revision with the IB-II modified system may be effective.

▶ Early designs of posterior stabilized knees had a central stabilizing eminence that allowed dislocation, with the femur going anteriorly and the tibia posteriorly. The authors of this paper reviewed 3,032 primary TKAs and report 15 such dislocations. They suggest that a modification of the tibial component has corrected the problem, and they have seen only 1 similar dislocation in 656 arthroplasties using the modified component. One should be aware of this complication with posterior stabilized designs, its diagnostic features, and the availability of a modified tibial component for recurrent cases.—C.B. Sledge, M.D.

Patellar Tilt and Subluxation in Total Knee Arthroplasty: Relationship to Pain, Fixation, and Design

Bindelglass DF, Cohen JL, Dorr LD (Orthopaedic Specialty Group, PC, Fairfield, Conn; Stanislaus Orthopedic Sports Medicine Clinic, Modesto, Calif; Univ of California, Irvine)

Clin Orthop 286:103–109, 1993   129-94-9–44

Objective and Method.—Because problems related to the patellofemoral joint remain significant in patients having total knee arthroplasty (TKA), patellar function was examined in 183 patients having a total of 234 primary TKAs. All procedures were done by or under the direct supervision of the same surgeon.

Series.—There were 142 Total Condylar knee prostheses and 92 Natural Knee implants in the series. The patients had an average age of 67 years. Osteoarthrosis was the predominant diagnosis, but 26 patients had rheumatoid disease. Patellar position and fixation were assessed with the use of a 45-degree merchant view.

Findings.—Eighteen percent of the patellas tilted more than 5 degrees, laterally, 13% tilted more than 5 degrees medially, and 14.5% were displaced more than 5 mm laterally from the center of the trochlear groove. Patellar tracking did not differ significantly with the type of prosthesis implanted (table). Lateral release did not significantly influence patellar tracking. No patient required revision for patellofemoral instability. Partial radiolucent lines were seen in 21.5% of knees, but they did not progress and loosening was not observed.

Conclusion.—Patellar tilt appears to be inevitable in some patients having primary TKA, even when a careful technique is used. Tilt results in increased loading at the periphery of the component, where most metal-backed implants have a thin layer of polyethylene.

▶ The patella remains the most frequent cause of complications after TKA, and the authors of this paper address the issues of tilt and subluxation of the patella after arthroplasty. They point out the relationship between the preoperative finding of tilt and displacement of the patella and the postoperative

Patellar Position Using Different Prostheses

Prosthesis Femoral/Patellar	Neutral (%)	Lateral Tilt (%)	Medial Tilt (%)	Displaced (%)
Total Condylar/dome	54.9	19.7	14.1	11.3
Natural knee/dome	54.5	11.4	13.6	20.5
Natural knee/congruent	56.3	18.8	8.3	16.7

Notes: *Neutral,* central tracking; *lateral tilt,* greater than 5 degrees; *medial tilt,* greater than 5 degrees; *displaced,* 5 mm or more displacement from central tracking.
(Courtesy of Bindelglass DF, Cohen JL, Dorr LD: *Clin Orthop* 286:103–109, 1993.)

finding of these same characteristics. In fact, only 55% of the patellae in this study tracked centrally without tilt or displacement. This finding was unrelated to the clinical score as long as it was not severe enough to produce either wear of metal-backed patellar components or frank dislocation.—C.B. Sledge, M.D.

Isolated Patellar Component Revision of Total Knee Arthroplasty
Berry DJ, Rand JA (Mayo Clinic and Found, Rochester, Minn)
Clin Orthop 286:110–115, 1993   129-94-9–45

Introduction.—With the frequency of extensor mechanism problems after total knee arthroplasty (TKA) and the use of patellar resurfacing, more and more isolated patellar component revisions are being performed. Several reports have described the results of femoral and tibial component revision after failed TKA, but none have focused on isolated patellar component revision. The results and complications of such revisions were reviewed.

Patients.—The review included 42 knees in 41 TKA patients undergoing isolated patellar component revision during a 10-year period. The mean age was 68 years, and most of the initial TKAs had been done for osteoarthrosis. The reasons for revision included loosening in 14 knees; wear to the metal backing in 13; fracture of the fixation peg in 7; and dissociation of the polyethylene from the metal backing, anterior knee pain, patellar instability, and component malposition with fat pad proliferation in 2 each. The patients were followed for a mean of 3.5 years after their initial TKA.

Results.—The revision surgery improved the average Hospital for Special Surgery (HSS) knee score from 71 to 81. Clinical results were rated as excellent in 18 knees, good in 12, fair in 4, and poor in 2. However, 14 patients had a significant complication, including late patellar fracture in 5 knees, patellar instability in 3, peroneal nerve palsy and polyethylene wear to the metal backing in 2 each, and infection and extensor lag in 1 each. Eight knees required further operation for problems directly related to the knee revision. The HSS knee scores improved by an average of 12 points in patients without a complication, compared with 10 points in those with a complication.

Conclusion.—In patients with TKA, isolated patellar component revision is an apparently straightforward procedure with good results. However, the occurrence of complications in one third of patients and the need for reoperation in one fifth is documented. Awareness of the potential for complications may prompt steps to avoid them.

▶ Revision of the patellar component as an isolated event was carried out in 42 knees with very good results overall. There was, however, a very high complication rate with major complications in 14 of the 42 knees. One should be aware of the frequency of complications after this procedure and make sure this fact is known by both surgeon and patient before undertaking an otherwise "simple" operation.—C.B. Sledge, M.D.

Failure of the Porous-Coated Anatomic Prosthesis in Total Knee Arthroplasty Due to Severe Polyethylene Wear
Tsao A, Mintz L, McRae CR, Stulberg SD, Wright T (Univ of Mississippi, Jackson; Maricopa Med Ctr, Phoenix, Ariz; Univ of Pennsylvania, Wyomissing; et al)
J Bone Joint Surg (Am) 75-A:19–26, 1993   129-94-9-46

Background.—Polyethylene wear, related to a number of different factors, is a well-recognized cause of failure in both hip and knee implants. The polyethylene becomes worn as the result of large contact stresses, creating debris within the joint and, thus, a synovitis that can be associated with significant pain and loosening of the implant. Relevant characteristics of patients whose porous-coated anatomical total knee replacements failed as a result of polyethylene wear were identified.

Methods.—Thirty-two patients whose total knee arthroplasty (TKA) failed as the result of severe wear of the tibial and patellar polyethylene components were studied. They represented 7% of 487 knee arthroplasties performed by a single surgeon with the use of a porous-coated anatomical prosthesis from 1982 to 1989. Characteristics of the failure

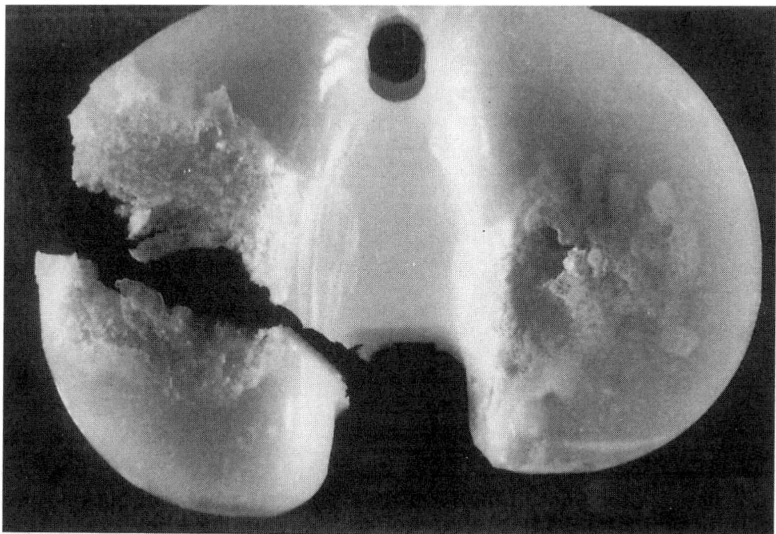

FIg 9–20.—Retrieved tibial component showing excessive polyethylene wear and delamination with a complete fracture through the medial plateau. (Courtesy of Tsao A, Mintz L, McRae CR, et al: *J Bone Joint Surg (Am)* 75-A:19–26, 1993.)

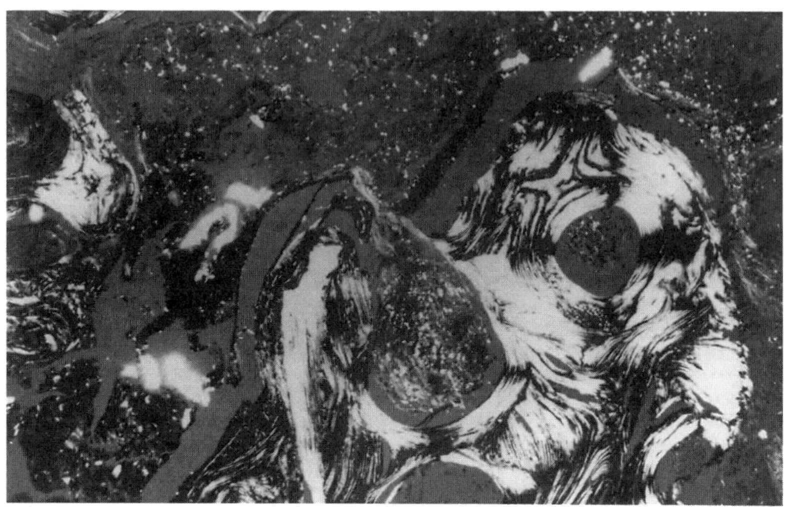

Fig 9–21.—Photomicrograph under polarized light. Mature lamellar bone and polyethylene debris are present in adjacent inflamed fibrous tissue. (Courtesy of Tsao A, Mintz L, McRae CR, et al: *J Bone Joint Surg (Am)* 75-A:19–26, 1993.)

group were compared with those of the group whose implants did not fail. Components retrieved from 12 patients with implant failure were also examined.

Findings.—Implant failure necessitated revision in 30 of the 32 patients. Implant failure occurred a mean of 4.5 years after TKA, the initial symptoms being painless effusion and decreased range of motion. The development of pain was considered an indication for surgery. Factors predicting an increased risk of failure were increased weight, younger age, and a thinner tibial component. The retrieved tibial components showed extensive delamination caused by fracture of the polyethylene about 1 mm below the surface (Fig 9–20). Light microscopy revealed signs of polyethylene-induced inflammation adjacent to mature lamellar bone (Fig 9–21). Many specimens showed cracks that spread inward from the medial and lateral periphery of the tibial component toward the center of the condyles. The projected 6-year failure rate from polyethylene wear alone was more than 20% (Fig 9–22).

Conclusion.—The development of mechanical failure of the polyethylene in porous-coated anatomical knee prostheses appears to result from both patient factors and implant design features. Risk of failure may be especially great in heavy, younger patients with a thin tibial component. The possibility of polyethylene wear should be considered in any young patient with a well-functioning implant who has an effusion.

▶ The porous-coated anatomical prosthesis has been the subject of several studies that demonstrate excessive wear of the polyethylene component. Risk factors appear to be the use of polyethylene inserts 6 mm or less in

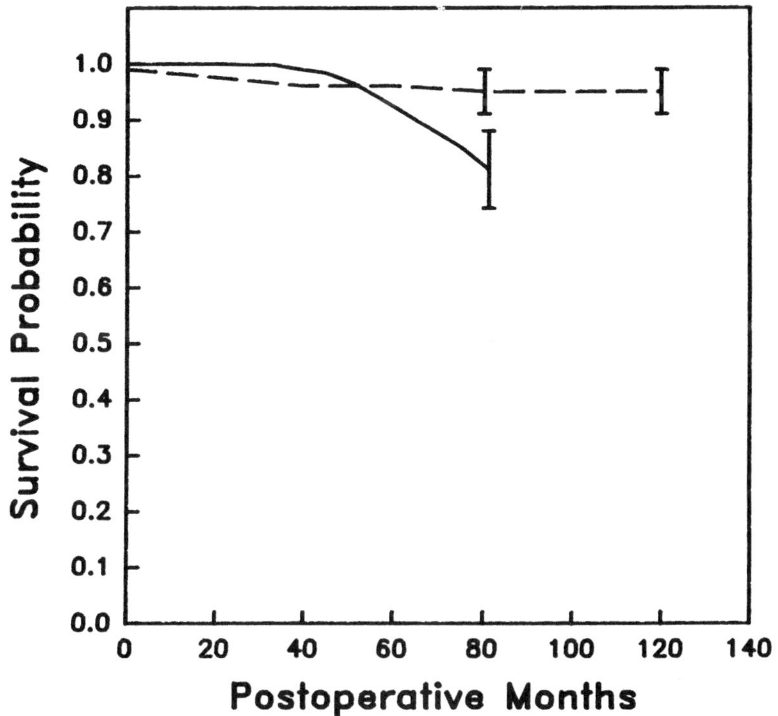

Fig 9–22.—Kaplan-Meier survivorship curves, with 95% confidence limits, for the patients in the current study who received a porous-coated anatomical prosthesis (*solid line*) and for another population of patients who received a total condylar-type knee replacement (*dashed line*). In both populations, the criterion for failure was loosening or revision. (Courtesy of Tsao A, Mintz L, McRae CR, et al: *J Bone Joint Surg (Am)* 75-A:19-26, 1993.)

thickness, heat pressure treatment of the polyethylene to improve surface finish, and the high unit stress imposed by the relatively flat contour of the tibial component. In this series of 487 arthroplasties, the failure rate caused by polyethylene wear was 7% at an average follow-up of only 4.5 years. This is in such striking contrast to the 15-year results of the Total Condylar reported by Ranawat et al. (Abstract 129-94-9–37) and numerous other series that one must look carefully at design characteristics to explain this incidence.—C.B. Sledge, M.D.

Difficulties With Bearing Dislocation and Breakage Using a Movable Bearing Total Knee Replacement System
Weaver JK, Derkash RS, Greenwald AS (Orthopaedic Assocs of Aspen and Glenwood, Glenwood Springs, Colo)
Clin Orthop 290:244–252, 1993   129-94-9–47

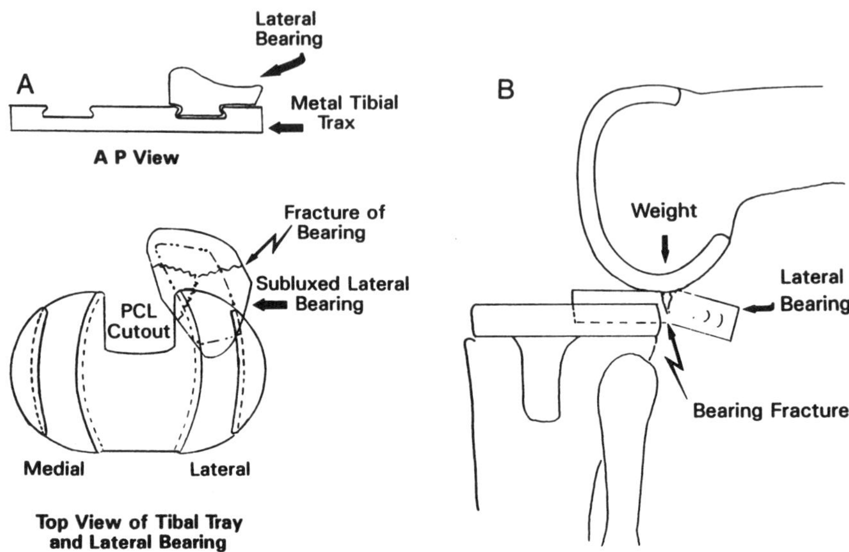

Fig 9–23.—Bearing fracture occurs when (**A**) the bearing is subluxated posteriorly and (**B**) cantilevered over the edge of the metal tray. (Courtesy of Weaver JK, Derkash RS, Greenwald AS: *Clin Orthop* 290:244–252, 1993.)

Background.—The low contact stress (LCS), or New Jersey, knee replacement system, has movable high-density polyethylene bearings between its metallic femoral and tibial components. The system was introduced in 1980 in response to concerns about loosening and wear with conventional knee replacements. A 4- to 10-year evaluation of the LCS system was conducted as part of a Federal Drug Administration review.

Methods.—The first phase of the study, conducted from 1981 to 1984, included 40 knees in which all components were cemented using low-viscosity cement and pressurization. In the second phase, 16 knees were selected for cementless fixation. The anterior cruciate ligament was spared in 23 of 40 cases in the cemented phase. The ligament was routinely excised in all patients in the cementless phase. Patients in the first phase were followed for an average of 7 years and in the second phase for an average of 5 years. Outcomes were evaluated in terms of pain, function, and deformity.

Results.—The rate of failure, as determined by the need for revision surgery, was 10% in the cemented group. This included 2 failures caused by tibial component loosening, 1 from bearing dislocation, and 1 from infection. A further 30% of knees had lucent tibial zones greater than 1 mm. In the uncemented group, the failure rate was 31%, including 4 failures from bearing fracture and 1 from knee pain of unknown cause. The bearing failures resulted from entrapment of the subluxed lateral bearing (Fig 9–23).

Conclusion.—Intermediate-term experience with the LCS knee replacement system suggests that it is no more effective than conventional systems in avoiding the problem of loosening. Sacrifice of the anterior cruciate ligament increases freedom of rotation, predisposing to subluxation and failure of the polyethylene bearings. These types of systems are, therefore, probably best designed for anterior cruciate ligament preservation.

▶ The concept of a movable bearing in total knee arthroplasty is attractive as a solution to polyethylene wear problems. This paper points out that movable bearings have their own problems, including breakage and dislocation. The operation appears to be technically somewhat more demanding than conventional knee arthroplasty, and the degree to which it reduces polyethylene wear has yet to be conclusively determined.—C.B. Sledge, M.D.

Exchange Arthroplasty for Infected Knee Replacements: A New Two-Stage Method
Scott IR, Stockley I, Getty CJM (Northern Gen Hosp, Sheffield, England)
J Bone Joint Surg (Br) 75-B:28–31, 1993   129-94-9–48

Introduction.—For patients who have deep infection after knee arthroplasty, aggressive local débridement and antibiotics are unlikely to be successful if delayed for more than 2 weeks. Another option is exchange arthroplasty, including meticulous débridement, antibiotic therapy, and implantation of a new prosthesis. This may be done either in a single stage or in 2 stages, with the new prosthesis implanted after a delay of weeks to months. The results of exchange arthroplasty in 17 patients with deep infection of knee replacements were evaluated.

Patients.—The operations were performed during an 8-year period in 13 women and 4 men (average age, 66 years). Five had overt sepsis, and the others had increasing pain in a previously successful arthroplasty. Ten patients underwent a 1-stage procedure; the other 7 had 2-stage procedures. In the latter group, a prosthesis was used as a spacer in the interval between operations. Acrylic cement beads containing an appropriate antibiotic were used to provide high local concentrations.

Outcomes.—Although all knees had some extensor lag after exchange arthroplasty, 15 had at least 90 degrees of flexion. The hospital stay averaged 16 days after a 1-stage procedure, 21 days after the first stage of a 2-stage procedure, and 12 days after the second stage. There were no serious complications other than 3 cases of infection after 1-stage exchange arthroplasty; all of these patients were successfully managed by further exchange operations.

Conclusion.—For surgically fit patients with infected knee arthroplasty, the modified 2-stage technique of exchange arthroplasty appears to be the optimum management approach. It can eradicate the local infection while restoring knee function and independent mobility. For patients who are unfit for surgery, incision and drainage plus antibiotics appear to be the only feasible treatments.

▶ Infected knee arthroplasty can be a disaster. The functional consequences—even if a successful arthroplasty is eventually achieved—can be devastating. In an attempt to avoid or shorten the functional consequences of revision, many have been tempted to carry out 1-stage revisions. This paper very clearly indicates the improved results achieved when the exchange is staged using a spacer and antibiotic-impregnated beads in the interval between removal of the infected prosthesis and reimplantation.—C.B. Sledge, M.D.

Gastrocnemius Muscle Flap Coverage of Exposed or Infected Knee Prostheses

Gerwin M, Rothaus KO, Windsor RE, Brause BD, Insall JN (Hosp for Special Surgery, New York)
Clin Orthop 286:64–70, 1993   129-94-9-49

Introduction.—Perhaps 1 in 5 patients undergoing total knee arthroplasty (TKA) will have wound-healing problems, whether or not the knee prosthesis is infected. Wound exposure places the prosthesis at risk of infection, the most common cause of failure of cemented knee implants. The most effective means of providing wound coverage is by using a rotational gastrocnemius muscle flap.

Series.—Data were reviewed on 12 patients who required flaps for coverage of knee prostheses. The indications for primary TKA included osteoarthrosis, traumatic arthritis, tumor, and rheumatoid disease. Two of the patients had revision of a TKA. Exposed prostheses underwent soft tissue coverage when the wound demarcated. Infected prostheses were removed, antibiotic treatment was given for 6 weeks, and muscle flap coverage was undertaken when bacterial counts were below 10.

Technique.—Necrotic tissue is débrided under epidural anesthesia, and a medial gastrocnemius flap is then developed through a posteromedial incision (Fig 9–24). The flap is based proximally on the sural artery. After the muscle has been divided distally at its musculotendinous junction and folded back on itself, the flap is passed beneath a medial skin bridge to the wound and sutured securely (Fig 9–25). The muscle is covered with a split-thickness skin graft, and the donor site is closed primarily.

Results.—Six patients had their prostheses exposed over an average of 7 cm² in the center to the distal third of the incision. Flap coverage was performed on average about 7 weeks after implant arthroplasty. All 5 patients who were followed for an average of 53 months had an excellent outcome with no signs of infection. Six patients whose soft tissue

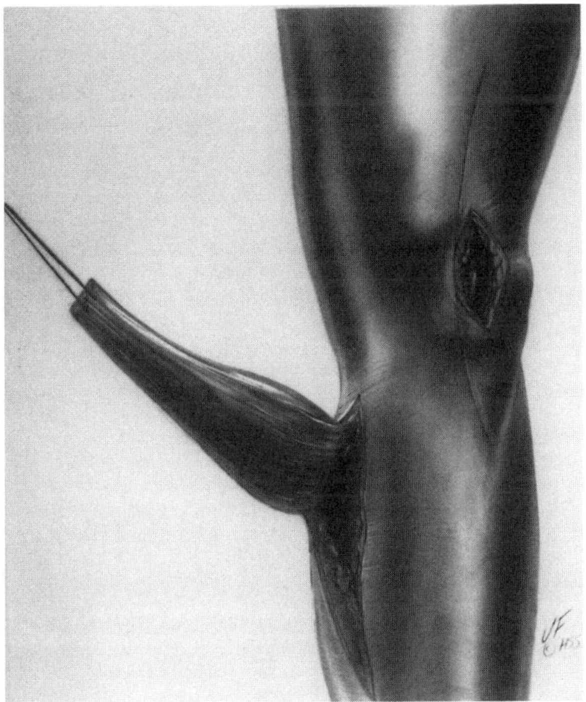

Fig 9–24.—The medial gastrocnemius muscle flap is elevated through a posteromedial incision and transected distally. (Courtesy of Gerwin M, Rothaus KO, Windsor RE, et al: *Clin Orthop* 286:64–70, 1993.)

defect was an average of 4 cm² had chronically infected prostheses. The prosthesis was reimplanted from 1 month to 1 year after flap coverage in 5 patients. One patient was awaiting revision of a contralateral prosthesis. All the wounds retained soft tissue coverage with no evidence of recurrent infection.

Summary.—Ten of 12 patients in this series (83%) had an excellent outcome, with adequate soft tissue coverage and a functioning total knee prosthesis, after gastrocnemius muscle flap coverage of an exposed or infected knee implant. No flap placed on a wound measuring less than 12 cm² failed.

▶ For the 20% of patients undergoing knee arthroplasty who have wound-healing problems, a low threshold for intervention must be maintained. This paper demonstrates that such early intervention in the form of a gastrocnemius muscle flap to improve coverage and blood supply can be extremely effective in such patients. Knee surgeons should be familiar with this procedure and quick to recognize potentially disastrous failure of healing of the incision after knee arthroplasty so that they can intervene before the wound breaks down and the implant is irretrievably infected.—C.B. Sledge, M.D.

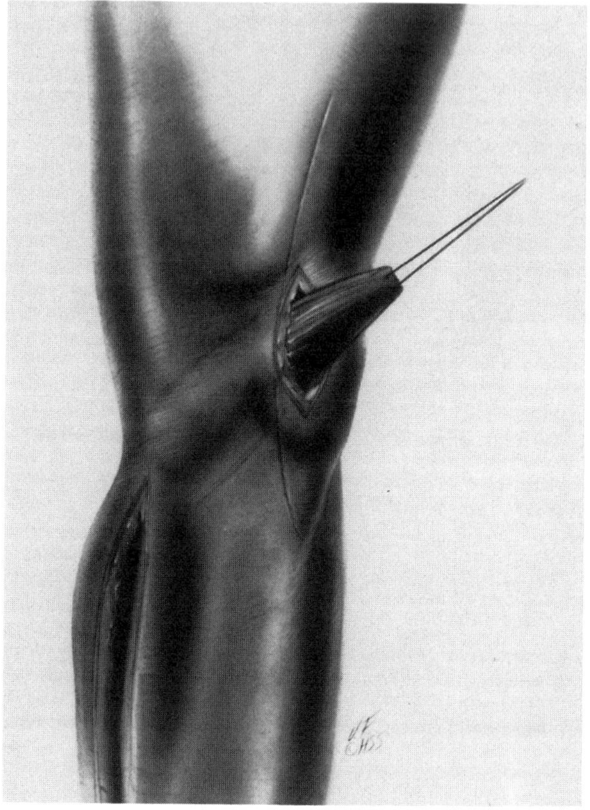

Fig 9–25.—The gastrocnemius muscle flap is passed through a skin bridge to the site of the previously débrided defect. The flap must lie easily over the defect and not be under tension. (Courtesy of Gerwin M, Rothaus KO, Windsor RE, et al: *Clin Orthop* 286:64–70, 1993.)

Massive Allografts Sterilised by Irradiation: Clinical Results

Hernigou P, Delepine G, Goutallier D, Julieron A (Univ of Paris XII; Hôpital Henri Mondor, Créteil, France)

J Bone Joint Surg (Br) 75-B:904–913, 1993   129-94-9–50

Background.—Irradiation is the most commonly used technique for sterilizing human tissue grafts for transplantation. One experience with massive allografts sterilized by irradiation with a follow-up of 3 years or more was reviewed.

Methods.—Between 1984 and 1988, a total of 127 allografts that exceeded 7 cm in size were implanted (Fig 9–26). All had been irradiated at a dose of 25,000 Gy. The grafts were obtained from 41 trauma victims. The recipients were 44 patients receiving allografts for revisions of joint arthroplasty or for a tumor, who received no adjuvant therapy, and

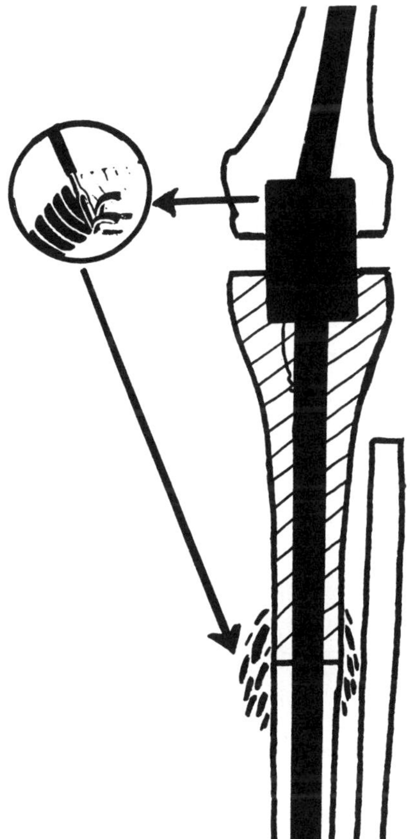

Fig 9–26.—Cancellous autograft is obtained from the healthy bone end during allograft-arthroplasty and packed around junction between allograft and host bone. (Courtesy of Hernigou P, Delepine G, Goutallier D, et al: *J Bone Joint Surg (Br)* 75-B:904–913, 1993.)

83 patients who also received chemotherapy or radiation therapy, or both, for bone tumor.

Findings.—None of the patients who did not receive adjuvant therapy had bacteriologic infections. In those needing chemotherapy or radiation therapy, or both, the infection rate was 13%. The major mechanical complications were nonunion in 7 grafts (5.5%) (Fig 9–27) and fracture in 8 (6%). These rates were not significantly different from rates reported for nonirradiated grafts.

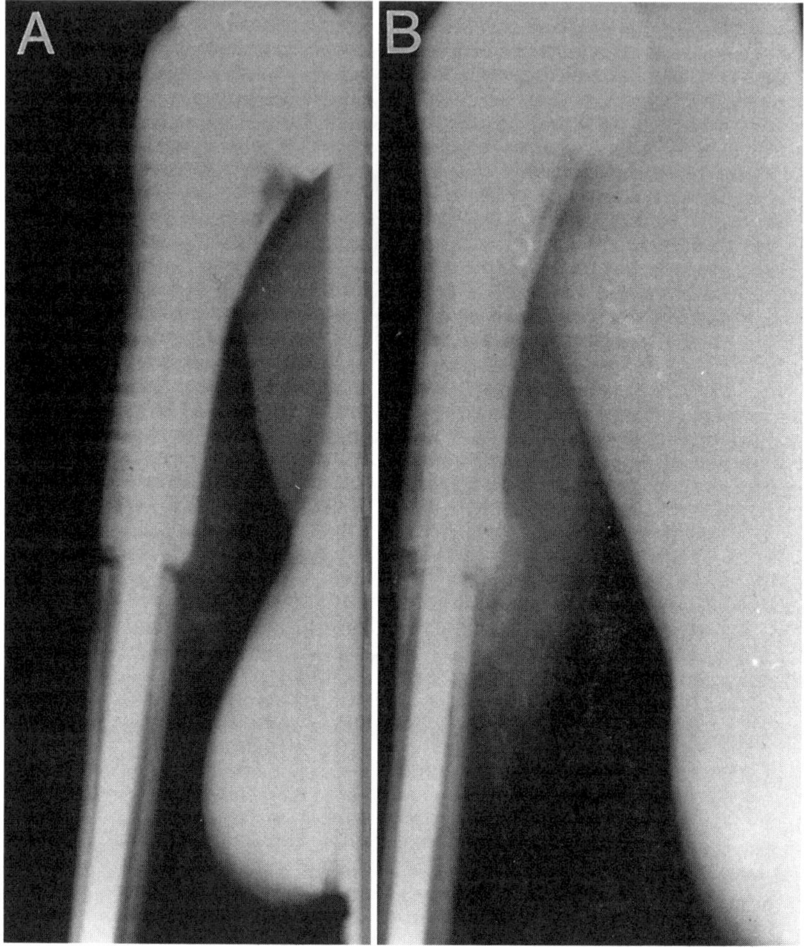

Fig 9–27.—A, nonunion at 8 months between allograft arthroplasty of the shoulder and the host bone. **B,** union 3 months after packing the junction with autograft from the iliac crest. (Courtesy of Hernigou P, Delepine G, Goutallier D, et al: *J Bone Joint Surg (Br)* 75-B:904–913, 1993.)

Conclusion.—Irradiation apparently does not jeopardize clinical results. This method of sterilization remains the most convenient and widely accepted technique.

▶ When there are major bony defects around the knee in patients who need arthroplasty, allografts are often the most effective, and sometimes the only, way of handling such massive defects. There are concerns, however, about the safety of such allografts with respect to transmission of diseases such as AIDS and other viral diseases. This paper demonstrates that massive bone grafts sterilized by high levels of radiation can be successfully used. These authors could not distinguish any untoward effects of such sterilization when compared with their earlier experience with nonirradiated grafts, and they certainly offer a margin of safety.—C.B. Sledge, M.D.

The Incidence of Deep-Vein Thrombosis After Upper Tibial Osteotomy: A Venographic Study

Turner RS, Griffiths H, Heatley FW (St Thomas' Hosp, London)
J Bone Joint Surg (Br) 75-B:942–944, 1993   129-94-9–51

Background.—The reported rates of deep-vein thrombosis after total knee replacement revealed on venography have ranged from 56% to 84%. After tibial fractures, the reported rate was 44.7%. The venographic findings in a group of patients undergoing Maquet barrel vault upper tibial osteotomies were reported.

Patients and Methods.—The study subjects were 81 patients having their first upper tibial osteotomy for medial compartment osteoarthritis between January 1985 and September 1992. The ages of the 28 women and 53 men ranged from 30 to 73 years. Heparin, 5,000 IU, was given subcutaneously twice a day, beginning 48 hours after surgery.

Findings.—Forty-one percent of the patients had thrombosis. One patient had a nonfatal pulmonary embolus. Twenty of the 47 thrombi were in the deep veins of the calf only. The diagnosis of thrombosis was made clinically in 7 cases. The incidence of deep-vein thrombosis increased with age but not significantly with weight. The incidence by site and sex is shown in the table.

Conclusion.—In this series, the incidence of deep-vein thrombosis after upper tibial osteotomy was 41%. The significance of thrombi in the deep veins of the calf has not been established definitively.

Distribution of Deep-Vein Thrombosis (DVT) by Sex and Site

Patients		DVT		Site		
Sex	**Number**	**Number**	*Percentage*	**Calf**	**Popliteal**	**Iliofemoral**
Male	53	24	*45*	21	3	6
Female	28	9	*32*	9	3	3
Total	81	33	*41*	30	6	9

(Courtesy of Turner RS, Griffiths H, Heatley FW: *J Bone Joint Surg (Br)* 75-B:942–944, 1993.)

Incidence of Pulmonary Embolism After Total Knee Arthroplasty With Low-Dose Coumadin Prophylaxis

Vresilovic EJ Jr, Hozack WJ, Booth RE, Rothman RH (Rothman Inst, Philadelphia)
Clin Orthop 286:27–31, 1993   129-94-9–52

Objective.—The risk of pulmonary embolism was determined in a prospective series of patients, aged 50–70 years, with osteoarthrosis who underwent primary cemented total knee arthroplasty (TKA) between January 1984 and July 1989 and received low-dose Coumadin as prophylaxis. A total of 852 arthroplasties were done in 755 patients.

Management.—A medial parapatellar approach was used to implant a posterior stabilized prosthesis in 92% of patients under general and spinal anesthesia and tourniquet control. Elastic compression stockings were used after operation. Continuous passive motion was undertaken in the recovery room, and patients walked the first postoperative day. Coumadin, 10 mg, was given the evening of surgery, and starting on the second postoperative day the daily dose was adjusted to maintain the prothrombin time at 1.2–1.4 times the control level. All patients had a chest roentgenogram on postoperative day 6 and a ventilation-perfusion scan the following day (or earlier, if indicated).

Results.—Pulmonary embolism developed in 5.6% of patients having TKA. No patient died as a result, and only 6 of the 48 patients were symptomatic. Pulmonary embolism was about twice as frequent in patients with a history of phlebitis, but a history of cardiac disease appeared to protect against pulmonary embolism. No operative or anesthetic factors could be related to the risk of pulmonary embolism. In particular, spinal anesthesia did not protect against pulmonary embolism.

The Incidence of Fatal Pulmonary Embolism After Knee Replacement With No Prophylactic Anticoagulation

Khaw FM, Moran CG, Pinder IM, Smith SR (Freeman Hosp, Newcastle upon Tyne, England)
J Bone Joint Surg (Br) 75-B:940–941, 1993   129-94-9–53

Background.—The incidence of fatal pulmonary embolism after total hip replacement ranges from 1.7% to 2.3% and may be reduced with prophylactic anticoagulation. The value of routine prophylactic anticoagulation in total knee replacement surgery, however, is less certain.

Methods.—The incidence of fatal pulmonary embolism after total knee replacement with no prophylactic anticoagulation was determined in 499 consecutive patients undergoing 527 knee replacements. Patients wore antithromboembolic stockings and were mobilized 48 hours after operation.

Findings.—Fatal pulmonary embolism occurred in 1 patient 22 days after surgery, for an incidence of .19%. No other deaths occurred within 3 months of operation. Seven other patients had clinical symptoms and signs of pulmonary embolism while hospitalized. The diagnosis was confirmed in all cases by isotope ventilation-perfusion scanning. All 7 recovered after treatment with anticoagulation.

Conclusion.—In this series, fatal pulmonary embolism was rare after total knee replacement without prophylactic anticoagulation. Previous studies have also reported a very low incidence. Thus, the value of routine anticoagulation in this patient population is questionable.

▶ Deep-vein thrombosis and pulmonary embolus occur after operations on the knee. The precise incidence detected depends on the method of detection chosen (clinical examination, ultrasound, or venography). The importance of clots in the veins distal to the knee is also unknown. Some maintain that such clots are innocuous and do not need treatment, whereas others express concern that distal clots might propagate proximally and produce fatal emboli. There is also some evidence that distal clots in the calf veins may themselves embolize with serious consequences, especially in patients who have a patent foramen ovale, allowing paradoxical embolization to the cerebral circulation.

Turner et al. (Abstract 129-94-9–51), using venography, showed that 41% of their patients had a deep-vein thrombosis after upper tibial osteotomy, and they had one nonfatal pulmonary embolus. The diagnosis was made clinically in only 7 of the 47 cases. The authors were unable to establish the importance of calf thrombi. Vresilovic et al. (Abstract 129-94-9–52) had a nearly 6% incidence of pulmonary embolism after TKA in spite of a routine of prophylaxis with warfarin. The only risk factor that they could identify was a history of previous phlebitis in the operated extremity.

Khaw et al. (Abstract 129-94-9–53) carried out 527 knee replacements without anticoagulant prophylaxis and had 1 fatal pulmonary embolism. They used this low incidence to support the practice of not using prophylactic anticoagulation based on an assumed cost-benefit ratio, but they ignored the consequences of nonfatal emboli and untreated thromboses; the former may lead to chronic pulmonary disease and the latter to stasis changes in the lower extremity. Clearly, a fatal pulmonary embolus is the complication most feared after arthroplasty, but one should not use its low incidence as the only argument against prophylaxis; the morbidity of nonfatal emboli is real and should be measured before deciding not to use routine prophylaxis.—C.B. Sledge, M.D.

Subject Index*

A

Abduction
  orthosis for Legg-Perthes disease,
    93: 26
    Scottish Rite, 93: 25
Ablation
  in duplicated thumb, 94: 38
Abscess
  spinal epidural, diagnosis and
    management of, 93: 161
Absorbable
  tacks, in arthroscopic repair of superior
    glenoid labral detachments, 94: 77
Absorptiometry
  dual-photon, current status of, 93: 148
  single-photon, current status of, 93: 148
  x-ray
    dual, after uncemented hip
      arthroplasty, 93: 134
    dual-energy, and bone remodeling
      after cementless hip arthroplasty,
      93: 131
    dual-energy, current status of, 93: 148
    dual-energy, for bone mineral loss
      after lower extremity trauma,
      94: 279
Accident
  department, knee radiography in,
    94: 364
Acetabular
  augmentation, slotted
    in childhood and adolescence, 93: 3
    in Legg-Perthes disease, 93: 30
  bone deficiency, revision arthroplasty
    with antiprotrusio cage for 93: 125
  component in total hip arthroplasty (*see*
    Arthroplasty, hip, total, acetabular
    component in)
  cup loosening after low-friction
    arthroplasty, 93: 111
  development after closed reduction of
    congenital hip dislocation, 94: 7
  fixation in total hip arthroplasty,
    93: 115
  fracture (*see* Fracture, acetabular)
  index after reduction in developmental
    dysplasia of hip, 94: 6
  protrusion in neurofibromatosis, 93: 11
Acetabuloplasty
  lateral shelf, for Legg-Perthes disease,
    93: 29
Achilles tendon
  allograft in static stabilizer for shoulder
    instability after arthroplasty, 94: 77

injuries, surgical repair vs. no repair in
  (in rat), 94: 203
rupture, healing process, ultrasound
  monitoring of, 93: 225
Acral
  paresthesias, permanent, after distal
    interphalangeal joint arthrodesis,
    93: 286
Acromioclavicular
  dislocation (*see* Dislocation,
    acromioclavicular)
  injuries, acute type-V, surgical treatment,
    in athletes, 94: 378
Acromion
  degeneration, relation to
    coracoacromial arch anatomy,
    93: 72
Acromioplasty
  open vs. arthroscopic, for subacromial
    impingement, 93: 75
Acrylic
  cement, hyperthermia during
    occipitocervical fusion with,
    93: 157
Activity
  physical, and bone gain in young adult
    women, 93: 147
Adductor
  hallucis release, plantar incision in,
    94: 205
Adolescent
  acetabular augmentation in, slotted,
    93: 3
  giant cell tumor of bone in, 94: 229
  knee hemarthrosis in, acute, 94: 23
  polyarthropathy in, debilitating, total
    arthroplasty for, 93: 395
  scoliosis in, idiopathic (*see* Scoliosis,
    idiopathic, adolescent)
  spondylolisthesis treatment in,
    operative, long-term evaluation,
    93: 14
Aerosols
  blood-containing, generated by surgical
    techniques, 93: 347
Age
  bone, in adolescent idiopathic scoliosis,
    94: 25
  complications early after anterior
    dislocation of shoulder and, 94: 63
  health status and elective surgery,
    94: 112
  median nerve sensory conduction in
    industry and, 93: 276
  morbidity and mortality after lumbar
    spine operations and, 93: 186

** All entries refer to the year and page number(s) for data appearing in this and the previous edition of the* YEAR BOOK.

S

X

X-ray
  (*See also* Radiography)
  absorptiometry (*see* Absorptiometry,
    x-ray)

Z

Zimmer hip prosthesis
  interface motion in, effect of femoral
    stem geometry on, 93: 138
Zimmer implant
  in knee arthroplasty, unicompartmental,
    94: 386
Zinc
  deficiency in osteoporosis, 94: 148

Author Index

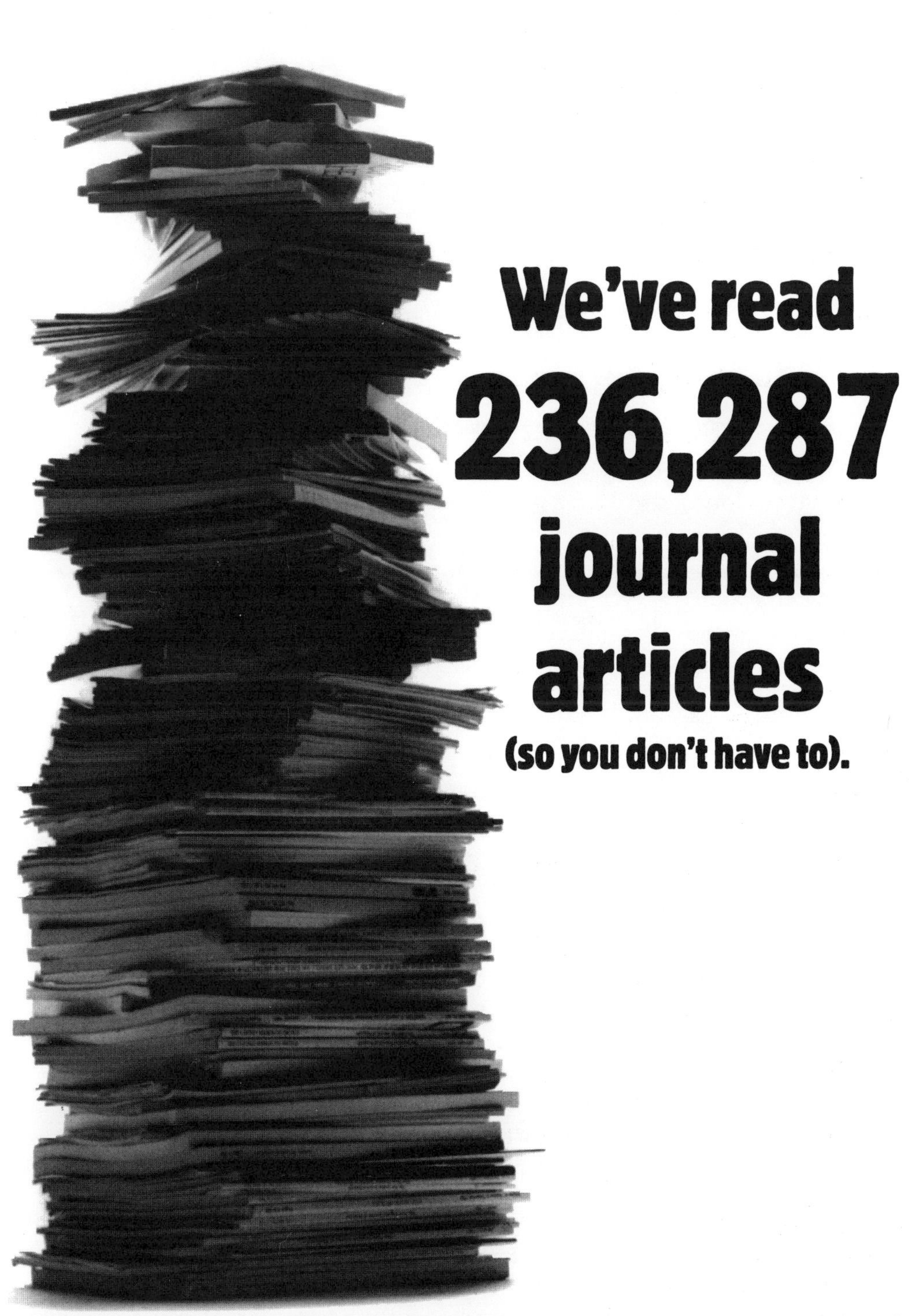
We've read
236,287
journal
articles
(so you don't have to).

The Year Books–
The best from 236,287 journal articles.

At Mosby, we subscribe to more than 950 medical and allied health journals from every corner of the globe. We read them all, tirelessly scanning for anything that relates to your field.

We send everything we find related to a given specialty to the distinguished editors of the **Year Book** in that area, and they pick out *the best*, the articles they feel *every practitioner in that specialty should be aware of*.

For the **1994 Year Books** we surveyed a total of 236,287 articles and found hundreds of articles related to your field. Our expert editors reviewed these and chose the developments you don't want to miss.

The best articles–condensed, organized, and with personal commentary.

Not only do you get the past year's most important articles in your field, you get them in a format that makes them easy to use.

Every article that the editors pick is condensed into a concise, outlined abstract, a summary of the article's most important points highlighted with bold paragraph headings. So you can quickly scan for exactly what you need.

In addition to identifying the year's best articles, the editors write concise commentaries following each article, telling whether or not the study in question is a reliable one, whether a new technique is effective, or whether a particular trend you've head about merits your immediate attention.

No other abstracting service offers this expert advice to help you decide how the year's advances will affect the way you practice.

With a special added benefit for Year Book subscribers.

In 1994, your **Year Book** subscription includes a new added benefit. Access to **MOSBY Document Express**, a rapid-response information retrieval service that puts copies of original source documents in your hands, in a little as a few hours.

With **MOSBY Document Express**, you have convenient, *around-the-clock-access to literally every article* upon which **Year Book** summaries are based. What's more, you can also order journal articles cited in references—or for that matter, virtually any medical or scientific article that can be located. Plus, at your direction, we will deliver the article(s) by FAX, overnight delivery service, or regular mail.

This new added benefit is just one of the enhanced services that makes your **Year Book** subscription an even better value—it's your key to the full breadth of health sciences information. For more details, see **MOSBY Document Express** instructions at the beginning of this book.